HAIR LOSS

Options for
Restoration & Reversal

Also by Gustavo J. Gomez:

HAIR LOSS: Options for Restoration & Reversal 1st Edition (Multi-Award-Winning Book)

Private Money Lending: Learn How to Consistently Generate a Passive Income Stream 1st and 2nd Edition (Multi-Award-Winning Books)

Balding: Hair Loss and Restoration

Terapéutica Respiratoria: Normas y Aplicaciones

Medical Necessity Guidelines for Ordering Respiratory Care Services: A Physician's Pocket Reference

HAIR LOSS

Options for Restoration & Reversal

GUSTAVO J. GOMEZ, PH.D.

Foreword by:
Manuel A. Soler-Perez, M.D.

Reviewed by:
Manuel A. Soler-Perez, M.D.
Margot C. Sarratea, MSN, ARNP, FNP-BC, NP-BC, CPN

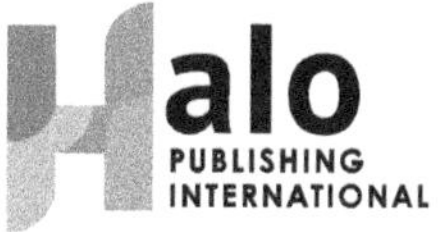

Revised Edition

Library of Congress Control Number (LCCN): 2017902450
Printed in the United States of America

ISBN-13: 978-1-63765-288-6 (Hardcover Edition)
ISBN-13: 978-1-63765-289-3 (Paperback Edition)
ASIN: B074TNDLR1 (eBook)

© Cover Design by Margot C. Sarratea &
JD & J Design, LLC
© Author Photograph by Manuel A. Soler

Author: Gustavo J. Gomez, Ph.D.
Book Title: HAIR LOSS: Options for Restoration & Reversal

Author's official website: https:// www.gustavojgomez.com
Amazon author's page: https:// www.amazon.com/author/gustavojgomez

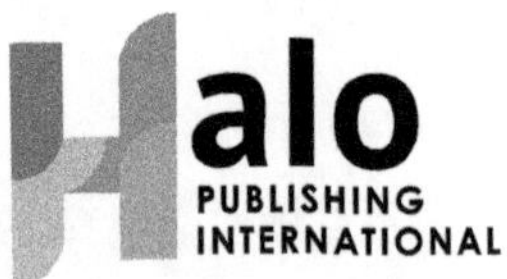

Halo Publishing International, LLC
www.halopublishing.com

Printed and bound in the United States of America

Disclaimer:

The information contained herein is specifically intended for informational purposes only. The hair products mentioned if any, and the information presented in this publication are based on the literature review by the author and his own experience with the majority of the treatment modalities that have been described. The author is a hair transplant recipient of the punch graft, strip/FUT, and scalp reduction methods. He has also experimented with low-level laser light therapy (LLLT), all the FDA-approved hair loss medications and numerous other topical solutions. The literature was meticulously researched, and it is believed to have come from reliable sources. Nothing within this publication should be construed as dispensation of medical advice, promotion, or endorsement of any particular treatment modality or product. The reader should use the information contained within this book to develop the educational foundation necessary to make safer, well-informed decisions before selecting any course of action as it relates to hair-loss issues. When selecting any kind of healthcare service, it is always a prudent practice to consult with a competent and skilled licensed healthcare professional who is knowledgeable about the field before committing to any medical treatment. No warranties or guarantees are expressed or implied by the publisher's choice to include any of the content in this volume. Neither the publisher nor the individual author(s) or reviewer(s) shall be liable for any physical, psychological, emotional, financial, or commercial damages, including, but not limited to, special, incidental, consequential or other damages. The consumers are ultimately responsible for their own choices, actions, and results.

Copyright Infringement Claims Disclaimer:

The author of this book honors the intellectual property rights of others and expects the same in kind. All the images that have been used in this book are either from creative commons, purchased from paid image vendors and/or used with permission from the copyright's owner. In accordance with the provisions of the Copyrights Act of 1976 and the Digital Millennium Copyright Act (DMCA) of 1998, 17 USC sec. 512, the author has designated an agent to receive notices of claims of copyright infringement: Copyright Agent, 2655 Le Jeune Rd., Suite # 808, Coral Gables, Florida, 33134; fax: 305-969-2917; Gobla1950@gmail.com. If you believe any of the images that appear in this book constitute copyright infringement on your work, please provide the copyright agent with the following information. Please be advised that to be effective, the notification must include ALL the requested information shown below:

1. A physical or electronic signature of a person authorized to act on behalf of the owner of an exclusive right that is allegedly infringed;

2. A description of the copyrighted image that is being claimed to have been infringed. Please provide the chapter and page number where the image is located to permit the author to identify the image in question.

3. Your address, telephone number, e-mail address, and all other information reasonably sufficient to permit the author to contact you;

4. A statement by you that you have a good-faith belief that the disputed use is not authorized by the copyright owner, its agent, or the law; AND

5. A statement by you, made under penalty of perjury, that the above information in your notification is accurate and that you are the copyright owner or are authorized on behalf of the owner of an exclusive right that is allegedly infringed. Notices of claimed copyright infringement should be directed to:

By Mail:
Copyright Agent
2655 Le Jeune Rd., Suite # 808,
Coral Gables, Florida 33134

By Fax: 305-969-2917
E-mail: Gobla1950@gmail.com

Dedication

To Margot, for taking this journey with me.

Acknowledgements

Hardly any book project is done in isolation. There are always individuals who encourage, support, recommend, suggest, and review these endeavors. The presence of these individuals in anyone's life makes the project much better because of the synergistic effects brought forth by these knowledgeable individuals.

Therefore, it is appropriate at this juncture to thank two such individuals. Firstly, I would like to express my gratitude and special thanks to Dr. Manuel A. Soler-Perez, M.D., for his valuable recommendations, suggestions, and careful review of this book. Dr. Soler's input substantially improved the quality of this project. Additionally, I would like to thank Margot C. Sarratea, MSN, ARNP, FNP-BC, an exceptional nurse practitioner whose knowledge, experience, and creative artistic talents unquestionably improved the content of this book and the design of its cover.

It is essential to understand that the quality of any book is attributed chiefly to its editor. Good editors make the work of the author that much better. HAIR LOSS: Options for Restoration & Reversal was substantially improved because of the excellence of its editor, Margot C. Sarratea. As always, I would like to express my sincere gratitude to Lisa Michelle Umina, an award-winning author, and publisher of Halo Publishing International, for her encouragement and support during this project.

Acknowledgments

Table of Contents

Chapter 12

Chapter 13

Chapter 14

Chapter 15

Chapter 19

Foreword

Hair loss affliction is a stressful experience for both men and women. However, it is substantially more distressing for women. From a historical perspective, the perceptions, and attitudes toward contracting the baldness condition have been overwhelmingly negative. Living with alopecia— hair loss— can be a stressful and challenging experience to endure, especially in cultures that view hair as a sign of youthful vitality and good health.

It is important to understand that hair loss has few physically harmful effects. However, for some, contracting the condition can result in psychological consequences, which can include high levels of anxiety and depression. Moreover, medical treatments for hair loss disorders have had limited effectiveness, and the failure to find a permanent cure can leave patients very distressed and disillusioned (Hunt, 2005).

It is my contention that given a choice, no one would want to lose their hair, especially at a young age. However, in today's contemporary society, shaving the head is a popular fad that— at least for the time being— can alleviate the psychological and emotional aspects of living with hair loss. It is a fact that living with the realization that we are losing our hair can be a challenging experience for most people.

Because hair loss can be a frightening experience for the afflicted, it renders these individuals vulnerable to an industry that thrives on the gullibility of individuals willing to pay for any product or service that claims to restore their hair-loss condition. Despite the negative stigma associated with the hair restoration industry, it is important to note that there are several reasonably safe, affordable, accessible, and effective hair-loss treatments currently available for most of the stricken. Therefore, to prevent being subjected to costly, ineffective, and even potentially dangerous hair restoration treatments, the solution is to become well-versed and educated on the subject matter. In fact, there is nothing more essential to mitigating risk in life than by becoming an educated consumer.

With that being said, the benefit for the consumer in search of reliable information about effective restorative hair-loss solutions is to purchase a copy of this valuable, essential, and informative book by Dr. Gomez. In fact, procuring a copy of this well-organized and researched book should be the first step for anyone afflicted with any of the forms of alopecia.

This book, essentially, will provide the consumer with a wealth of information about what is important to know about the field of hair loss and its many restorative treatment modalities. In essence, the book will explain what works and what does not work. Only after being armed with the excellent information that permeates the pages of this well-organized and researched book will the consumer be sufficiently educated to make a sound and informed decision about selecting the right course of action.

Your purchase of this book will be a worthwhile investment of time and money to learn how to select the correct treatment modality for your hair-loss condition in a safe way. I encourage every individual experiencing hair loss that has been fortunate enough to discover this informative book to embrace the teachings that Dr. Gomez presents and explains in its pages. The information will build your knowledge, which will help safeguard your health and financial resources when deciding on a course of action.

Manuel A. Soler-Perez, M.D.

Preface

The condition of hair loss is a topic of significant public interest, and understanding the pathophysiology and treatment of the different types of alopecia (hair loss) will surely have an impact on the men and women afflicted by this condition. This book aims to disseminate reliable factual information to the consuming public regarding the various causes of hair loss, the numerous hair restoration programs, and the multitude of treatment modalities available in the marketplace to address the problem of baldness.

Contemporary society places great emphasis on looking and feeling good due to the increased awareness about nutrition, exercising, anti-aging programs, and personal grooming practices. This environment of health-conscious consumers is fertile ground for the proliferation of deceptive and corrupt marketing schemes. These fraudulent schemes only increase the financial well-being of the individuals who cater to these markets without any benefits to the consumer.

An integral part of this looking-and-feeling-good philosophy is hair-loss restoration programs. These programs can be based on the topical application of various substances to the scalp, systemic medications, nutritional supplementation, low-level laser therapy (LLLT), Platelet-Rich Plasma (PRP) therapy, hair transplantation surgery, or a combination of two or more of these treatment modalities. Some of these programs can be helpful to the consumer, but others are designed to separate people from their hard-earned money. Most of these treatment modalities are extremely expensive; however, no matter how costly they might be, a large number of people will invest whatever is required in the hope of regrowing some of the hair they have lost throughout the years.

In this book, the author explains how hair grows, why it falls out, and the different types of alopecia. The book will also address the scientific basis of why certain treatment modalities cannot possibly work and why others can. The book will also explain hair's nutritional requirements, how hormones, age, and heredity affect hair loss, and many other related topics of interest. In essence, everything that is pertinent to the understanding of hair loss will be addressed throughout the book to create consumer awareness about hair loss and what can or cannot be done about it.

Finally, the author wants the readers to understand that the book is based on an extensive literature review of existing hair-loss research and the author's personal experiences with the majority of these hair restoration programs over the past thirty years. The author contends that it is possible to improve, restore, and in some cases, reverse the hair loss condition. However, to accomplish this objective, a multi-faceted strategic approach is required. This multi-faceted approach will require the use of several or all of the following modalities:

- Hair transplantation surgery.
- Topical minoxidil application.
- Systemic or topical finasteride (Propecia) therapy.
- Low-level laser therapy (LLLT).
- Platelet-Rich Plasma (PRP) therapy.
- Platelet-Rich Fibrin Matrix (PRFM) therapy.
- Scalp massage.
- Proper scalp and hair hygiene practices.
- Appropriate nutrition.

By employing this incremental approach of using the appropriate modality, the afflicted consumer will successfully maintain and retain a substantial amount of their hair. Moreover, with all the promising research studies currently being performed, the future for the prevention and regeneration of hair loss looks very promising. It is the sincere hope of the author that consumers armed with the information from this publication will be better prepared to make educated and well-informed decisions when selecting or evaluating any of the numerous hair restoration programs available today.

Gustavo J. Gomez, Ph.D.

1

Anatomy and Physiology of Hair Growth

As mentioned in the preface, the objective of this book is to provide a sound educational foundation for the reader who might be experiencing some degree of alopecia or is merely curious about discovering the various solutions available to treat hair loss. However, to accomplish this objective, it is essential for the reader to understand the anatomy and physiology of hair growth before delving into the specifics regarding the different theories and programs of hair loss restoration.

After understanding this foundational material, the consumer will be sufficiently knowledgeable regarding the various myths behind the different hair-loss treatment modalities addressed throughout this book. By merely understanding the physiology of hair growth, the reader will be able to discern why many of the treatments associated with hair-loss restoration programs cannot possibly work.

In humans, hair is a unique characteristic of mammals, which serves several functions. Hair is a special and cherished feature in humans, especially for females. However, the primary function of hair is protecting the skin from mechanical (traumatic) insults and facilitating a homeothermic environment (i.e., a stable internal body temperature). For example, the eyebrows and eyelashes can prevent foreign objects from entering the eyes, while scalp hair prevents sunlight, cold, and physical damage to the head and neck. Furthermore, the hair also has a sensory function. It increases the perception of the skin surface for tactile stimuli and additionally subserves important roles in human sexual and social communication (Buffoli et al., 2013).

Hair is composed of keratin (a sulfur-rich protein), which is the end product of a living structure called the hair follicle. Therefore, hair is simply the unification of dead cells in the form of threads or keratin filaments. The visible part of the hair is the shaft, while the root is the part embedded in the dermis (inner layer of the skin). The root, together with its covering, forms the hair follicle (Fig.1.1). At the bottom of the hair follicle, there is a loop of capillaries enclosed in a connective tissue covering called the hair dermal papilla. Human hair is a complex organ composed of two different types of cells: epithelial cells and dermal papillae cells. The clusters of epithelial cells lying over the papillae are the ones that reproduce themselves through the mitotic process, which makes the hair shaft.

Fig. 1.1: The Hair Follicle and its many parts

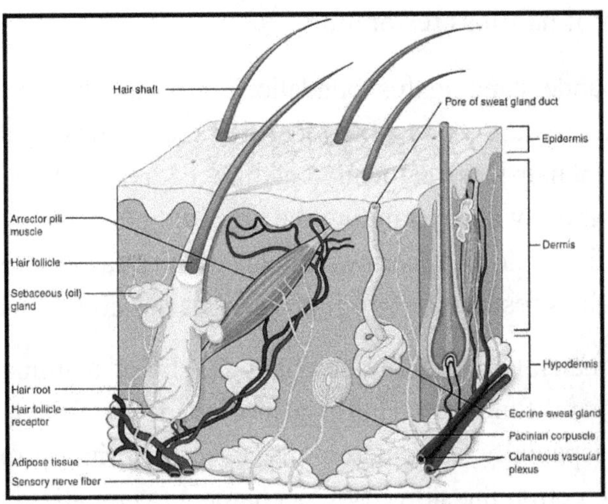

Image Source: By OpenStax College [CC BY 3.0 (http://creativecommons.org/licenses/by/3.0)], via Wikimedia Commonshttps://upload.wikimedia.org/wikipedia/commons/4/4f/501_Structure_of_the_skin.jpg

The hair shaft is the only part of the hair follicle to exit the skin's surface. Hair fibers are not continuous in their full length; instead, they result from compact groups of cells within the fiber follicle, from which three basic morphological components of hair structure originate. The hair shaft consists of a cortex, cuticle cells, and in some cases, a medulla in the central region (Fig.1.2). The medulla is the central part of the hair, whereas the cortex is on the periphery. The cortex represents the majority of the hair-fiber composition and plays a vital role in the physical and mechanical properties of the hair. Approximately 50-60% of the cortex is made up of ***macro-fibrils***, which consist of rods of ***micro-fibrils*** (keratinized filaments) embedded within a protein matrix (Fig.1.3). The cortex comprises the bulk of the hair shaft and is what gives hair its strength and most of its pigmentation (Buffoli et al., 2013).

Fig. 1.2: Human Hair Shaft Cross-Section

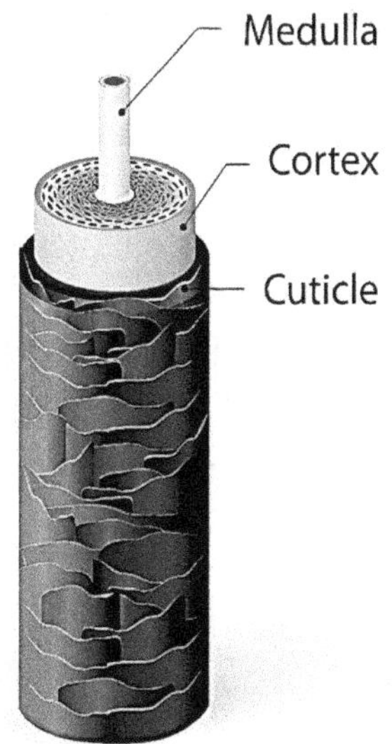

Image Source: http://www.istockphoto.com/vector/diagram-of-a-hair-follicle-in-a-cross-section-of-skin-layers-gm522128164-91529079

The dermal papillae cells regulate the proliferation of epithelial cells and influence hair growth. Men with male pattern baldness lose both types of cells, thus causing follicular miniaturization. This miniaturization process gradually makes the hair follicle smaller and smaller until it becomes a vellus-type hair (Yang & Xu, 2013;

Johnson, 2014). According to Drs. Yang and Xu, hair loss is difficult to treat because epithelial stem cells localized in a stem-cell-rich area of the hair follicle known as the bulge— are required for hair to grow. If these cells are absent, hair growth cannot occur.

The hair goes through a normal shedding (exogen) period during which up to 150 hairs per day are shedded. Hair loss (alopecia) will not occur as long as these cells remain alive and continue to reproduce, thereby replacing the shed hairs (Cheng & Bayliss, 2008). The individual hairs are kept soft and pliable by the glands that secrete varying amounts of an oily substance (sebum) onto the shaft of the hair follicle, which also lubricates and protects the epidermis, the outermost layer of skin (Fig. 1.1). These glands that secrete sebum— which is the hair's natural conditioner— are called the sebaceous glands. If for any reason, these sebaceous glands become overactive, more sebum will be secreted, which can cause a condition known as alopecia seborrheica. The term alopecia seborrheica is credited to the research studies of famed French physician Dr. Raymond Sabouraud and will be addressed more extensively in a subsequent chapter.

1.3: A cross-section of the hair follicle with its micro- and macro-fibrils structure

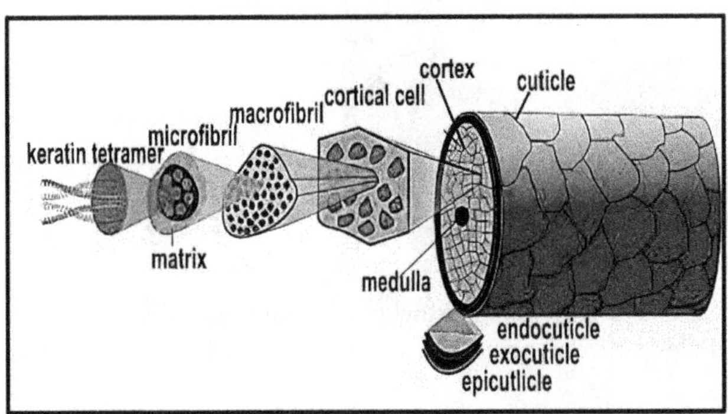

Image Source: Cruz, C.F., Costa, C., Gomes, A.C., Matamá, T., Cavaco-Paulo, A. Human Hair, and the Impact of Cosmetic Procedures: A Review on Cleansing and Shape-Modulating Cosmetics. Cosmetics. 2016; 3(3):26. http://www.mdpi.com/20799284/3/3/26/htm http://link.springer.com/chapter/10.1007/978-3-540-46911-7_1#page-1. Open Access License Image CC BY 4.0 International.

Ethnicity Hair Variations

Hair also has racial variations, which are believed to result from the asymmetric formation of the inner root sheath. Everyone is unique, and hair production rate, size, and shape differ for everyone. However, in general, there are some variations in the hair fiber for people of different ethnic backgrounds. If one looks at the cross-section of the inner root sheath, the shape is elliptical— shaped like a flattened circle— in Africans, round in Asians, and oval in Europeans (Fig.1.4). The shape of the follicle determines the shape of the hair shaft as it grows from the follicle. Since the hair shaft grows out of the hair follicle, the hair fiber diameter will be the same as the diameter of the inside of the follicle (Rook, 1975; Harris, 2015).

Fig. 1.4: Racial Hair Growth Variations

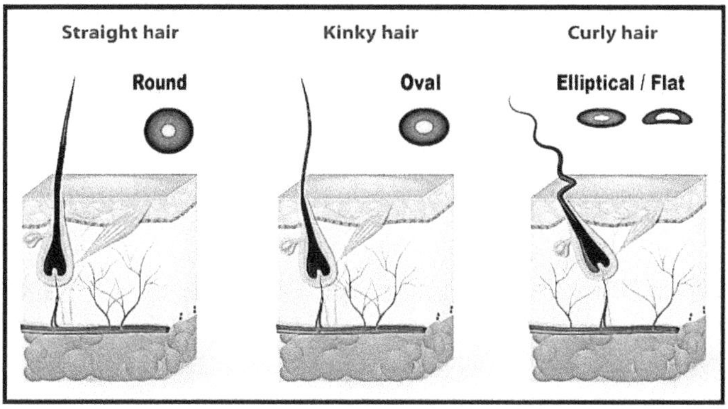

Image Source: http://www.istockphoto.com/vector/shape-of-the-hair-and-hair-anatomy-gm499580931-42594606. Modified image.

It has been observed that in straight or wavy hair, the hair follicles are almost vertical to the scalp's surface, with a slight angle. The angle of the hair follicle will determine the natural flow or wave pattern of the hair. In other words, the greater the curvature, the tighter the curl pattern. The follicle in straight or wavy hair is typically round or oval. In tightly curled hair, the hair follicles grow from the scalp almost parallel to the surface of the scalp. The hair follicle that produces tightly curled hair has a flattened, elliptical shape (Harris, 2015).

Hair-Growth Cycles Mechanism

The development of the hair is a dynamic, cyclic process in which many hormones and cytokines coordinate the duration of the hair-growth cycle. These cytokines are chemical messengers that mediate intercellular communication. This process depends not only on where the hair is growing but also on other factors, such as the individual's age, stage of development, nutritional habits, and environmental alterations like day-length (Buffoli et al., 2013; Wolfram, 2003).

Hair serves the functions of camouflage, communication, and protection from heat loss, trauma, infestation, and sunlight (Stenn, 2005). Moreover, it is a well-known theory that the functional activity of the hair follicle is a cyclical phenomenon in many species, including humans, which involves periods of active growth and periods of apparent inactivity (Chase, 1954; Flesh, 1954). The nature of this control mechanism is unknown. However, according to Hardy (1949, 1951), the mechanism controlling this cycle is cutaneous since hair growth can be seen to occur in vitro. Essentially, in-vitro (Latin for "within the glass") study or experimentation is a process that takes place in a test tube, culture dish, or elsewhere outside a living organism. This contrasts to with in-vivo (Latin for "within the living") studies, which are done on living organisms.

The following four steps represent the mechanisms of hair growth:

1. At the base of the hair follicle, there are living epithelial cells that go through an active mitotic process (multiplication or replication of cells).

2. As this mitotic process continues, the cells form a compact column, which eventually extends toward the surface of the skin.

3. This replication of epithelial cells (mitotic process) passes through an area where they are keratinized (covered by the protein keratin). This keratinizing region is located directly above the actively dividing cells.

4. As the cells become keratinized, they dehydrate and die, simply becoming a mass of keratin filaments (micro-fibrils) that are cemented together by a matrix rich with the amino acid cysteine. After this process is completed, the resulting structure is what is known as hair.

Hair-Growth Cycles

The hair follicle has the unique capacity to undergo periods of growth, regression, rest, and shedding before regenerating itself to restart the cycle. This dynamic cycling capacity enables mammals to change their coats and allows hair length to be controlled at different body sites. The timing of the hair-cycle phases and the overall duration of each phase varies depending on body site, gender, species, and race. Therefore, the hair follicle has been described as a cutaneous mini-organ that undergoes a continuous, self-organized, cyclical regeneration, and regression process. During each hair-growth cycle, a hair shaft is produced and shed. Thus, this event repeats cyclically for the individual's entire lifetime (Higgins et al., 2009).

Hair-growth cycles have been generally recognized as following specific growth phases with three distinct, concurrent stages. In other words, all three phases occur simultaneously, with each phase having a precise characteristic that determines the length of the hair. For example, one strand of hair may be in the anagen (growth) phase, while another is in the catagen (regression or transitional) phase, while still another is in the telogen (resting) phase. These terms were first suggested in 1926 by F.W. Dry to describe the growth phases of fur in mice.

It is important to note that, until recently, the hair-shedding function was assumed to be part of the telogen (resting) phase.

However, according to Milner et al. (2002), shedding actually occurs as a distinct phase. Therefore, instead of three hair-growth cycles, Milner contends that there are four phases, the fourth being the exogen (shedding) phase or cycle. In fact, Milner's research—with the use of the electron microscope—uncovered that the moored (anchored) cells of the exogen root show intercellular separation, suggesting a proteolytic process in the final shedding step of the exogen cycle. Milner's research is the first to describe a distinct shedding, or exogen, phase of the hair-growth cycle. Their study supports the notion that the exogen phase is uniquely controlled and that the final step in the shedding process involves a specific, proteolytic step. Thus, Milner contends is that there are four hair-growth stages, as listed below and schematically demonstrated in Figure1.5.

- Anagen Stage (growing phase).
- Catagen Stage (regression/transition phase).
- Telogen Stage (resting phase).
- Exogen/Teloptosis Stage (shedding phase).

Fig. 1.5: The Four Hair-Growth Cycle

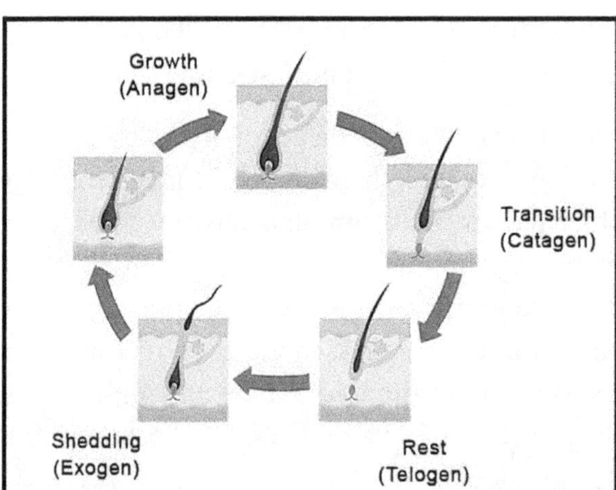

Image Source: By Suneticslasers (Owner). Modified image. (Use with Permission). http://www.suneticslasers.com/how-it-works/

Anagen Stage (growth phase)

Anagen is the stage or period when the hair is actively growing. As previously mentioned, this is the time when the cells actively divide and go through the keratinizing area. This stage, which is the longest, begins in the papilla and can last from two to six years, though the average length of time is three years. The span of time that the hair remains in this stage of growth is determined by genetics. The longer the hair stays in the anagen stage, the faster and longer it will grow. It has been observed that the anagen stage is longer for Asians, lasting approximately seven years. Therefore, Asian hair can grow longer than hair from other ethnicities. Asian hair can grow as much as one meter. It is estimated that approximately 85-90% of all the hairs on the scalp are in this anagen stage (Ferriman, 1971).

Catagen Stage (regression/transition phase)

The catagen phase starts when the anagen (growth) phase comes to an end. This is the stage of the hair-growth cycle that responds to an unknown trigger. The hair follicle begins to change rapidly, with the base of the hair becoming keratinized to form a club-like shape. The middle region of the hair bulb shrinks, cellular growth stops, and the hair root is pushed toward the surface of the skin.

The catagen stage is also known as the regression or transition phase. This stage, in essence, allows the hair follicle to renew itself. The stage lasts approximately one to three weeks before the hair goes into a complete resting stage, the telogen stage.

Telogen Stage (resting phase)

In this stage, the papilla of the hair is released from the hair bulb, making the hair go into a resting period. This phase in the hair growth cycle lasts approximately two to four months, which means that hair growth ceases since the hair follicle is inactive during this period.

During this stage, the hair is still attached to the follicle's base, but if this attachment is weakened, the hair is shed. It is estimated that approximately 10%-15% of the hairs on the human scalp are in this telogen, or resting, stage. At the end of the telogen stage, the hair follicle reenters the anagen (growth) phase. The dermal papilla and the base of the follicle join together again, and a new hair begins to form. If the old hair has not already been shed, the new hair pushes the old one out, and the growth cycle starts all over again.

Exogen Stage/Teloptosis (shedding phase)

"Exogen" is a term coined by Kurt Stenn (2005) and indicates the moment the club-like hair is shed from the follicle that is already occupied by a new, terminal, anagen hair. Thus, the exogen phase is a part of the resting phase in which the old hair detaches and sheds, and new hair continues to grow. As the term suggests, Exogen is a new phase of the hair cycle. However, according to researchers C. Piérard-Franchimont and G. E. Piérard (2001), the term has created a controversy. These researchers contend that since the duration of the exogen cycle is too short, it should not deserve the recognition of being classified as a cycle.

In fact, researchers Piérard-Franchimont and Piérard (2001) contend that the exogen cycle might more appropriately suggest a biological, exogenous process rather than a distinct hair cycle. Hence, they instead proposed the term "Teloptosis" as a more appropriate term. These researchers felt that the word teloptosis, which is derived from the Greek word τελος πτωση, which means falling off, is more relevant to indicate the same phenomenon.

Hair is shed at a rate of approximately 50 to 150 hairs per day or an average of 100 hairs, with roughly the same number being regenerated (Milner et al., 2002; Cheng & Bayliss, 2008; Stenn, 2005). If this process is not balanced, meaning that if hair loss is greater than the rate of regeneration, thinning of the scalp will begin to occur. The end result will be hair loss, or alopecia, as it is medically called. Thinning or balding will not be apparent until approximately 25% of the hair is lost (Cheng & Bayliss, 2008). Everyone sheds hair; however, the presence of a large number of hairs on the comb, in the sink, in the tub, or on the bed pillow can be a sign of hair loss caused by traumatic grooming practices, poor nutrition, medications, or an underlying disease process (Harris, 2015).

The ratio between the hairs that are in the anagen and the telogen stage can be a useful diagnostic tool in evaluating if there is excessive hair loss. This test is convenient because the anagen or telogen stage possesses distinct characteristics in their histological appearances, which can be observed with the aid of a microscope. If there is a high telogen count— hairs having a club-like appearance— in proportion to the anagen count, it is an indication that an abnormal amount of hair is being shed or permanently lost.

At this juncture, it is important to state that scientists have observed a novel phenomenon in hair cycling research. This new discovery was the observation of the existence of yet another hair-growth cycle that has been named the ***kenogen cycle.*** The author will describe this new hair-growth cycle in the next section.

Kenogen Cycle (empty phase)

As mentioned above, more recently, another important concept has been introduced in human trichology by Rebora and Guarrera (2004)—the kenogen cycle, which, in essence, is the fifth hair growth cycle. Trichology is the science that deals with the study of hair and its diseases. Rebora and Guarrera, while researching hair-growth cycles with the use of phototrichogram, observed an interesting phenomenon in the hair-cycling mechanism. The phenomenon they observed was the emptiness of the follicle after the exogen/teloptosis cycle. Rebora and Guarrera called this phenomenon "kenogen," which, according to the researchers, is a word derived from the Greek word "kappaepsilonnuóvarsigma" which means "to empty out." However, it could also be derived from κενόω (kenóo), which also means "to empty out" or "emptied."

Kenogen indicates the physiological interval of the hair cycle in which the hair follicle remains empty after the telogen hair has been ejected or shed and before a new anagen hair emerges. Kenogen frequency and duration are greater in men and women with androgenetic alopecia (AGA), which possibly could account for baldness (Rebora & Guarrera, 2004). Therefore, exogen is the release of telogen fibers from hair follicles. Kenogen is the lag time between exogen and the new anagen fiber development. It is postulated that in kenogen, the hair follicle may follow an alternative route during which the telogen phase, not accompanied by a coincident or concurrent, new, early anagen hair, ends with teloptosis, leaving the follicle empty (Fig. 1.6). In other words, whenever a telogen hair is shed, there is an anagen hair already present in the follicle to replace the ejected hair. However, occasionally the follicle will stay empty after the telogen hair has been shed.

Fig. 1.6: Kenogen Hair Cycle

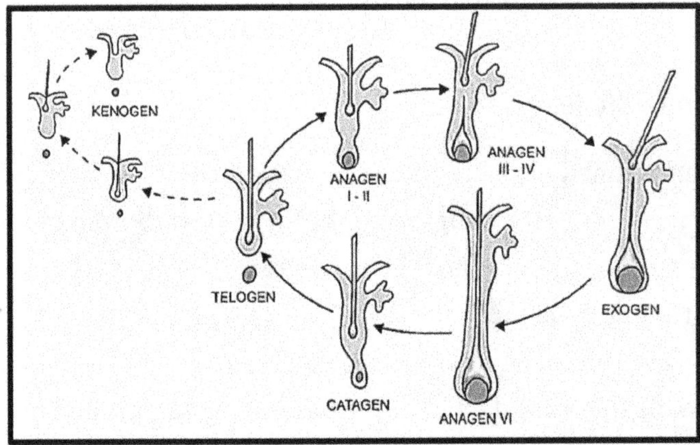

Image Source: Cruz, C.F., Costa, C., Gomes, A.C., Matamá, T., Cavaco-Paulo, A. Human Hair, and the Impact of Cosmetic Procedures: A Review on Cleansing and Shape-Modulating Cosmetics. Cosmetics. 2016; 3(3):26. http://www.mdpi.com/2079-9284/3/3/26/htm http://link.springer.com/chapter/10.1007/978-3-540-46911-7_1#page-1. Open Access journal. License Image under CC BY 4.0 International.

Researchers have observed this new kenogen cycle using the phototrichogram (photographic trichogram), which is a non-invasive method that provides an accurate qualitative and quantitative assessment of the hair. The phototrichogram was first introduced by Saitoh et al. in 1970. This technology allowed for the in-vivo study of the hair-growth cycle. The phototrichogram can also be used to quantify shed hair and to determine the rate of hair growth, the size of hair fibers, and the frequency of telogen hair follicles. Several variants of the phototrichogram have become popular for evaluating hair in restoration clinics and clinical research trials. The TrichoScan® and the FolliScope® are the two-main automated phototrichogram systems available.

It is estimated that the human scalp holds approximately 100,000 hairs, with blond people having slightly more and redheads having slightly less. These hairs do not emerge individually from the scalp but are arranged in small groups of one to four hairs each. These one-to-four hair groupings are called follicular units (FUs). There are approximately 50,000 to 65,000 FUs on the human scalp (Harris, 2015.). Approximately 10,000 to 15,000 hairs are in the Telogen (resting) stage, and 85,000 to 90,000 are in the anagen (growth) stage (Cotsarelis & Millar, 2001; Garza et al., 2012; Ferriman, 1971; keratin.com, 2013).

Hair undergoes these four stages of growth every two to six years on average. Scalp hair grows faster in men than in women. In men, it grows approximately 0.44 millimeters per day on the crown and 0.39 millimeters per day on the temple— in other words, about half an inch every month. The rate of growth is slightly less for women. Each hair follicle goes through the hair cycle 10 to 20 times in a lifetime (Ferriman, 1971; keratin.com, 2013). All body hair undergoes a similar life cycle. However, the extent and the duration of its growth phases and the length of individual shafts vary between different body areas and between individuals depending on genetic programming, genre, age, and health status (Araújo, Fernandes, Cavaco-Paulo, & Gomes, 2010).

Types of Human Hair Classification

Human hair can be classified in two ways—as androgen-independent hair, such as the eyebrows and the eyelashes, and as androgen-dependent hair in body regions such as the scalp, beard, chest, axilla, legs, and pubic area (Buffoli et al., 2013). Biologically, there are only three main types of human hair that are naturally formed by the body. They are:

- Lanugo Hair.
- Vellus Hair.
- Terminal Hair.

Lanugo Hair

This type of hair is known as fetal hair. It is the first hair that begins to form by the third month in the womb. Lanugo hair has a downy texture that is unpigmented and unmedullated. It is found in fetuses and sometimes in malnourished children and adults (Menton, 2007). This type of hair is rather long and silky and is usually shed in the womb a few weeks before birth. Subsequently, it is replaced with vellus hair, which grows out of the same hair follicles (Menton, 2007).

However, lanugo hair can be seen on premature babies because they are born before the lanugo hair is shed. Therefore, the growth of lanugo hair is a normal physiologic occurrence for practically all infants while in the womb; and it is not uncommon for premature babies to be born with lanugo hair still covering their entire bodies (Fig.1.7). Moreover, the growth of lanugo hair is also a symptom of deep starvation. In fact, the growing of fine, white hair all over the body is a phenomenon almost exclusively related to anorexia.

Fig.1.7: Premature baby with unshed lanugo hair

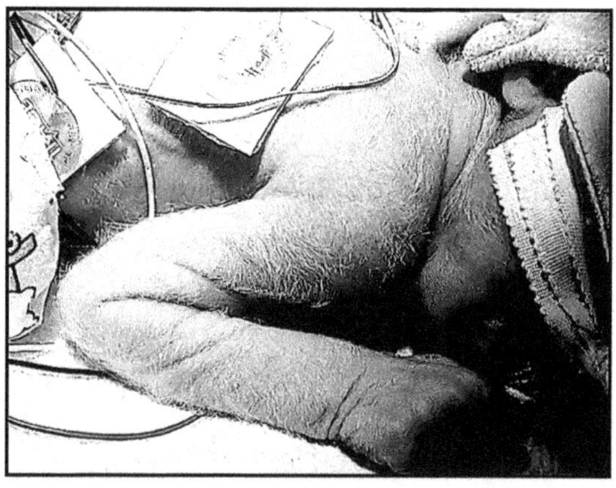

Image Source: https://cdn assets.answersingenesis.org/img/articles/am/v2/n3/Human_Hair1. License under Creative Commons (CC) Attribution Share-Alike 3.0. file:///C:/Users/MyPC/Documents/Downloads/Integumentary-System---of---EPISD-Anatomy-and-Physiology_ch_v52_lz5_s1.pdf

The reason why the body grows lanugo hair in the anorexic or malnourished individual is as a compensatory mechanism to maintain the body temperature. When an anorexic loses too much weight and no longer has sufficient body fat for insulation to help maintain an adequate thermal environment, the body takes over and produces lanugo hair. These hairs grow thickly in an attempt to trap heat that is lost from the body before it dissipates. Lanugo hair is almost like a blanket that the body grows itself (Morrisey, 2016).

Vellus Hair

Vellus hair replaces lanugo hair in the postnatal period (following birth), and it covers the entire surface of the body, with the exception of certain areas. For example, vellus hair is not typically found on the lips, eyelids, backs of the ears, palms of the hands, soles of the feet, or navel. Vellus hair remains on the body throughout life and is later joined by darker, coarser terminal hair, especially after puberty. In fact, humans are usually born with approximately 5 million follicles, and it is believed that no new follicles are added after birth. Thus, in the womb, the body develops all the hair follicles it will ever have (Wolff et al., 2009; Habif, 2010). Vellus hair is soft, fine, and unmedullated like lanugo hair; however, it may be pigmented (Fig. 1.8 and 1.9). A true vellus hair does not have an attached arrector pili muscle. Only the miniaturized vellus-like hairs found in androgenetic alopecia have arrector pili muscle.

Fig. 1.8: Vellus Hairs "Peach Fuzz"

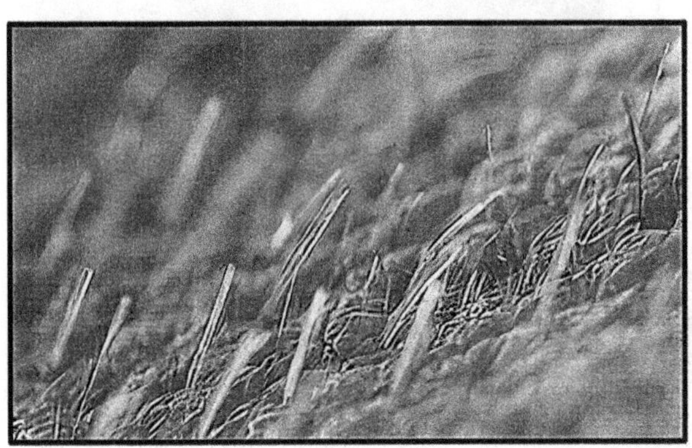

Image Source: By Svdmolen (Self-published work by Svdmolen) [GFDL (http://www.gnu.org/copyleft/fdl.html), CC-BY-SA-3.0 http://creativecommons.org/licenses/by-sa/3.0/) or CC BY 2.5 https://commons.wikimedia.org/wiki/File:Huid.jpg#/media/File:Huid.jpg

Fig. 1.9: Vellus and Terminal Hairs

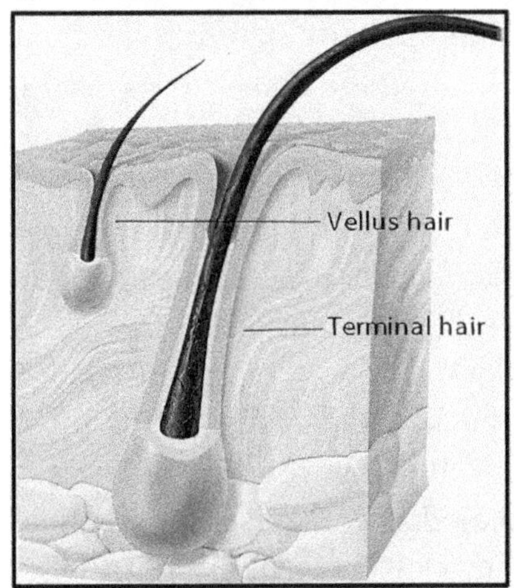

Image Source: https://drentezari.com/wp-content/uploads/2015/01/Velus-terminal-hair.jpg. Modified image.

According to some researchers, vellus hair has a dual function. It can provide both thermal insulation and cooling of the body, which helps regulate body temperature. In fact, vellus hair functions as a wick for sweat. For example, while a skin pore is open, sweat wets a strand of vellus hair, which then evaporates. This continuous process of wetting and evaporating of the vellus hair is the process of perspiration. Thus, vellus hair— though it may seem small and unimportant— serves an essential function in thermoregulation.

Another useful function of vellus hair is that it serves as an extension of the skin's sensory functions. It can alert an individual to the presence of goosebumps or insects crawling on the skin. Therefore, vellus hairs extend our sense of touch beyond our skin into the air around us, detecting puffs of breeze and even the vibrations of the wings of passing insects, with no direct contact required (Menton, 2007).

Vellus hair is the scientific name for what has been called "peach fuzz." The bulb of a vellus hair follicle is found in the upper dermis region of the skin; therefore, the vellus follicle is not connected to a sebaceous gland, as seen with terminal hairs. However, there is some research that indicates that a relationship between sebaceous gland activity and vellus hair growth does exist (Kligman & Strauss, 1956). Vellus hairs are very short, rarely exceeding .03 millimeters in diameter or greater than 1to 2 millimeters in length (Fig. 1.9). Notwithstanding their small size and proclivity for going unnoticed, vellus hairs are essential for a person's general well-being.

Terminal Hair.

Terminal hair begins its development as peach fuzz or vellus-type hair. Subsequently, during puberty, because of the introduction of androgenic hormones such as testosterone, it continues to grow and finally begins to develop color (pigmentation) and some degree of coarseness. The end result of this process is the development of terminal-type hair (Fig.1.10). Therefore, terminal hair is thick, strong, and pigmented. These hairs have fully matured and have a medulla. This type of hair grows from the scalp, eyebrows, underarms, pubic area, and other parts of the body.

Fig. 1.10: The development of the terminal hair process

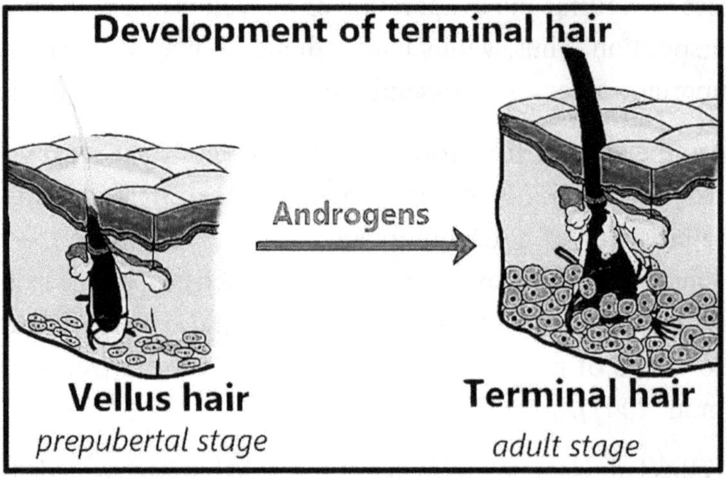

Image Source: By Kubek15/Slave (File: Androgensensibilitaet. JPG) [GFDL (http://www.gnu.org/copyleft/fdl.html) or CC BY-SA 4.0-3.0-2.5-2.0-1.0 https://commons.wikimedia.org/wiki/File%3AVellushaarTerminalhaar-translation.JPG (http://creativecommons.org/licenses/by-sa/4.0-3.0-2.5-2.0-1.0)], via Wikimedia Commons

This type of hair is created in the anagen stage of the hair-growth cycle. In fact, all terminal hair is finer and shorter at some point as it comes out of the telogen cycle and enters the anagen stage, where it thickens, enlarges, darkens (becomes pigmented), and subsequently matures. This process, or change, occurs in both males and females. However, because males have a higher level of testosterone than females, they tend to grow a denser amount of mature terminal hairs throughout the body. This growth can be typically seen around the face, under the arms (axilla), and sometimes on the chest. It is important to remember that not all vellus hair becomes terminal. Moreover, both types of hair, terminal and vellus, can be found on the body at all times.

The Hair Miniaturization Process in Hair Loss

When male and female baldness begins to appear, thinner and thinner hair replaces the terminal hair until the hair follicle eventually is returned to a primitive, embryonic state. In other words, terminal hair essentially undergoes a process of miniaturization. This hair miniaturization process is strongly believed to be due to the influence of the hormone dihydrotestosterone (DHT). During the hair miniaturization process, the hair shafts become thinner over time until the hair is returned to a vellus-type hair that becomes dormant and static in its ability to grow (Figs. 1.11 and 1.12). This process of miniaturization continues until partial or complete baldness results.

As previously stated, the miniaturization process is initiated by the influence of the hormone DHT on genetically predisposed hair. When these genetically predisposed follicular units are affected by DHT, there is a gradual decline in the hair's diameter, which results in thinner, shorter, and weaker hairs with each successive hair-growth cycle. When enough terminal hair is in a state of miniaturization, there appears to be a visible thinning of the hair in the affected areas. As more hairs in each follicular unit become miniaturized, the process may eventually lead to complete baldness in that area of the scalp (Bernstein, 2013).

Fig. 1.11: Genetic hair loss by the process of miniaturization (schematic I)

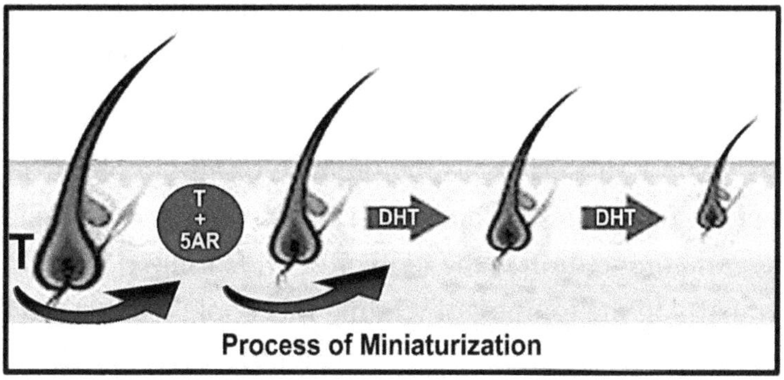

Image Source: Gustavo J Gomez. Modified image. Testosterone-5-AR-DHTconversion process.

Fig. 1.12: Genetic hair loss by the process of miniaturization (schematic II)

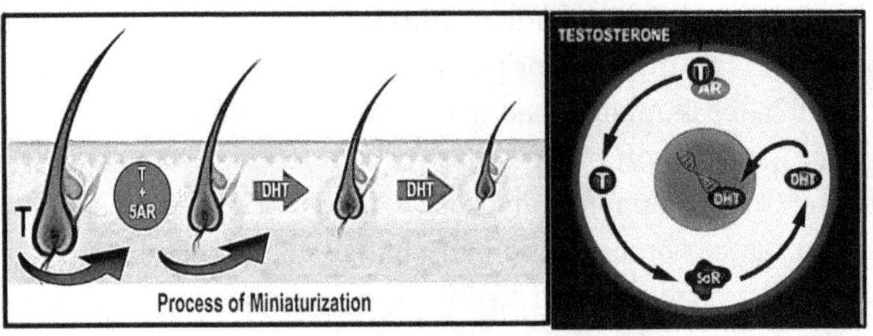

Image Source: http://www.istockphoto.com/vector/treatment-of-hair-thinning-and-shedding-gm656040416- Gustavo J Gomez. Modified image. Testosterone-5-AR-DHTconversion process.

Therefore, the gradual process of follicular miniaturization is essentially considered the primary cause of androgenetic alopecia (AGA) or male pattern baldness (MPB). In fact, identifying hair miniaturization is an excellent diagnostic tool or marker that can be used as a key identifier when visually inspecting the scalp for signs of hair loss. When hair miniaturization is identified, it almost always means that future hair loss can be expected.

A parting note to the reader before proceeding to all subsequent chapters, it is possible you will encounter a certain degree of repetition in some sections. I assure you this repetitiveness was intentional. The objective of any book is to teach the reader something of value—hopefully. Thus, the author decided to use some repetition to emphasize specific points that are considered necessary.

The author subscribes to the premise of an old philosophical Latin phrase that states, ***"Repetitio est mater studiorum."*** What this means is that repetition is the mother of all learning. Therefore, as you embark on the journey of reading this book, understand that a degree of redundancy is necessary for learning. It is especially crucial when learning about medical concepts and terminology essential to understanding this topic. Thus, repetition helps to improve speed, increases confidence, and strengthens the brain's connections that support the learning process. In essence, it ensures reception by the audience. Enjoy the journey.

2

Male Pattern Hair Loss Classifications

Androgenetic alopecia, or pattern hair loss, is the most common cause of hair loss experienced by both men and women after puberty. This type of hair loss typically manifests as progressive thinning, miniaturization, and loss of hair at the affected sites. To date, there have been numerous pattern hair-loss classification systems proposed by various researchers for grading hair-loss patterns of both men and women. These systems vary from simpler systems based on hairline recession to more advanced, multifactorial systems based on the morphological and dynamic parameters that affect the scalp and the hair itself (Gupta & Mysore, 2016).

The pattern hair-loss classifications for men are described below, followed by the female hair-loss classifications in Chapter 3. Below is a historical sequence of the most important hair-loss classification systems for men that have been proposed to date.

Hair-Loss Classification Scales

- **Beek Classification (1950)**

  In 1950, Dr. C. H. Beek developed what is considered a simple hair-loss classification system. He essentially evaluated 1000 Caucasian subjects who had male pattern baldness. Beek's system classified these patterns into two stages of hair loss based on the stage of evolution: frontal and frontovertical. Despite the simplicity of Beek's approach, the scale is considered significant because this was essentially the first attempt to classify hair loss.

- **Hamilton Classification (1951)**

  The Hamilton hair-loss classification scale set the benchmark for all future male pattern hair loss classifications because it elaborately described the various evolutionary stages of hair loss. However, Hamilton did not describe a few rare hair-loss patterns, which Dr. O'Tar Norwood subsequently added to his hair-loss classification scale. The addition of these new hair loss patterns by Norwood contributed to today's most commonly used scale, the Hamilton-Norwood scale. Hamilton's research is described in more detail later in this chapter.

- **Ogata Classification (1953)**

  In 1953, Dr. T. Ogata identified 15 different subtypes of pattern hair loss and classified them into six distinct subtypes based on a study of Japanese men. Ogata's scale is somewhat different from other classification systems that are based on Caucasian men, suggesting that the development of pattern baldness in Japanese men may be different from Caucasians.

- **Feit Classification (1969)**

  In 1969, Dr. L. J. Feit developed a hair-loss classification system that was more detailed than Dr. Hamilton's 1951 version. Feit characterized 12 different varieties of hair-loss patterns with 16 categories.

- **Setty Classification (1970)**

  Dr. L. R. Setty, in 1970, developed a classification system that was an improvement over Hamilton's classification because it incorporated patterns of hair loss seen in black males. However, Setty's scale lacked the detailed staging of hair loss evolution of hair loss. Thus, it failed to find much favor with practicing clinicians.

- **Norwood Classification (1975)**

  Dr. O'Tar Norwood revised Hamilton's hair-loss classification system in 1975 after studying pattern hair loss in 1,000 males. The Norwood classification, combined with Hamilton's, is the most widely used hair-loss classification system for men. However, as previously mentioned, the Norwood scale further defined two major patterns and several less common types. Despite being the most widely used classification system, it is considered too detailed, divided, and complicated to be used for various surgical procedures. Norwood's research is described in more detail later in this chapter.

- **Bouhanna and Nataf Classification (1976)**

  Dr. P. Bouhanna's 1976 scale was a simplified classification system based on the observations of European Caucasian men. This classification determined the extent of hair loss as well as allowing for a precise evaluation of the surgical indications for hair transplantation. However, this classification system was not helpful in deciding the type of surgical procedure required; thus, it had a usefulness limitation. This initial limitation was later addressed by Dr. Bouhanna himself in 1996 when he developed a dynamic classification system with Dr. Dardour (Gupta & Mysore, 2007).

- **Blanchard and Blanchard Classification (1984)**

  In 1984, Drs. G. Blanchard and B. Blanchard proposed a different classification system that considered six evolutionary stages that were determined by six measurements. These measurements were: glabella-frontal, superciliary-frontal, interparietal, frontovertical, helicon-vertical, and nucho-vertical distances. This classification system was not a commonly used scale because it was difficult to apply. It required multiple measurements from every patient in order to classify the various patterns of hair loss, which was a tedious and time-consuming process.

- **Bouhanna and Dardour Dynamic Classification (1996)**

  This classification was more detailed than the previously described system by Bouhanna and Nataf in 1976. The various parameters included in this system considered the stage of hair loss, the density of hair, laxity or looseness of the scalp, aspect of hair, color and thickness of the hair, and the rate of hair growth.

  Moreover, this dynamic classification system considered varying parameters that were not contemplated by Hamilton, such as the covering power of hair, density in each region, and rate of hair growth. However, this system was too complicated and difficult to apply in routine practice because it involved many scalp measurements and parameters.

- **Koo Classification (2000)**

  The research team of Koo et al. (2000), in their study of more than 1,700 Korean male participants with pattern hair loss, proposed a new, simpler, more straightforward classification method. In this classification, male pattern baldness was classified into six subtypes. For example, type M, type C, type O, type U, type MO, and type CO. These classifications used English alphabetical letters that reflected or resembled the shape of the area of baldness. The primary advantage of Dr. S. H. Koo's classification over previous systems was that it claimed to be a simpler and easier-to-apply scale that did not require any complex scalp measurements and was also useful for planning surgery.

Despite all these proposed hair loss classification scales, the Hamilton and Norwood hair-loss scales are currently the two most-used classification systems for determining men's baldness patterns.

Typically the terms male pattern baldness, male pattern hair loss, androgenetic alopecia, hereditary alopecia, and common baldness are all synonymous terms that follow a well-defined and distinct hair-loss pattern.

Both Dr. James B. Hamilton in 1951 and Dr. O'Tar Norwood in 1975 performed extensive studies relating to the classification of various types of baldness patterns seen in men. The work of these two researchers provided a standardized guide for physicians or anyone interested in hair restoration to compare patterns of baldness with the standard classified pattern.

Development of Hamilton's Hair-Loss Classification Scale

Dr. Hamilton, an anatomist, developed his male pattern hair-loss scale by recording his observations of 312 men and 214 women, ranging in age from 20 to 89 years old. All the study participants were Caucasian except for 77 Chinese males. Hamilton used a classification system that involved eight separate hair-loss patterns—types I through VII, with an additional type-III-vertex pattern. In types I through III of Hamilton's classification system, including type III vertex, there was minimal hair loss. However, classification types IV through VII manifested progressively more extensive hair loss (Fig. 2.1).

Hamilton contends that his study demonstrated that up to 96% of men and 79% of women would develop at least a type-II hair-loss stage once the individual reaches full pubertal sexual maturation. He further claimed that 58% of men over the age of 50 manifested a type-V to a type-VII hair-loss pattern, which appeared to subside once the subject reached the age of 70. The progression for women indicated that by 50 years of age, 25% of women had developed a type-IV hair-loss pattern, which stabilized once women were past the age of 50. According to Hamilton, his classification scale was 99% accurate.

Fig. 2.1: Hamilton's classification of male pattern baldness by types of hair loss

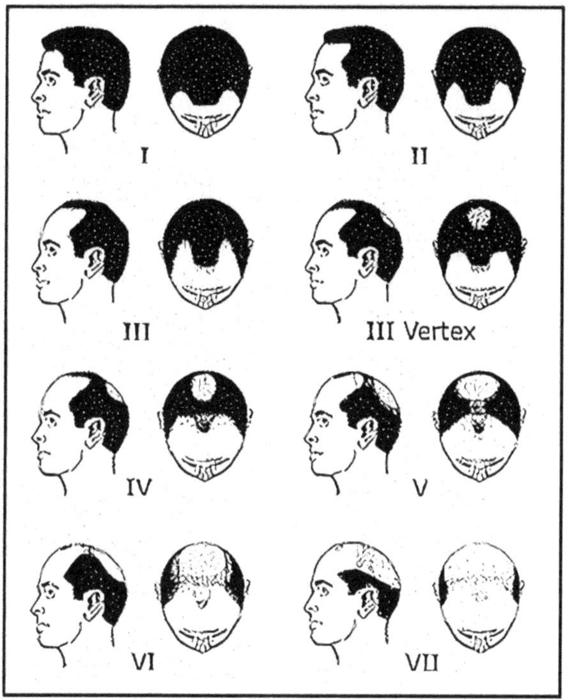

Image Source: http://www.thehealthsite.com/beauty/what-are-the-causes-of-male-pattern-baldness-k915/

To validate or prove his classification scale's ease of use and effectiveness, Hamilton recruited four attendants at a mental institution who had no scientific training. He gave each attendant a copy of his sketches and a brief description of the various hair-loss classifications. The four attendants briefly studied Hamilton's information and then used his sketches or drawings to classify 125 subjects who Hamilton had previously examined correctly. The validation study results showed that 98% of the time, attendants could replicate the same classifications that Hamilton had assigned to the study participants. This rudimentary evaluation process yielded simple but persuasive evidence that the classification scale was accurate and could be reliably used in dermatology clinics by anyone with some basic training.

What follows is an explanation of Hamilton's various types of hair-loss classification, as shown in Figure 2.1.

- TYPE I

This hair-loss pattern indicates a minimal amount or no recession in the fronto-temporal area. Therefore, no treatment is required. Unless there is a familial genetic predisposition identified for baldness, there is no need to worry. However, if there is a family history of hair loss, then the situation should be monitored in order to take the appropriate steps if it becomes necessary.

- TYPE II

This pattern manifests as a triangular and typically symmetrical area of recession in the fronto-temporal area, with no recession in the mid-frontal border. Hair loss remains ahead of a line several centimeters in front of the ears. Hair falls out and may become less dense in the central- front part of the scalp. Initial signs of baldness are becoming evident.

- TYPE III

This pattern indicates a deep recession of the fronto-temporal area, with a moderate recession of the mid-frontal area. This classification is considered the point of sufficient hair loss and can be called true baldness.

- TYPE III Vertex

This pattern is a variation of the type-III classification. In this type of baldness, the loss of hair is mainly in the vertex area, with a minimal fronto-temporal recession.

- TYPE IV

This pattern indicates a severe recession in the fronto-temporal area, with concomitant baldness in the vertex area. It can also be observed that a wide band of moderately dense hair separates the area of the vertex from the frontal area.

- TYPE V

This pattern indicates a more advanced degree of baldness, with a narrower hairband separating the vertex area from the frontal area. When classification types V through VII are viewed from above, the remaining hair at the sides and back are a distinct horseshoe shape.

- TYPE VI

This pattern indicates a more severe or complete type of baldness in both the frontal and vertex areas. The bridge of hair that once crossed the crown is now lost, with only sparse hair remaining. In essence, the fronto-temporal and vertex areas are coalescing or merging into one region. Additionally, the hair loss from the sides has extended further.

- TYPE VII

This hair-loss pattern is called calvities Hippocratica, or Hippocratic baldness, named after the Greek philosopher Hippocrates. It is the most severe type of baldness, creating a horseshoe-type appearance. It is possible to see this type VII classification without the hairband that separates the fronto-temporal area from the vertex.

Development of Norwood's Hair-Loss Classification Scale

In 1975, Dr. O'Tar Norwood, a dermatologist and distinguished hair transplantation surgeon expanded Hamilton's classifications after conducting his own study of 1,000 male subjects. To develop his hair-loss classification chart, Norwood took Hamilton's classifications from 1951 and improved upon them by adding more detail. Norwood added more classification stages and included 474 more participants in his study. Norwood's hair-loss classification chart would eventually become known as the *Norwood Chart of Male Pattern Baldness* (Fig.2.2). As previously mentioned, Norwood's hair-loss classification chart is currently the most widely used scale for determining the pattern of hair loss in men.

Fig. 2.2: The Norwood-Hamilton combined hair loss scale with type-A variants (or the Norwood chart of male pattern baldness)

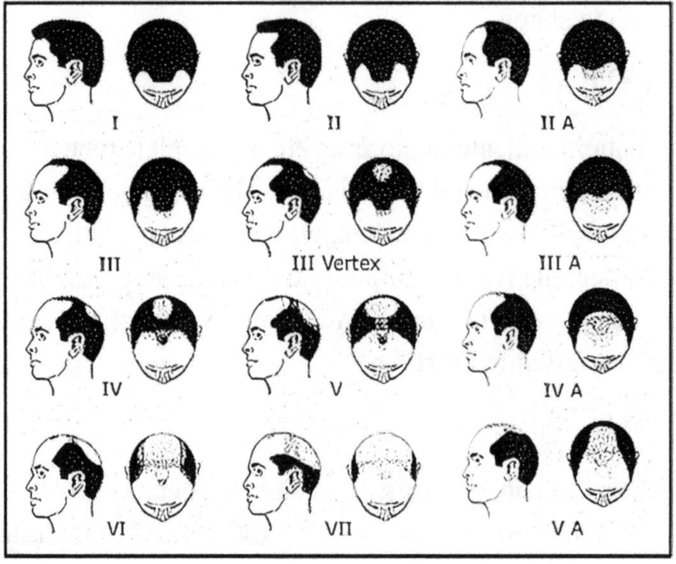

Image Sources: http://prescottgenomics.wikispaces.com/androgenetic+alopecia. Contributions to http://prescottgenomics.wikispaces.com/ are licensed under a Creative Commons Attribution-Share-Alike 3.0 License.

Dr. Norwood's research determined that there were two major hair-loss patterns: the common baldness pattern and the type-A variant pattern. The common pattern was the predominant type of hair loss that affected 97% of the men who participated in the study. This common alopecia pattern showed significant hair loss at the classification level of type-III. Norwood observed that in this common hair-loss pattern, thinning began in the temples and in the crown-vertex area, which slowly but progressively encompassed the entire top of the scalp. To learn about the various regions of hair loss, see Figure 2.3.

Fig. 2.3: Baldness map to determine the area of hair loss

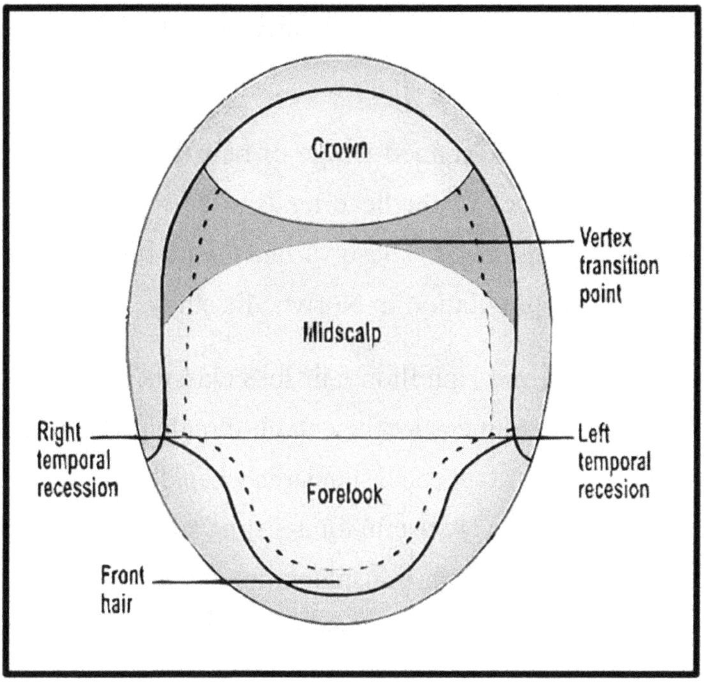

Image Source: http://www.hairtransplantkochi.com/fue-hair-transplant.php

Type-A Variant Hair-Loss Classification Patterns

The second type of hair loss that Norwood classified was the type-A variant, which constituted the remaining 3% of the study participants. Dr. Norwood contends that type-II through type-V hair-loss patterns may be designated as type-A variants. To warrant a type-A variant classification, the following major and minor features must be present:

Major features of alopecia type-A variants

- The entire anterior hairline border recedes in unison without leaving the mid-frontal peninsula of hair.
- There is no simultaneous balding of the crown-vertex.

Minor features of alopecia type-A variants

- Scattered, sparse hairs frequently persist in the entire area of balding.
- The horseshoe-shaped fringe of hair that remains on the sides and back of the head tends to be wider and reaches higher on the head. These variants were observed in only 3% of the population in Norwood's study.

The Norwood and Hamilton hair-loss classification scales are standardized ways to measure the extent of male pattern baldness. They are generally the accepted standards when describing hair loss (Fig. 2.2). These scales are useful for assisting surgeons in screening candidates for possible hair transplantation surgery. They can also help guide the selection of the hair transplant procedure that will lead to the best results for the client.

Norwood's type-A variants are typically characterized by a predominantly front-to-back progression of hair loss. These type-A variants tend to lack the connecting bridge across the top of the scalp. They usually have less hair loss in the crown, even at an advanced stage. However, these variants are important to recognize because when the hair loss is in the front, patients can appear balder than they are, even though their hair loss might be minimal.

Moreover, as previously explained, one of the minor features of the type-A variant is the horseshoe-shaped fringe of hair that remains on the sides and back of the head, which tends to be wider and reaches higher on the head. This inherent characteristic of the type-A variants makes them good candidates for hair transplantation surgery because of the excellent donor area that exists (Figs. 2.4- 2.7).

Norwood's hair loss type-A variants explained

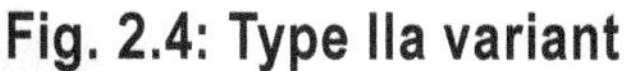

Fig. 2.4: Type IIa variant

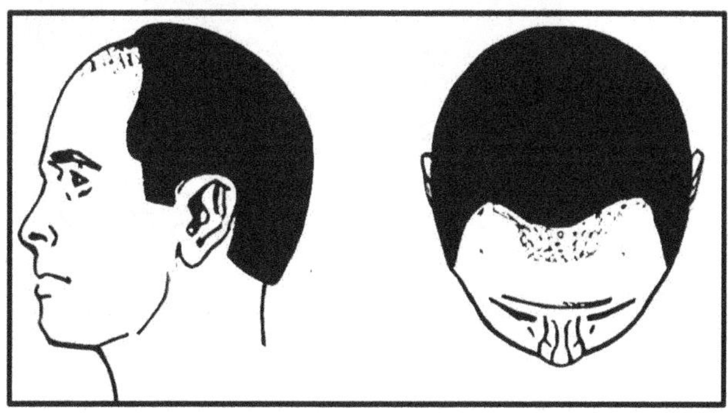

The type-IIa variant shows that the entire frontal border, including the temples, lies high on the forehead. The mid-frontal peninsula, or peak, of hair on the forehead is gone and is only represented by a few fine vellus hairs. Typically, the recession is less than one inch.

Fig. 2.5: Type IIIa variant

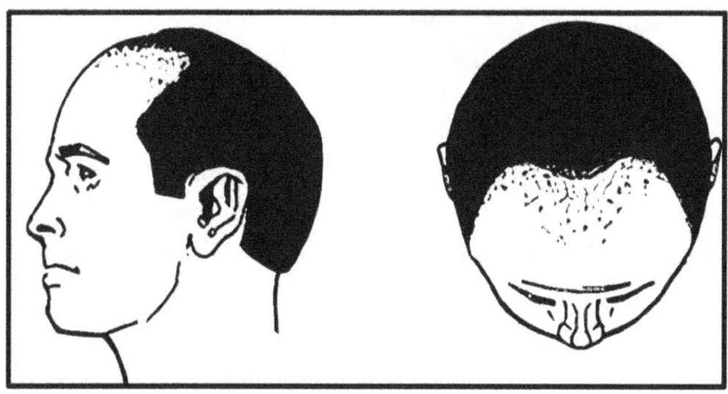

The type-IIIa variant shows an area of recession in the fronto-temporal region, which is almost vertical with the front portion of the ear.

Fig. 2.6: Type IVa variant

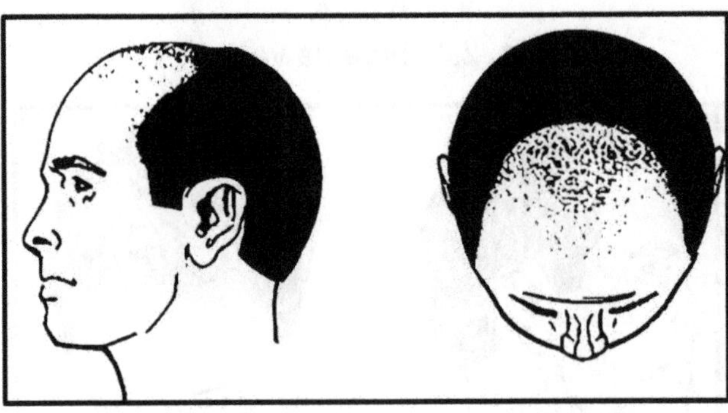

Image Source: http://prescottgenomics.wikispaces.com/androgenetic+alopecia. Contributions to http://prescottgenomics.wikispaces.com/ are licensed under a Creative Commons Attribution-Share-Alike 3.0 License.

The type-IVa variant shows that the hairline has receded beyond the front portion of the ear but has not reached the vertex. The area behind the hairline may show thinning and fine vellus hair.

Fig. 2.7: Type Va variant

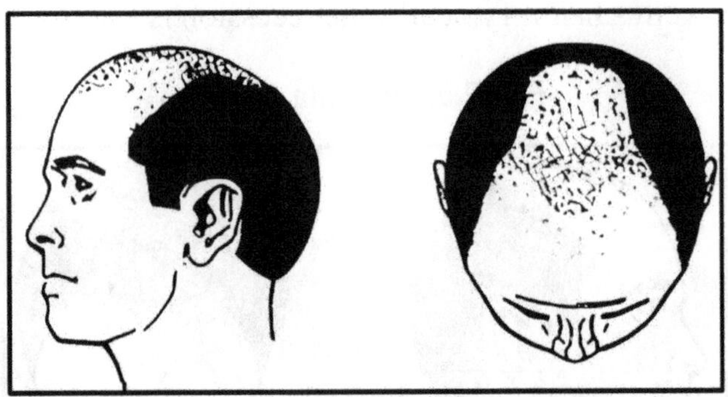

Image Source: http://prescottgenomics.wikispaces.com/androgenetic+alopecia. Contributions to http://prescottgenomics.wikispaces.com/ are licensed under a Creative Commons Attribution-Share-Alike 3.0 License.

The type Va variant shows an area of alopecia that includes the vertex. Hair loss more severe than type Va cannot be distinguished from types VI or VII in Hamilton's scale. The more advanced types of baldness, especially types V, VI, and VII, usually occur during the sixth decade of life. This fact validates the premise that two-thirds, or 67%, of all men, will be bald or will show some degree of baldness by the time they reach the age of 60. In fact, according to the Mayo Clinic, approximately 80% of men show signs of male pattern baldness by the time they reach the age of 70. Furthermore, the Mayo Clinic contends that the rate of hair loss depends on heredity and race. They claim that white males are the most affected by baldness, while men of Asian, Native American, or African heritage are more immune to the affliction (Mayse, 2010).

Ebling and Rook Ethnicity Pattern Baldness

Researchers Ebling and Rook originally developed a female pattern hair-loss scale that comprised a five-stage classification system used to determine the degree of hair loss in women. The Ebling and Rook scale essentially expanded Ludwig's female three-stage scale by taking into consideration that women can have both a diffuse form of hair loss as well as a male hair-loss pattern with recession of the fronto-temporal hairline. The reader can find a complete description of this scale in Chapter 3 that addresses female pattern hair loss.

However, in 1997, Ebling and Rook further expanded their hair-loss classification system to include male ethnicity hair-loss patterns. This ethnicity classification system is mainly used by European dermatology clinics. The Ebling and Rook ethnicity hair-loss classification patterns are of particular interest to ethnic groups for classifying their type of hair loss. The ethnicity hair-loss scale may be more relevant for diagnosing some ethnic patients than the combined Norwood-Hamilton *"catch-all"* type of classification.

This system is rarely used in medical research as it is not detailed enough, but the five-stage classification is useful for explaining hair loss to patients. Some of the ethnic classifications scales developed by Ebling and Rook are:

- Mediterranean or Latin Scale.
- Semitic (Jewish, Arabian) Scale.
- Nordic Scale.

Mediterranean or Latin Scale.

The *Mediterranean or Latin* hair-loss pattern manifests itself by showing recession of the frontal hairline, with the eventual development of vertex baldness (Fig. 2.8). These two regions of hair loss expand and coalesce (unite) into the extensive type-V baldness pattern.

Fig. 2.8: Mediterranean or Latin Scale

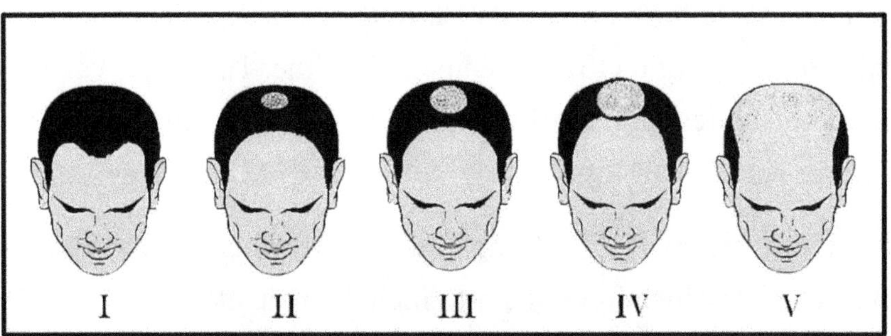

Image Source: Gustavo J. Gomez. Modified from Ebling and Rook ethnic hair-loss scale.

Semitic (Jewish, Arabian) Scale.

According to Dr. Ebling, the Semitic (Jewish, Arabian) presentation of pattern hair loss involves progressive recession of the frontal hairline; however, there is no associated thinning on the vertex (Fig. 2.9).

Fig. 2.9: Semitic (Jewish, Arabian) Scale

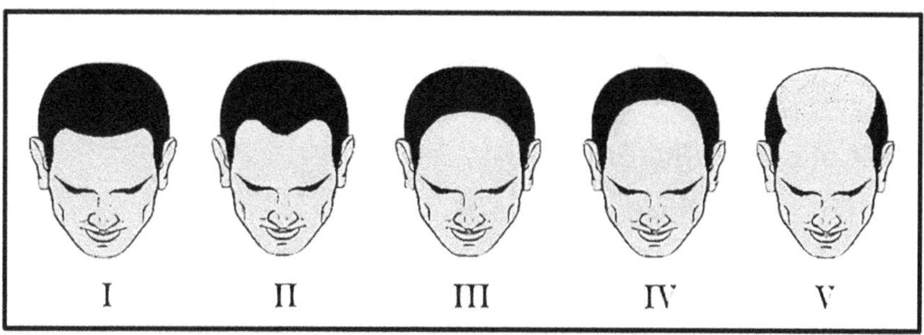

Image Source: Gustavo J. Gomez. Modified from Ebling and Rook ethnic hair-loss scale.

Nordic Scale.

According to Dr. Ebling, the Nordic hair-loss pattern evolves in its presentation as a central lock of surviving hair (Fig.2.10). This baldness pattern was also noted by Norwood in the development of his hair-loss classification system. The image below shows Ebling's suggested five-stage system for the Nordic scale.

Fig. 2.10: Nordic Scale

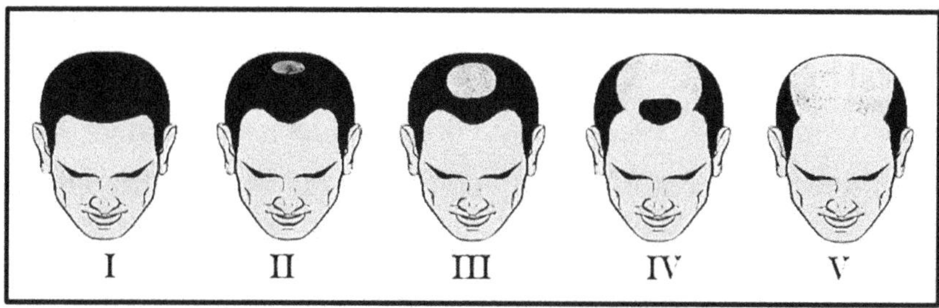

Image Source: Gustavo J. Gomez. Modified from Ebling and Rook ethnic hair-loss scale.

A large number of the hair-loss classification systems were developed to assist physicians in diagnosing the various degrees of pattern hair loss. However, the reader should also be mindful of the fact that all these preexisting hair-loss classifications have some inherent limitations. They either do not explain the complete evolutionary stages of hair loss or are too detailed and complicated to be of any practical use to the physician.

Basic and Specific (BASP) Hair-Loss Classification Scale

It has been previously mentioned that the combined Hamilton-Norwood hair loss classification system for men and the Ludwig grade or stage system for women are the most commonly used scales to describe the various patterns of hair loss. However, because of the inherent limitations of these scales, Won-Soo Lee et al. (2007) conducted a study entitled *"A New Classification of Pattern Hair Loss That Is Universal for Men and Women: Basic and Specific (BASP) Classification.*" The primary objective of Dr. Lee's study was to establish an acceptable, universal, and accurate standard for both male and female pattern hair loss and to report its use in determining the incidence of pattern hair loss (PHL) (Fig. 2.11).

The BASP classification study was essentially based on the observation of numerous patterns of hair loss. The study included a total of 2,213 participants, of which 1,768 were male and 445 were female. The research was conducted as a multicenter study at thirteen different university dermatologic centers throughout South Korea. The study classified the participants according to the pattern of hair loss they manifested in accordance with the BASP classification system, which includes four basic types of hair-loss patterns, two specific types, and a final type decided by a combination of identified basic and specific types (Lee et al., 2007).

Fig. 2.11: BASP Hair-Loss Classification System

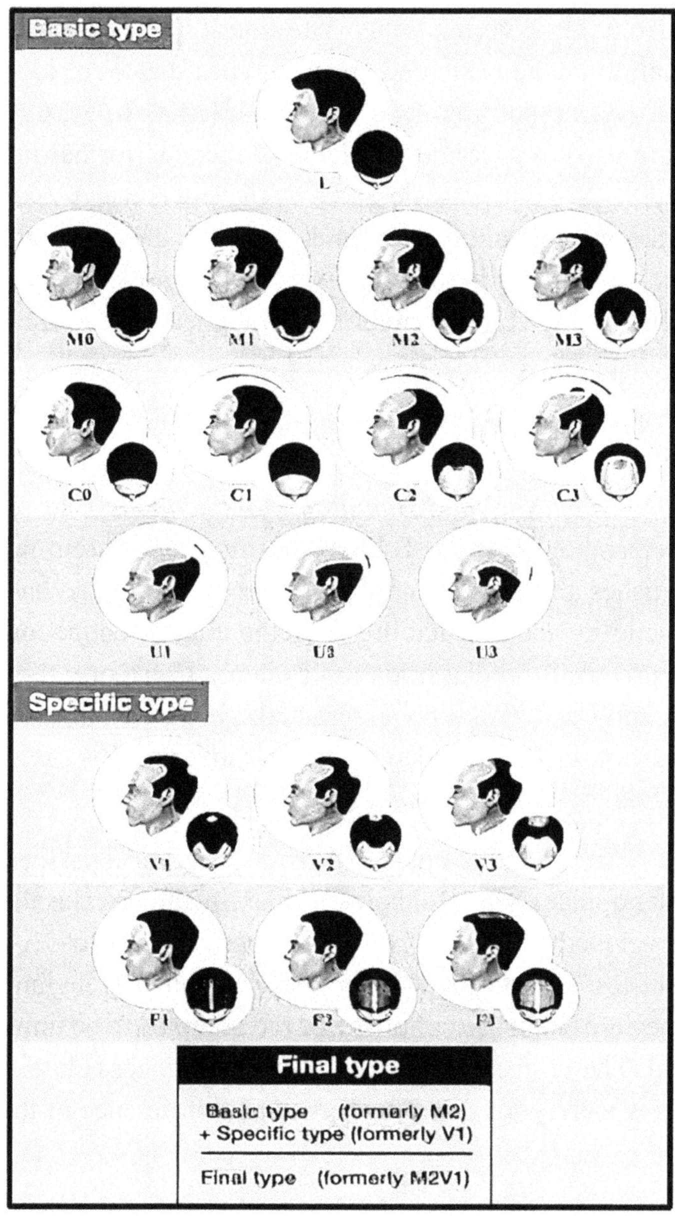

Image Source: By Drs. Paulo Müller Ramos, Hélio Amante Miot and Anais Brasileiros de Dermatología (Owners). Female pattern hair loss: a clinical and pathophysiological review; vol.90 no.4 Rio de Janeiro July/Aug. 2015 http://dx.doi.org/10.1590/abd1806-4841.20153370. Modified image (Use with Permission).

The basic (BA) patterns represent the shape of the anterior hairline, and the specific (SP) patterns represent the density of hair on the frontal and vertex areas. The final type is essentially the combination of the basic and specific types that were identified. The four (BA) types are identified by the letters L, M, C, and U, which are used to describe the shape of the anterior hairline. The two specific (SP) types are identified by the letters F and V, and each of the various types are further subdivided into three or four grades (subtypes) according to the severity of the hair loss. The final type is decided by the combination of the assigned or identified basic (BA) and specific (SP) types selected.

In a comparative study by Hong et al. (2013) entitled *"Reliability of the Pattern Hair Loss Classifications: A Comparison of the Basic and Specific and Norwood-Hamilton Classifications,"* the research team determined that the BASP classification system not only distinguishes all kinds of hair-loss patterns, but it also has better reproducibility and repeatability than the quintessential combined Norwood-Hamilton classification system. Therefore, the BASP classification system is a novel, gradual, systematic, and universal classification system for identifying hair loss patterns regardless of sex (Lee et al., 2007; Agarwal et al., 2013).

This chapter has attempted to provide a historical perspective of the most popular and useful hair-loss classification scales that have been developed to date. It should be apparent to the reader that all these hair-loss classification systems have certain inherent limitations since they are either too simplistic or too complex to be universally practical. Therefore, the use of any of these hair-loss classification systems is merely for the convenience and preference of the user.

3

Pattern Female Hair Loss Classification

Even though hair loss is frequently thought of as a strictly male affliction, evidence shows that 25% of women, or one in every four, will suffer some degree of hair loss. However, unlike for men, where a certain degree of hair loss is often considered inconsequential and more socially acceptable, for women, the psychological distress caused by hair loss, including feeling unattractive, can be devastating for their self-image and emotional well-being (Hunt, 2005).

Hair research investigators concur that there are other types of hair-loss patterns than those described in Chapter 2, especially in women, but these rarely occur to the same degree as seen in male pattern baldness. While it is a fact that some women lose their hair in a similar manner as men, this is not true for all women. Women tend to have a more diffuse type of hair loss, causing hair to become sparse, but rarely does the hair fall out completely. To assist in the classification of female hair loss, various scale classification systems have been proposed to identify the degree or type of hair loss in women.

There are five well-known female hair-loss classification scales used by most hair restoration specialists to determine the type of hair loss pattern in women. They are presented here in the order of their development according to the literature review, which is believed to have come from accurate and reliable sources. These female hair-loss classification scales are:

- The Ludwig Scale.

- The Ebling and Rook Scale.
- The Savin Scale.
- Olsen Female Hair Loss Stages.
- The Gan-Sinclair Scale.

The Ludwig Scale

In 1977, Dr. E. Ludwig arbitrarily developed his hair-loss classification scale and arranged it into three basic stages, or grades of severity, to describe genetic female hair loss (Fig. 3.1). These hair loss patterns are based on Ludwig's study of 468 female participants. In Grade I, there was a perceptible degree of hair thinning (rarefaction) on the crown, typically located one to three centimeters (1-3 cm) behind the frontal hairline. This diffuse hair loss is the most common form of female hair loss, with up to 80% of affected women presenting with this mild form of alopecia. In Grade II, the diffuse hair thinning is more pronounced than in Grade I, which is also limited to the crown area (Dinh & Sinclair, 2007).

In all three of Ludwig's hair-loss stages, there is a certain degree of hair loss on the front and top of the scalp, with minimal hair loss in the hairline area. However, in Ludwig's scale, hair loss on the back and sides of the head may or may not be involved. Ludwig's Grade III classification is a rare form of female baldness, which is found in approximately less than 5% of women afflicted with androgenetic alopecia (AGA). Ludwig's scale emphasized preservation of the frontal fringe despite the progressive, centrifugal loss over the top of the scalp. However, his classification scale did not incorporate the accentuation of frontovertical hair loss, which was later included in a scale developed by Dr. Elise Olsen. Moreover, another limitation of Ludwig's scale was that females who also presented with male pattern hair loss (MPHL) could not be classified with this system (Gupta & Mysore, 2016).

If one is considering hair transplantation surgery, the same protocol holds true for both male and female patients. This means that regardless of the degree of hair loss, the client must have a stable donor area on both the back and side of the scalp to be a good candidate for the procedure. In other words, the transplant candidate must have an abundant or robust "*safe donor zone* " (see Fig. 9.5, 9.6, and 9.7).

Fig. 3.1: Ludwig Women's Hair Loss Scale

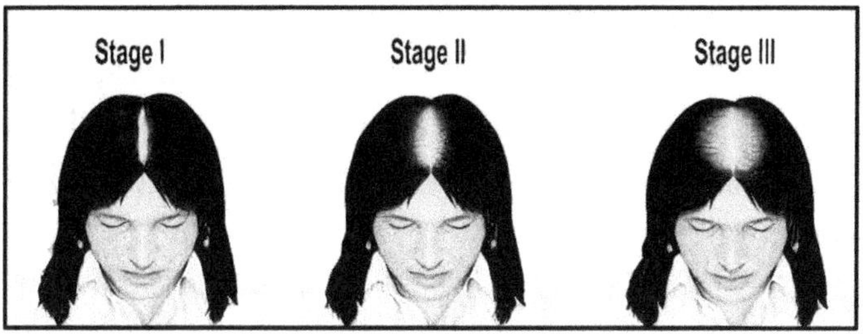

Stage I Stage II Stage III

Image Source: John P. Cole, M.D. (Owner). Modified image. (Use with Permission). https://www.forhair.com/hair-loss/female-pattern-baldness/

Stage I.

In this female pattern hair loss (FPHL) classification stage, there is perceptible early thinning of the hair on the crown, which is limited by a line situated one to three centimeters behind the frontal hairline. This degree of hair loss is so minimal that it can easily be camouflaged with proper grooming or the application of some keratinized hair-fiber concealer, such as Toppik (Figs. 15.2 and 15.3).

Stage II.

This alopecic stage is considered moderate hair loss. This stage or grade shows a more pronounced rarefaction (decreased density) of the hair on the crown within the area seen in stage I. Moreover, there is also a visibly significant widening of the midline part.

Stage III.

In this FPHL classification, total denudation (complete baldness) can be detected within the area seen in Grades I and II.

The Ebling and Rook Scale

The Ebling and Rook female pattern hair-loss scale was developed in 1975 and is comprised of a five-stage classification system. The Ebling and Rook Scale is quite similar to the Ludwig Scale. The main difference between the two scales is that the Ebling and Rook scale measures both overall thinning as well as the hair loss density. Therefore, despite the fact that the scale was developed to determine the degree of female pattern baldness, Ebling and Rook also considered that women could have both a diffuse form of alopecia (hair loss) as well as a male pattern recession of the fronto-temporal hairline.

Conversely, the Ludwig scale measures most levels of female pattern baldness or androgenetic alopecia, but it does not incorporate the accentuation of the fronto-temporal hairline. Thus, the Ebling and Rook scale essentially expands Ludwig's three-stage scale by considering that women can have both a diffuse form of hair loss and a male hair-loss pattern with a recession of the fronto-temporal hairline (Fig. 3.2).

Fig. 3.2: Ebling and Rook Female Pattern Baldness Scale

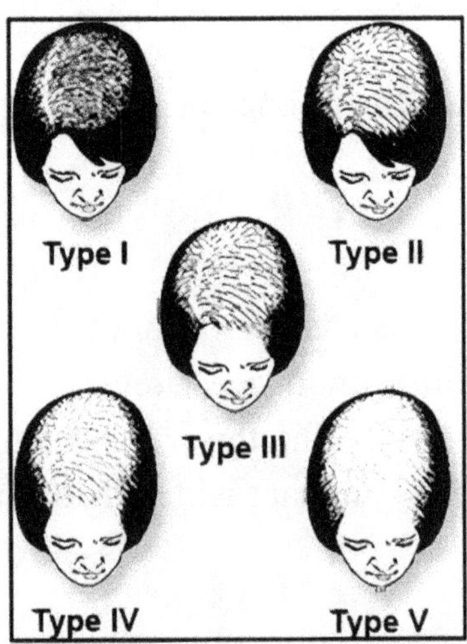

Image Sources: http://www.dubrules.com/female-pattern-baldness.html http://ihrshair4me.blogspot.com/2015/07/common-reasons-for-hair-loss-in-women.html

The first two baldness types on the Ebling and Rook scale are essentially the same as the Ludwig classification system. Type I show perceptible thinning of the hair on the crown. Type II shows a more pronounced rarefaction (less density) of the hair on the crown within the same area seen in Type I. Type III shows continued, diffuse hair loss in the same region identified in stages Types I and II but also the initial loss of hair from the fronto-temporal hairline. Type IV shows a continuation of this diffuse hair loss and some fronto-temporal recession. In Type V, there is a complete loss of hair on the top of the scalp, resembling a male pattern of baldness.

Types III, IV, and V are quite rare and generally occur in post-menopausal women. When hair loss manifests itself in a male-type pattern in pre-menopausal women, this strongly suggests an abnormal, or excessive, androgen production that generally occurs in polycystic ovarian syndrome (PCOS) and other conditions that increase the production of androgen (Venning & Dawber, 1988; keratin.com, 2013). It also suggests, as contended by researchers Dinh and Sinclair (2007), that FPHL is an androgen-dependent condition.

In fact, androgen excess affects mainly the pilosebaceous unit (PSU) and the reproductive system. The PSU secretes sebum and is the unit from which hair grows. Androgen prolongs the anagen (growth) phase of hair promotes conversion from vellus to terminal-type hair. For example, excess of androgen production can result in hirsutism, which affects 70%-80% of women with an excess of androgen. Sebum production from the PSU is also increased by androgen excess (Yildiz et al., 2009, 2010). Moreover, FPHL is considered the most common form of hair loss in women, the prevalence of which increases with advancing age or senescence. According to Dihn and Sinclair (2007), fewer than 45% of women go through life with a full head of hair.

In 1997, Ebling and Rook further expanded their hair-loss pattern classification system to include male ethnicity hair-loss patterns, such as the *Mediterranean (Latin) scale, the Semitic (Jewish, Arabian) scale, and the Nordic scale.* These classification systems are mostly used by European dermatology clinics. These hair loss scales will be described more extensively in Chapter 2, which addresses male pattern hair loss (MPHL).

The Savin Scale

The Savin classification scale for women was developed in 1992 by Dr. Ronald C. Savin of Yale University in association with his colleague, Dr. Ronald J. Trancik, an Upjohn Company pharmaceutical researcher. Initially, Dr. Savin proposed nine computer images demonstrating varying degrees of female pattern hair loss (FPHL). Subsequently, these nine images became the hair loss classifications that Dr. Savin incorporated into the Savin scale (Fig. 3.3). Dr. Savin developed this pictorial hair-loss classification scale to clinically quantify pattern hair loss in women.

Fig. 3.3: Savin Female Hair Loss Scale

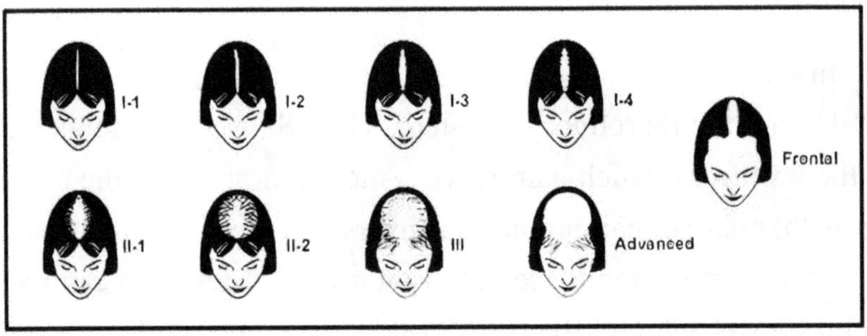

Image Source: http://prescottgenomics.wikispaces.com/androgenetic+alopecia. University of New Hampshire Contributions to http://prescottgenomics.wikispaces.com/ are licensed under a Creative Commons Attribution-Share-Alike 3.0 License.

The nine images the Savin scale classifies FPHL into eight stages of increasing crown hair loss or balding. Additionally, for classification number nine, Savin developed a special subcategory to determine the degree of recession of the frontal-anterior area. These nine illustrations provided a finer visual gradient of hair-loss pattern and density than previous classification scales for women with pattern hair loss. The usefulness of the Savin scale was validated by a study that demonstrated its accuracy, ease of use, and consistency, which could be used to evaluate women with hair loss (Savin, 1992; androgeneticalopecia.com, n.d.).

As shown in Figure 3.3, the Savin Scale shows that FPHL occurs along the hair part, and it acknowledges three different stages of hair loss, just like the Ludwig Scale stages I, II, and III (Fig. 3.1). However, the Savin scale further differentiates nine different hair loss stages: I-1, I-2, I-3, I-4, II-1, II-2, III, advanced, and frontal (Fig. 3.3). The first image in Figure 3.3, labeled I-1, shows the central parting of a woman's hair with no hair loss. The second through fourth images, I-2, I-3, and I-4, illustrates that the part's width gets progressively wider, indicating thinning hair along the center of the scalp.

Images II-1 and II-2 show a pattern of diffuse hair thinning on top of the scalp (crown), while image III represents extensive, diffuse hair loss on top of the scalp, with some hair still surviving. The *"advanced"* image shows a woman with extensive hair loss and little to no surviving hair in the alopecia affected area. Very few women ever reach this stage, and if they do, usually it is because they have a condition that causes significant, abnormally excessive androgen hormone production. The frontal image on the Savin scale is somewhat different. It shows a woman with a pattern of hair loss that is described as "frontally accentuated." In this type of alopecia, there is more hair loss at the front and center of the hair part instead of just in the top-middle of the scalp.

Female pattern hair loss (FPHL) has emerged as the preferred term to identify androgenetic alopecia (AGA) in females. FPHL is a chronic, progressive condition that is histologically identical to male androgenetic alopecia (Dinh & Sinclair, 2007). According to most hair-loss researchers, FPHL is a rapidly growing phenomenon. The only significant difference between male and female hair loss is that the female hairline does not recede in the majority of cases.

Some investigators believe that the reason for the increase in hair loss experienced by women in today's society is that women are exposed to the same stressors as men. Conversely, other researchers believe that the major factor for female hair loss is a genetic, androgen-dependent condition, at least in the majority of cases (Dinh & Sinclair, 2007).

Olsen Female Hair Loss Stages

Dr. Elise A. Olsen (2001) is the founder and director of the Duke University Hair Disorders Research and Treatment Center. Additionally, she is the past president of the North American Hair Research Society and the author of the textbook *Hair Disorders: Diagnosis and Treatment*.

According to Olsen, much less is known about FPHL than MPHL, partly because of fewer recognizable hair loss patterns in women. In developing her female hair-loss scale, Dr. Olsen classified female pattern hair loss as a three-stage pattern based on a *frontal accentuation pattern.* In this type of classification, hair loss was more profound in the frontal region and gradually tapered back toward less hair loss in the back part of the head (occiput), which gave the impression of a *Christmas tree-type pattern* (Figs. 3.4 and 3.5). The Christmas-tree pattern is a term that Olsen coined to describe this type of hair loss.

In order of frequency of occurrence, the hair-loss stages in Olsen's classification are as follows:

- Frontal Accentuation.
- Diffuse Central.
- Vertex/Frontal (male hair-loss-type pattern).

FPHL is a condition clinically characterized by a decrease in hair density in the central scalp and histologically, by a progressive miniaturization process of the hair follicles with an increased percentage of hair in the telogen (resting) phase in the affected area (Olsen, 2001). According to Dr. Olsen (1999), the frontal accentuation stage accounts for 70% of female hair loss. In stage I, there is mild to moderate frontal accentuation loss. In stage II, the frontal accentuations can be more severe than in stage I and mixed with diffuse hair loss. In stage III, the loss of hair is so severe that only diffuse thinning is principally noted (Fig.3.4).

Fig. 3.4: Olsen Frontal Accentuation FPHL

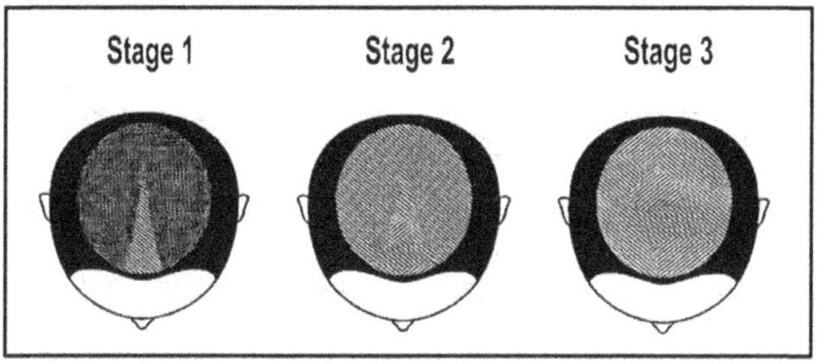

Stage 1 | Stage 2 | Stage 3

Image Source: http://www.blogtricologiamedica.com.br/2014/04/pacientes-e-conflitos-como-isso-impacta_23.html

Fig. 3.5: An actual photo of a Christmas-tree hair-loss pattern

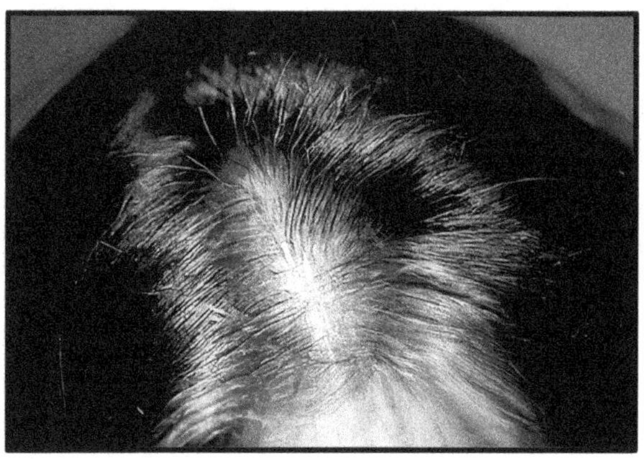

Image Source: http://www.barterweb.net/Christmas-tree-hair-loss-pattern/. http://hairthinningremedies.org/wp-content/uploads/2014/12/Female-Hair-Thinning-2.jpg

The Gan-Sinclair Scale

The occurrence of androgenetic alopecia (AGA) can be observed in both men and women. The determining factors associated with hair loss appear to be a genetic predisposition, coupled with the presence of sufficient circulating androgens (Gan & Sinclair, 2005). According to Professor Sinclair of the University of Melbourne in Australia, FPHL manifests itself quite differently from the more typically recognizable male pattern baldness, which usually begins with a receding frontal hairline and progresses to a bald patch on top of the head. To describe this female pattern of hair loss, Drs. Gan and Sinclair developed a modified, five-point, visual analog grading scale that they used to score the degree of female pattern hair loss (Fig.3.6).

It is uncommon for women to go bald by following the typical pattern of male hair loss unless there is an excessive production of androgens in the body. However, it is common for some women to develop hair thinning at the frontal hairline with normal aging (senescence). In fact, as stated before, fewer than 45% of women go through life with a full head of hair. The prevalence of hair loss in women increases with age, from approximately 12% of women ranging in age from 20 to 29 years old to over 50% of women over the age of 80 (Gan & Sinclair, 2005).

Fig. 3.6: Gan-Sinclair Five-Point Grade Hair-Loss Scale

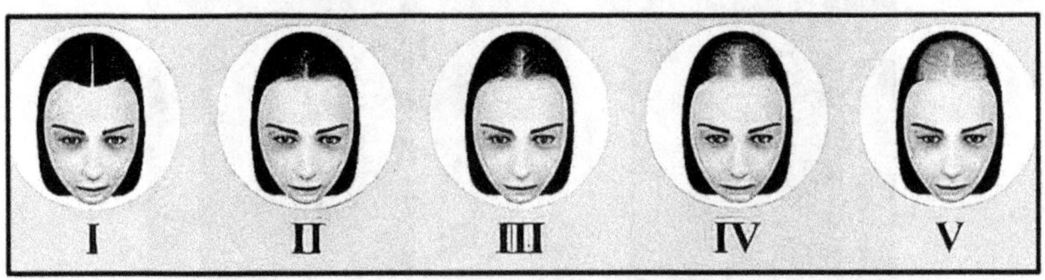

Image Source: By Drs. Paulo Müller Ramos, Hélio Amante Miot and Anais Brasileiros de Dermatología (Owners). Female pattern hair loss: a clinical and pathophysiological review; vol.90 no.4 Rio de Janeiro July/Aug. 2015 http://dx.doi.org/10.1590/abd1806-4841.20153370. Modified image (Use with Permission).

Unlike in men, hair loss in women is associated with significant psychological morbidity (distress) because women generally place greater emphasis than men on their physical appearance and outward attractiveness. In fact, societal norms dictate that having a full head of hair is an essential component of a woman's sexuality and gender identity. Therefore, any hair loss that occurs generates feelings of low self-esteem and anxiety from a perception of diminished attractiveness. Moreover, women are not only more likely than men to have a lower quality of life, but they are also more likely to restrict social contacts as a result of hair loss (Cash, Price, & Savin, 1993; Van Neste & Rushton, 1997). It is essential to understand that the emotional distress that occurs from losing one's hair is a legitimate concern that should be effectively addressed and should not be ignored.

4

Hair Loss Treatments: A Historical Perspective

Now that we have reviewed the anatomy and physiology of hair growth topics and the various hair-loss classification scales used to diagnose both male and female pattern hair loss. It is appropriate at this juncture to pause and look back at the history of hair loss and its preventative and therapeutic treatment modalities before we enter our discussion of contemporary hair loss theories and their possible solutions. It will be an illuminating and amusing topic before continuing to learn about the promising and exciting future trends and discoveries that are currently being made. It is an exciting and bright future for hair-loss research.

As far back as 4000 B.C., Egyptian papyruses (records) have revealed countless recipes or remedies for curing hair loss in both men and women. There are records indicating that there were physicians who specialized in treating male pattern baldness in ancient Egyptian times. Some of the remedies used by Egyptians to treat their hair-loss conditions were a mixture of dates, dog paws, and donkey hooves that were grounded into a powder and then slowly cooked in oil. This blend of ingredients produced a topical concoction that was rubbed on the scalp of balding areas. However, there is no evidence that this concoction had any effect in improving hair loss.

Four thousand years later, science still lacks a genuinely effective hair-loss treatment—short of hair transplantation surgery—for growing hair on a bald scalp or preventing hair loss in any significant way. Notwithstanding this lack of success, some encouraging research studies currently may yield impressive results. The findings of these promising research studies will be thoroughly examined in a later chapter.

It is important to note that the Egyptians were not the only ones concerned with hair-loss issues. The Greeks and the Romans were as well. These ancient civilizations postulated numerous theories to explain the etiology (cause) of male pattern baldness (MPB). Some of these archaic theories are listed below:

- Roman superstition held that the fumes of snake poison occasionally present in the air were detrimental to hair growth.

- Claudius Galen was a prominent Greek physician, surgeon, and philosopher who went to Rome and revived the ideas of Hippocrates and other Hellenic doctors. Galen was arguably the most accomplished of all medical researchers of antiquity. Moreover, he also contributed extensively to understanding numerous scientific disciplines, such as anatomy, physiology, pathology, pharmacology, neurology, philosophy, and logic.

- Galen believed that noxious or harmful elements in the air—possibly referring to air pollution of the time—were detrimental to hair growth because they obstructed the passages by which hair received its nourishment.

- During the Renaissance, some scientists believed in a theory similar to Galen's.

- Around 400 B.C., Hippocrates invented numerous topical concoctions to prevent hair loss, none of which grew a single hair on his bald scalp. He was the first scientist to recognize a link or connection between baldness and testosterone— the male sex hormone. He concluded by observing that castrated men (eunuchs) did not lose their hair.

- Aristotle, just like Hippocrates, believed that there was a link between baldness and sex hormones. Since these observations were made centuries ago, both Aristotle and Hippocrates did not fully realize how correct their observations and conclusions were. It wasn't until 1960 that a Yale doctor named James B. Hamilton discovered the connection or link between hair loss and testosterone while studying 21 boys who were undergoing castration.

- Hamilton's findings suggested that high levels of testosterone might lead to baldness. However, it is currently known that testosterone levels are not as important as the conversion of testosterone to dihydrotestosterone (DHT). This testosterone conversion to DHT gave rise to the term *"androgenic, or androgenetic alopecia."* Aristotle further observed that babies, most women, and castrated men (eunuchs) never became bald. It is important to note that the following terms, male pattern baldness, alopecia prematura, common baldness, androgenic and androgenetic alopecia, are all synonymous and are used interchangeably within this book.

- There were many other treatments used for hair loss, which included the topical application of ibex (goat) fat, chicken manure, cow dung, alligator grease, pigeon droppings, and castor oil, to name a few.

Raymond Sabouraud

During the late 1800s and early 1900s, famed French dermatologist and mycologist— a specialist in the study of fungi— Dr. Raymond Sabouraud conducted extensive scientific investigations on the role of fungal infections as a cause of skin disease. Sabouraud is credited for the discovery of at least 50 species of fungi causing skin diseases, as well as the development of agars for culturing and observing these fungi.

Additionally, Dr. Sabouraud also conducted studies on the hyperactivity of the sebaceous glands. From the findings of these studies, Sabouraud postulated the theory that hair loss was the result of overactive sebaceous glands. Because of this finding, Sabouraud is credited with coining the term *"alopecia seborrheica."* This condition of seborrheic overactivity of the sebaceous glands was believed by most dermatologists of that period to be the primary cause of common male pattern baldness (MPB). Furthermore, many other theories were proposed during this period to explain why seborrheic type hair loss could develop. Below are some of these proposed theories:

- Metabolic Disorders.
- Environment of the Individual.
- Excessive Exposure to Stress.
- Race and Occupation.

Metabolic Disorders.

During Sabouraud's time, some authorities believed that seborrheic dermatitis could result when metabolic disorders were present, such as stomach diseases, hypothyroidism, iron deficiency, and hyperglycemia (diabetes). Seborrheic dermatitis, or dandruff, is a common, chronic, superficial, inflammatory disease of the scalp, face (especially the eyebrows and nasolabial folds), ears, and central chest, affecting 2-5% of the population. Clinically, this disease is characterized by thin, erythematous (redness of the skin) plaques, often with fine, greasy scales. The pathophysiology of this phenomenon is still not completely understood; however, some authorities believe the cause may be genetic. The condition is not contagious and is not caused by poor or inadequate hygiene practices (Grandinetti & Tmecki, 2010; Giron, 2015).

Other authorities believe that seborrheic dermatitis is a combination of different factors, such as a weak immune system, poor nutrition, unstable hormone levels, or nervous system complications. However, what is essential to understand is that as this seborrheic condition progresses, hair loss is experienced as a side effect of the inflammation associated with the disease process. The hair loss resulting from this condition can be permanent because of the possible damage to the hair follicles. This permanent hair loss, according to researchers, is caused by the scalp irritation produced from Malassezia, which is a yeast-causing agent associated with seborrheic dermatitis (Giron, 2015).

The Environment of the Individual.

During Dr. Sabouraud's time, it was also believed that individuals who lived in cold climates had a higher predisposition toward developing a seborrheic condition than people living in warmer climates. This belief was based merely on the idea that people from warmer temperatures would wash their hair more frequently due to the hot weather, thus preventing a dirty scalp and promoting a healthier environment in which hair could thrive.

In contemporary times, Dr. Nilofer Farjo (2016), a hair transplantation surgery expert and a founding member and past president of the British Trichological Society, contends that an excess of free radicals triggered by pollution, radiation, cigarette smoke, and herbicides' causes damage to hair cells. Therefore, Dr. Farjo's contention could be confirmation that environmental influences can result in hair loss problems.

Excessive Exposure to Stress.

In Sabouraud's time, dermatologists believed that exposure to the stress and strain of daily life could result in seborrhea. During this period, researchers thought that a seborrheic condition correlated with the nervous makeup of the individual. In contemporary times, the link between stress and hair loss has been confirmed. In fact, there are three types of hair-loss conditions associated with high-stress levels. These conditions are telogen effluvium (TE), trichotillomania, and alopecia areata (AA), which are more extensively explained in Chapter 8. It is important to understand that hair loss attributed to stress does not have to be a permanent condition in most cases. According to Dr. Daniel K. Hall-Flavin (2016), he contends that it is quite possible to regrow the lost hair completely if the stressful situation is improved or controlled.

Race and Occupation.

Additionally, during Dr. Sabouraud's time, some authorities within the field believed that people who engaged in the pursuit of knowledge had a higher predisposition for developing a seborrheic condition than people not involved in such activity. It was also believed that Latin races had less of an inclination towards the condition than Nordic races. Both observations presumed that the underlying cause of hair loss had to do with hygiene practices. However, in a study conducted by Davis et al. (2012), entitled *"Top Dermatologic Conditions in Patients of Color: An Analysis of Nationally Representative Data,"* Dr. Davis dispelled this view.

While all these theories during Sabouraud's time were postulated to address the reasons for the occurrence of a seborrheic condition, which they felt led to hair loss, at present, it is difficult to conceive that they are the only causes of common or premature baldness. This historical review of the various proposed hair-loss theories has been presented at this juncture as an illustration so that the reader can perceive the progression of hair-loss research.

The author hopes that as this educational journey continues, the reader will soon discover that many other factors influence hair loss besides seborrheic conditions. In fact, throughout history, there have been other proposed hair-loss theories. Some theories have been discredited, and others remain relevant today. However, no one theory can adequately explain the reasons behind the development of common male pattern baldness or androgenetic alopecia. Some of the other hair-loss theories that have been proposed are as follows:

- Hereditary (genetic) predisposition.
- Androgenetic (hormonal) influence, especially the conversion of testosterone to DHT.
- The aging (senescence) process.
- The theory that each hair has its own biological time clock for falling out.
- Tight scalp muscles.
- Mental stress.
- Too frequent or infrequent shampooing.
- Localized skin conditions.
- Diminished scalp circulatory blood flow.

The author will explain all these theories in subsequent chapters, in addition to delving into and addressing the most promising new scientific discoveries in hair-loss research. However, before continuing to the next chapter, it is appropriate at this juncture to mention that at the moment, what is available to treat hair loss—besides hair transplantation surgery—are just a few medications. Of these few drugs, only two have been approved by the FDA to specifically treat hair loss, minoxidil (Rogaine®) and finasteride (Propecia®). Primarily, these two drugs are used to slow the progression of hair loss, and in some cases, they can regrow some hair. These drugs are familiar names for most hair-loss sufferers since they are the leading hair-loss medications on the market today. These two hair-loss medications will be extensively discussed in subsequent chapters.

PUVA Therapy

Another drug that is not that well-known to treat hair loss is PUVA therapy. PUVA therapy is a combination treatment regimen that stands for Psoralen (P) plus ultraviolet radiation of 320–400 nm wavelength, commonly referred to as UVA; hence, the use of the acronym PUVA. The PUVA treatment modality has been explicitly used to treat alopecia areata (AA) since 1974. This type of alopecia is characterized by sudden hair loss occurring in individuals who have no apparent skin disorder or systemic disease. Alopecia areata is considered an autoimmune skin disease that results in the loss of hair on the scalp and elsewhere on the body. It usually starts with one or more small, round, smooth patches on the scalp or beard (Figs. 8.1 and 8.2). It is important to note that before its application for alopecia areata, PUVA therapy was mainly used to treat skin disorders. Some of the skin disorders treated with PUVA are psoriasis, vitiligo, mycosis fungoides (cutaneous T-cell lymphoma), localized scleroderma, photodermatoses, atopic dermatitis, and pruritus (itching).

Essentially, PUVA is a *photochemotherapy* that involves either a topical or oral application of psoralen followed by a measured dose of ultraviolet-A radiation. Psoralen is a drug that, in its natural state, is found in many plants. It contains a chemical called 8-methoxy psoralen, or 8-MOP, which is sensitive to ultraviolet rays. What 8-MOP does is enhance the effect of ultraviolet rays on the skin by making the skin photosensitive. It remains a mystery as to why psoralen plus UVA works for the conditions previously mentioned. Still, it has been postulated that the reason relates to the modulation of the skin's immune system (Wolf et al., 2006).

However, it is essential to note that most of the medications used to treat hair loss are only effective if used continuously—in essence, over the users' lifetime. If the drug is stopped, any hair growth that was gained will gradually be lost, and within six to twelve months, the scalp will revert to its previous, pre-treatment condition. As the reader will discern, in the world today, aside *from* Rogaine® and Propecia® and some exciting and promising research studies, things have not changed significantly from ancient times in relation to topical hair-loss treatment solutions. This fact will be evident to the reader as they progress to chapter 15 that describes the numerous *topical hair loss treatment modalities*. We are still treating hair loss with every conceivable topical concoction in the hope of regrowing some of the hair that has been lost due to health conditions or normal senescence (aging).

This behavior is understandable because, according to Jimenez et al. (2014), male and female pattern hair loss are common, chronic, dermatologic disorders with limited therapeutic options to resolve the condition. Consequently, because of the zeal to find a solution for hair loss, people are more susceptible than ever before to scams and deception by hair-restoration advertising. In fact, it is important to note that presently, with the advent of the Internet as a domestic and international marketing distribution channel, scamming and swindling of the public is more prevalent, dangerous, and far-reaching than ever before.

Moreover, because of the lack of FDA oversight for many types of promoted products, it is very easy for anyone to set up a website to sell any kind of hair product—from anywhere in the world—to unsuspecting consumers. It is improbable that any of the products or substances being sold to the uninformed public will grow any hair. Because the cause of premature baldness still remains a mystery—although not as much as before—it is a fertile marketplace for charlatans aiming to deceive gullible individuals afflicted by hair-loss problems. The only recourse available to protect the consuming public against these types of deceptive, shameful, and corrupt marketing practices is education, which, in essence, is one of the objectives of writing this book.

In closing this chapter, it is appropriate to reference a statement from the Washington Post that confirms why scamming and deceptive marketing practices are so prevalent; "Americans suffering from alopecia spend more than 3.5 billion dollars yearly in an attempt to treat their hair loss. Moreover, the Washington Post further claims that 99% of the products marketed to the unsuspecting consuming public are totally ineffective in resolving hair loss (americanhairloss.org, n.d.)." Due to this lack of product efficacy, which is why the *American Hair Loss Association (AHLA)*— a privately held consumer organization— recommends against purchasing any hair-loss product that has not received FDA approval.

5

Heredity and Its Effects on Hair Loss

Following the brief historical perspective from the previous chapter regarding various hair-loss theories and treatments, it is appropriate at this juncture to begin to explain the contemporary, accepted, scientifically-based theories of hair loss. Although the hair-loss theories being described are based on sound medical research, not all of them have withstood the test of time.

It is essential to understand that accepted theories are the best explanations available so far for how specific theories work. They have been thoroughly tested, are supported by acceptable research, and have been proven useful in generating plausible explanations on the subject. Moreover, they facilitate new opportunities for new areas of research. However, it is a well-known fact that science is always a work in progress, and even previously accepted theories can change. It is not uncommon to see many theories fall out of favor as new discoveries are uncovered.

According to researchers Montagna and Uno (1968), one of the reasons for the resistance to accepting baldness in its true perspective as a normal biological process is that baldness is still not viewed today as a disorder or disease process. Because male pattern baldness is not seen as life-threatening, doctors often disregard the condition. This view is an unfortunate attitude because hair loss can cause severe distress and some far-reaching psychological effects on the afflicted. Montagna and Uno, in their 1968 research entitled *"Baldness in Nonhuman Primates,"* discovered that hair loss in nonhuman primates seemed to share a similar trait with human hair loss. For example, the same hair-loss process of miniaturization observed in human androgenetic alopecia was also observed in nonhuman primates.

Montagna and Uno contend that this observation points out that human hair loss has some phylogenetic (evolutionary) significance and is not to be considered a disorder or disease. As a result of this view, the true nature of the origin of male pattern baldness has been a slow concept to accept. Moreover, Jackson and McMurty (1912) describe the process of common baldness as a form of hair loss that begins at any time before middle age and arises uninfluenced by any previous, concomitant, local, or general disease process.

For this reason, these researchers felt that baldness in many cases was *hereditary*, or passed on from father to son for many generations. Conversely, other investigators believed that baldness could be passed on from the mother's side of the family. However, despite these theories, any individual could become the first family member to acquire hair loss. In reality, there are no clear-cut answers to the hair-loss dilemma or problem. The myth that hair loss is passed down from a specific side of the family originated from a paper published by Dr. Dorothy Osborne in 1916. Osborne believed that a particular pattern of baldness was inherited from only one parent, typically the mother. Nevertheless, this theory has since been proven false (Bernstein, 2013).

The scientific investigation of three researchers, Montagna and Ellis (1958) and Hamilton (1942, 1946), is especially important in providing a better understanding of common pattern baldness. In 1942 and 1946, Hamilton published the results of two studies entitled *"Male Hormone Stimulation is Prerequisite and an Incitant in Common Baldness,"* and *"The Relationship Between Common Baldness and Male Sex Hormones,"* respectively. These research studies emphasized three factors that Hamilton believed were influential in the progressive development of common pattern baldness or alopecia prematura. The tenets that Hamilton emphasized in those two research papers are still applicable today. They are:

- Hereditary (genetic) predisposition.
- Hormonal or endocrine stimulus.
- Aging (senescence).

Dr. Hamilton further contended that these three factors were *interdependent.* Evidence of this interdependency is that no matter how strong the inherited (genetic) predisposition to hair loss is, baldness will not result if inciting agents such as androgens—explicitly testosterone—are not present. The same holds true for androgenic (hormonal) inciting agents; even though these agents might be present, if the inherited predisposition is not there, baldness will not occur (Hamilton, 1942, 1946).

Hair loss due to aging or senescent or senile alopecia is a specific type of age-related hair loss that occurs in both men and women as we pass the age of 50 and over. This type of hair loss occurs even though there is no family history of hereditary (genetic) hair loss. As we age, senile changes in physiology and immunity may influence the onset and course of hair loss (Chen et al., 2010).

Furthermore, as we age, hair growth decreases naturally in two fundamental ways. First, the total time the hair remains in the anagen or growth stage decreases. Staying in the anagen stage longer than usual means that hair follicles spend an increasing amount of time in the telogen or resting stage, producing no new hair. Second, the diameter of each strand of hair gets thinner and thinner over time. Consequently, this process leads to the appearance of diffused thinning, which makes the scalp increasingly visible, making the hair loss more evident over the years.

Donor Dominance Theory

Hamilton also cited that hair loss appears to be controlled by factors residing in localized areas of the scalp. This suggestion gives rise to another of Hamilton's theories, which is the theory that each hair follicle possesses its own inherited time clock for falling out. This theory is the precursor of the principle of *donor dominance,* as contended by renowned New York hair transplant surgeon Dr. Norman Orentreich in 1952. The principle of donor dominance maintains that in common pattern baldness, or androgenetic alopecia, the transposed skin graft will maintain its integrity and characteristics independent of the recipient site.

In other words, this principle established the theory that hair could safely be transplanted from the bald resistant donor areas of the scalp to the recipient balding areas. This bald resistant donor area is called *"the safe donor area or zone."* It was observed that hairs extracted from the donor area would continue to grow in its new recipient area for a lifetime because the transplanted donor hairs retained the genetic or hereditary characteristics that preclude them from hair loss. The concept of donor dominance essentially laid the foundation for the development of modern hair transplantation surgery. Thus, for the past 70 years, donor dominance has been the dominant principle in the field of hair transplantation.

Recipient Dominance Theory

Notwithstanding the importance of the donor dominance principle, it is important to note that the principle of *recipient dominance* is also an important concept to embrace and understand. In fact, researchers have been paying more attention to this principle lately. The reason for this renewed interest has to do with the observation that transplanted hair can take on the characteristics of the recipient site. For example, surgeons have observed that transplanted hair took on the characteristic wave of the hair that originally grew at the recipient site. Another interesting discovery was that eyebrow hair transplants were observed to be influenced by the native skin in the eyebrow region so that over time the hairs transplanted began to grow slower and finer than when first transplanted. Similarly, it was also observed that hairs transplanted from the body, such as from the chest, could grow faster and finer when moved from the body to the scalp. Therefore, it appears that the recipient site has a certain degree of influence over the transplanted hair (Lam, 2012).

In concluding this chapter on heredity and its effects on hair loss, it is essential to understand that an inherited predisposition for hair loss is absolutely necessary to develop any degree of male pattern baldness. In fact, some authorities on the topic hold that 95% of all hair loss is genetic in origin (Jackson & McMurty, 1912; Montagna & Ellis, 1958; Hamilton, 1951). It has been observed that in some non-Caucasian races and some Caucasian families, there exists an inherited predisposition for specific patterns of hair loss. This observation was confirmed by Ebling and Rook (1997) with the development of the classification of their *ethnic hair loss patterns* (Figs. 2.8, 2.9, and 2.10).

As previously mentioned, the influence of a hereditary predisposition has been proven by the fact that a castrated individual (eunuch) whose male relatives do not show a propensity to male pattern baldness will not acquire hair loss after treatment with testosterone. However, a castrated individual whose relatives do possess the hereditary predisposition for hair loss will also become bald when treated with testosterone.

Currently, it is a well-accepted fact that male pattern baldness, or androgenetic alopecia, is genetically based. That common baldness cannot occur without the presence of specific, inherited genes. It is also known that these genes can be passed on to offspring from either parent. What is still unclear is the exact mode of inheritance and the relative importance of each parent.

Several theoretical models have been proposed that focus on one particular dominant gene. However, what has become apparent is that hereditary hair loss most likely encompasses a variety of genes or *polygenic traits* (Heilmann et al., 2013). In other words, it is a complex genetic condition that most probably involves many different genes. It is now known that hereditary hair loss is a complex trait that may have contributing factors from both sides of the family. Gene expression is related to several other factors, such as age, stress, and hormone levels. Just because a person has the genes for baldness does not mean the trait will manifest itself (Hamilton 1942, 1946, 1951). Therefore, understanding the genetics of hair loss has practical implications for diagnosing and treating baldness.

6

Hormones and Their Effects on Hair Loss and Research Trends

Until recently, very little progress had been made in discovering the causes of male pattern baldness following Hamilton's research. Bruchovsky and Wilson (1968) observed that testosterone was converted to dihydrotestosterone (DHT) in the prostate gland of rats. Because of this discovery, these researchers proved that DHT, not testosterone, was the active androgen in rat prostate enlargement.

The term *"androgen"* is a generic term used for an agent— usually any steroid hormone, such as androsterone and testosterone— that stimulates the activity of the accessory male sex organs, which encourages the development of male sex characteristics. Androgens are a large class of steroidal hormones, some of which are also called anabolic steroids because they undergo anabolism conversion into other components of the body's biochemistry. Androgen is used synonymously with the term male sex hormone, but it also includes male sex hormones produced elsewhere in the body besides the testes.

Dihydrotestosterone (DHT)

The discovery by Bruchovsky and Wilson (1968) that testosterone was converted to DHT spurred an interesting hair-loss theory that suggested that high levels of DHT can also cause androgen-related disorders of the hair follicles. It is important to understand that DHT is an endogenous (originating within the body) androgen sex steroid and hormone that is also known as 5α-dihydrotestosterone

(5α-DHT), or as 5α-androstan-17β-ol-3-one. The conversion of testosterone to DHT is controlled by the enzyme 5-alpha-reductase (5AR). This discovery gives rise to the theory that if the activity of 5-alpha-reductase could be blocked or inhibited— at the scalp level— it might be possible that the onset of male or female pattern baldness or androgenetic alopecia could be prevented or improved. However, it is essential to understand that when testosterone is bound to sex hormone-binding globulin (SHBG)— also known as testosterone-estradiol binding globulin (TeBG)— it cannot be converted to DHT via the enzyme 5-alpha-reductase.

Sex Hormone-Binding Globulin (SHBG).

Essentially, SHBG is a glycoprotein or a molecule that consists of a carbohydrate plus a protein. SHBG is primarily produced by the liver and, to a lesser degree, by other sites, such as the brain, uterus, testes, and placenta. SHBG binds tightly to three sex hormones found in both men and women. These three hormones are testosterone, dihydrotestosterone (DHT), and estradiol (a form of estrogen). In this bound state, SHBG's function is to transport these hormones in the blood as biologically inactive forms. Thus, SHBG performs the function of transporting these three sex hormones to different parts of the body and ensuring their availability to the tissues that require them.

SHBG has a stronger affinity for testosterone and DHT than it does for estrogens. Although SHBG binds these three hormones, the critical hormone is testosterone. Essentially, SHBG controls the amount of testosterone that the body tissues can use. Too little testosterone in men and too much testosterone in women can cause imbalance problems. Therefore, SHBG plays a significant role in maintaining the delicate balance between testosterone and estrogen. Consequently, changes in SHBG levels can affect the amount of hormones bioavailable for use by the body's tissue.

It has been observed that balding men usually have lower levels of sex hormone-binding globulin (SHBG). Consequently, these decreased levels of SHBG results in a greater amount of unbound testosterone (free testosterone). This larger amount of available free testosterone facilitates the conversion of testosterone to DHT via the enzyme 5-alpha-reductase. A higher level of circulating DHT has been observed to cause male and female pattern baldness or androgenetic alopecia (AGA). Therefore, higher levels of SHBG results in lower levels of circulating DHT and less effect on hair loss. Conversely, lower levels of SHBG results in higher levels of circulating DHT, resulting in hair loss.

As men age, their levels of SHBG increase. As a result, more binding of testosterone occurs, reducing its bioavailability to the body tissues. Furthermore, through the process of aromatization, which is the conversion of testosterone to estrogen by way of the aromatase enzyme, concomitantly with an increased production of 5-alpha-reductase, local tissue expression of these enzymes affects hair and androgen levels alike (see Fig. 6.2).

Compared with men, women typically have higher levels of SHBG, which means lower levels of circulating DHT and thus less hair loss. However, the aging process, particularly for women, decreases their SHBG levels, which means higher levels of circulating DHT inducing hair loss. Conversely, younger women tend to have higher SHBG levels than postmenopausal women, resulting in lower levels of circulating DHT, thus less effect on hair loss. Therefore, the SHBG level is an important biomarker used in managing hair loss because it helps health practitioners assess the free (unbound) bioavailable testosterone. This free form of testosterone is the amount subjected to conversion to DHT by 5-alpha-reductase, which can incite the process of hair miniaturization (Hammond & Bocchinfuso, 1996). Figures 6.1 and 6.2 show a representation of the testosterone-5AR-DHT conversion interaction as it supposedly occurs in the target cell and the testosterone-aromatase conversion process, respectively.

Fig. 6.1: Testosterone-5α-Reductase-DHT Conversion Interaction

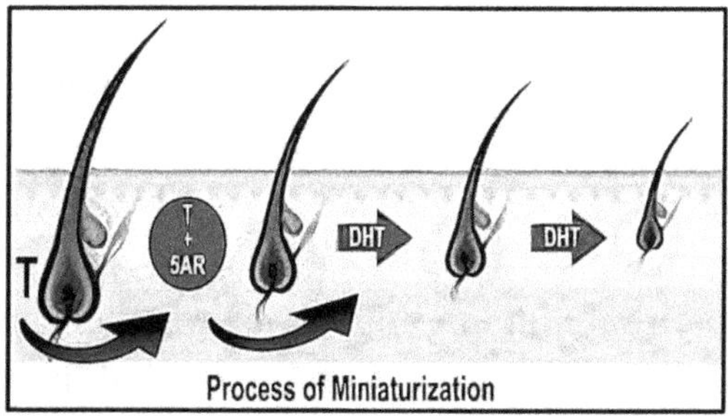

Image Source: By Gustavo J. Gomez. Modified image. Testosterone-5AR-DHTconversion interaction

Fig. 6.2: Testosterone-Aromatase-Estradiol Conversion Process

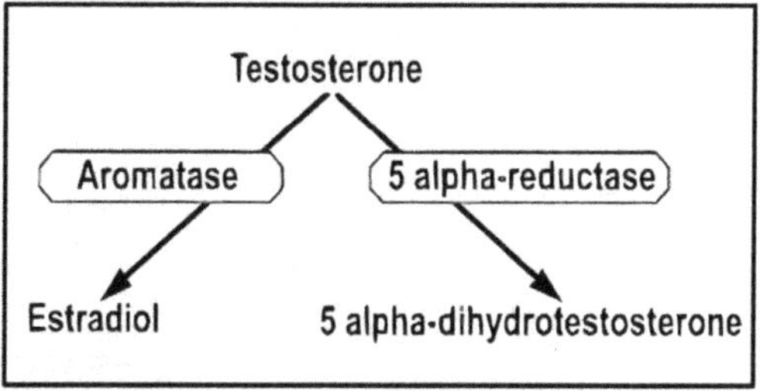

Image Source: http://jur.byu.edu/?p=10988

Hirsutism

It has also been shown that the response of the hair follicles, when brought into contact with DHT, is paradoxical, possessing two roles: hirsutism and male pattern baldness. Hirsutism is not considered a disease process. It is a condition that results in excessive hairiness in women on those parts of the body where terminal hair does not typically occur or is minimal. For example, areas where hirsutism can be seen, are the beard, sideburn, mustache, chest, stomach, or back (Figs. 6.3, 6.4, and 6.5). The condition usually develops during puberty and becomes more pronounced with passing age. However, hirsutism can also be seen at any age if there is an inherited predisposition, an overproduction of male hormones (androgens), medication, or a disease process such as polycystic ovarian syndrome (PCOS).

This paradoxical response results from response differences by the receptor cells in the hair follicle. According to Dr. Ferriman (1971), it is impossible to determine whether the difference in body hair growth can be accounted for solely on a biochemical basis. For example, based on response differences by the receptor cells in the hair follicle to circulating androgens, or whether there is also the involvement of a sex difference in sensitivity of the hair follicle to circulating androgen.

Fig. 6.3: Female hirsutism of the mustache and chin

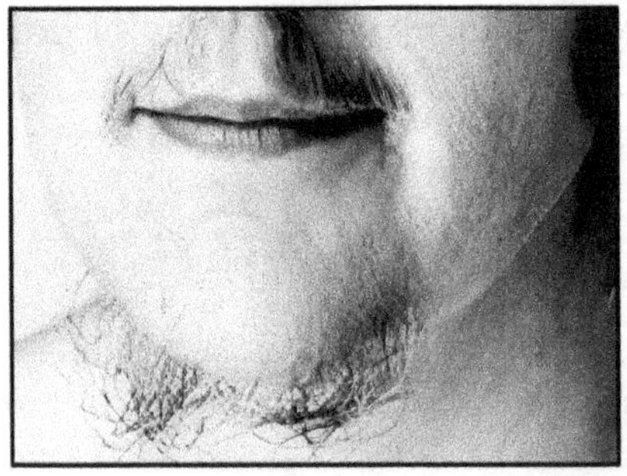

Image Source: http://www.digestground.com/hirsutism-or-excess-facial-hair-in-women-prevention-treatment-management

Fig.6.4: Female hirsutism of the sideburn and beard

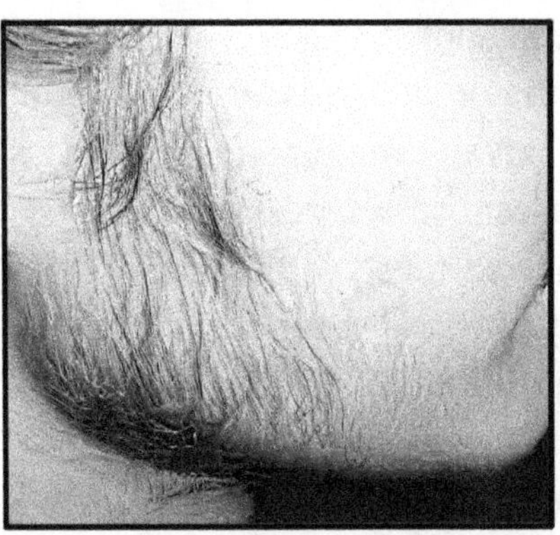

Image Source: http://www.digestground.com/hirsutism-or-excess-facial-hair-in-women-prevention-treatment-management.

Fig. 6.5: Other areas of female hirsutism

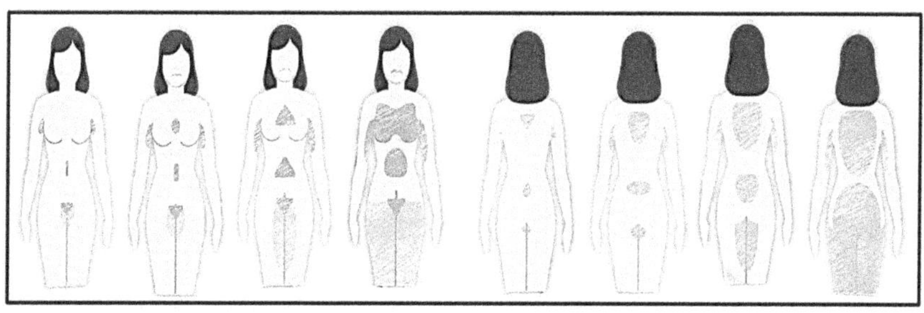

Image Sources: http://permanence.com.au/our-treatments/pcos/atribution

Dr. Ferriman was inclined to believe that a sex difference in sensitivity exists. This local sensitivity to circulating androgens was also demonstrated by French et al. (1966); Gwinup et al. (1966); and Morris and Mahesh (1963) by noting the condition of testicular feminization, where the absence of pubic, axillary, and body hair occurs in the presence of normal male levels of testosterone. Other investigators have also been successful in demonstrating these paradoxical responses. For example, Scheweikert and Wilson (1974) showed that hair in the anagen (growth) stage taken from the frontal area of balding scalps in men had a higher level of DHT than hair taken from the same area of the scalp that was not balding.

The research team of Mowszowicz et al. (1983) demonstrated that hirsute (hairy) women also manifested higher levels of DHT. However, their study concluded that the increased androgen-binding capacity seen in hirsutism could not be held responsible for the hypersensitivity to androgens. Mowszowicz observed that the level of androgens in the human skin of men, women, and hirsute patients was very similar. From this observation, the researchers concluded that the androgen receptor is not regulated by the androgens found on the skin. What the researchers found was the importance of the isoenzyme 5-alpha-reductase (5AR) as an amplifier of androgen action in areas where it is stimulated by androgens.

New Trends in Hair Loss Research Discoveries

In 1977, Dr. Norman Orentreich's research concluded that male pattern baldness was not a loss of hair follicles as was evident from biopsies of bald sites that showed intact, miniaturized hair follicles. Instead, what was found was a time-dependent, steroid, genetic expression with a diminution in the anagen (growth) phase of the hair cycle that progressively turns into a vellus-like hair.

The medical research team of Garza et al. (2011), in collaboration with Professor George Cotsarelis, chairman of the dermatology department at the University of Pennsylvania, discovered that the secret to a cure for baldness might just be found in the scalp. These researchers initially believed that balding men must have fewer of the necessary stem cells that produce hair. However, they were surprised to learn that the number of stem cells in bald men was actually the same as in men with full heads of hair. The discovery by Garza and Cotsarelis seems to validate the 1977 research by Dr. Orentreich that claimed that the miniaturization process of the hair rather than the actual loss of hair follicles characterized male pattern baldness.

The Garza's team was surprised to discover a totally normal number of stem cells in the hair follicles in the bald scalp. Dr. Cotsarelis stated that this discovery could raise hope that individuals afflicted by hair loss might be able to regrow their hair. The findings of this study support the notion that a defect in the conversion of hair-follicle stem cells to progenitor cells plays a role in the development (pathogenesis) of androgenetic alopecia (AGA), or common male pattern baldness.

Garza et al. (2011) also contended that it was necessary to find a way to activate the dormant stem cells. The researchers stated that they needed to get the stem cells already present in the scalp to produce the progenitor cells so they could start growing hair again. Often confused with adult stem cells, progenitor cells are early descendants of stem cells that can differentiate themselves to form one or more kinds of cells. However, they cannot divide and reproduce indefinitely. A progenitor cell is often more limited than a stem cell regarding the kinds of cells it can become. These researchers contend that if they could figure out a way to wake up (reactivate) those existing stem cells (i.e., get them to make hair from progenitor cells), it would go a long way toward developing an effective hair-growth treatment. Although the findings of Garza et al. (2011) appear very promising, any potential significant results lie many years in the future.

In 2012 Garza's research team made an additional promising discovery in a study entitled *"Prostaglandin D2 Inhibits Hair Growth and Is Elevated in Bald Scalp of Men with Androgenetic Alopecia."* In this study, the research team examined gene expression and other PGD_2-related factors in both bald and haired-scalp areas of individuals with common male pattern baldness or AGA. Gene expression essentially means the conversion of the information encoded in a gene first into messenger mRNA via transcription and then into a protein via translation resulting in the gene's phenotypic manifestation. In other words, genes themselves cannot be used by an organism. Instead, they must be turned into a gene product. Therefore, gene expression is how the information contained within a gene becomes a useful product (Compton, 2016).

The Garza 2012 study demonstrated that elevated levels of PGD_2 in the skin lead to the development of alopecia, follicular miniaturization, and sebaceous gland hyperplasia. All these features are the hallmarks of human androgenetic alopecia. These results define PGD_2 as an inhibitor of hair growth in androgenetic alopecia (AGA) and suggest that the PGD_2-GPR44 pathway is a potential target for hair loss treatment.

These researchers also identified a receptor molecule, a protein called GPR44, that binds with PGD_2 on the surface of cells in the hair follicle. Such binding is required to produce the condition of limited hair growth, which is symptomatic of AGA. According to the researchers, several inhibitors of the GPR44 receptor have already been identified and could eventually prove useful in reducing binding activity to treat the condition of AGA. Notwithstanding this new potential hair loss treatments discovery, currently, there are only two FDA-approved drug treatments that help prevent hair loss or stimulate new hair growth in balding areas. These drugs, as previously mentioned, are systemic Propecia® (finasteride) and topical Rogaine® (minoxidil).

Below are some of the findings from Garza's research describing the significant role PGD_2 might have in treating androgenetic alopecia (AGA).

- Among the genes most highly expressed in bald areas was prostaglandin D2 synthase, an enzyme that produces PGD_2.
- Higher PGD_2 levels were found in bald areas than in non-balding areas. According to Milner et al. (2002), the normal hair cycle has four phases: active growth (anagen), regression or transition (catagen), resting (telogen), and shedding (exogen). The study showed that in mice, PGD_2 levels were at their highest before or during the regression or transition (catagen) phase.
- Researchers observed that PGD_2 inhibited hair growth in cultured human hair follicles.
- Mice subjected to application of PGD_2 to their skin manifested decreased hair growth.
- A mouse that was genetically engineered to have elevated levels of PGD_2 in the skin developed symptoms of human androgenetic alopecia (AGA). The mouse also manifested hair follicle miniaturization and hyperplasia of the sebaceous cells, which, as previously stated, are all hallmark features of androgenetic alopecia.

According to Dr. Garza, all their findings point to a significant role for PGD_2 in hair-growth inhibition associated with androgenetic alopecia. Garza contends that by studying the disorder directly, they have been able to hone in on gene and lipid abnormalities that may explain the causes of AGA, which could lead to new treatment targets. *It is quite possible that developing a PGD_2-inhibitor medication could be the third FDA-approved medication in the limited medical arsenal available to combat androgenetic alopecia or common male pattern baldness.*

Garza and Cotsarelis have filed for numerous patents to protect their inventions, which essentially are owned by the trustees of the University of Pennsylvania. Some patents have already been granted, and others are still pending. For example, Garza and Cotsarelis, on February 9, 2016, received patent number US9254293 for their discovery of the prostaglandin D2 (PGD_2) receptor.

The fortunate opportunity for the PGD_2 discovery is that a few drugs are available in the market that already targets this receptor. Thus, there should already be a good deal of safety information on these products. Some of these drugs with PGD_2-inhibitory effects are Setipiprant, Fevipiprant, and Ramatroban. Setipiprant is a clinical-stage oral antagonist/inhibitor to the prostaglandin D2 (PGD_2) receptor. Actelion originally developed this drug but is currently owned by Allergan. Allergan purchased the rights by a licensing agreement with the University of Pennsylvania to evaluate the efficacy of Setipiprant on hair loss. This drug, in particular, is believed to affect this hair-loss pathway directly, and the preclinical and in-vitro human-hair models have confirmed this effect.

Since Setipiprant is a well-characterized molecule that already has a large safety database of over 1,000 subjects, the researchers believe that they can quickly initiate a development program to study its effect on hair loss. Setipiprant has already undergone numerous clinical trials that include:

- A Phase III study in patients with seasonal allergic rhinitis.

- A Phase IIa proof-of-concept study in asthma patients.
- A Phase IIa study to evaluate Setipiprant versus placebo for scalp hair growth in men with androgenetic alopecia (AGA).

The first phase IIa study was conducted from July 2016 to May 2018 at 18 sites in the United States. This study aimed to evaluate drug safety and demonstrate meaningful efficacy. The study was sponsored and funded by Allergan Aesthetics and conducted by Dr. Janet DuBois et al. (2021). The study was entitled "*Setipiprant for Androgenetic Alopecia in Males: Results from a Randomized, Double-Blind, Placebo-Controlled Phase 2a Trial.*" The conclusion of this first study demonstrated that Setipiprant at an oral dose of 1000 mg twice daily (BID) was safe and well-tolerated but did not demonstrate statistically significant efficacy versus placebo for scalp hair growth in men with AGA. This study assessed the effects of Setipiprant on hair loss in men only with AGA and not in women with female-pattern hair loss (FPHL).

Notwithstanding the initial lack of success during the first phase IIa trial does not mean that the drug will not ultimately be efficacious with more investigation. It is possible that the theorized role of PGD_2 signaling in hair loss does not directly translate to clinical outcomes in androgenetic alopecia, or higher doses of Setipiprant may be required. It may also be worth considering whether delivering the drug by topical administration might yield higher drug concentrations compared with oral dosing. Successful topical delivery will depend on the system used to provide therapeutic levels of Setipiprant across the dermal barrier to the target site (DuBois et al., 2021).

In yet another study, Dr. Cotsarelis, in collaboration with colleague Dr. Oh Sang Kwon, were also granted patent number US8871711 for their research on Fibroblast Growth Factor-9 (FGF-9). According to the patent abstract, the FGF-9 invention provides methods for treating, inhibiting, or suppressing degenerative skin disorders. It also provides methods for treating androgenetic alopecia (AGA), generating new hair follicles, and increasing the size of existing hair follicles.

These investigators identified a molecular pathway—the Wnt/β-catenin signaling pathway—that can be manipulated to generate new hair follicles. They postulated that the Wnt/β-catenin pathway could either be activated to prompt hair growth of dormant hair follicles or blocked to prevent unwanted hair growth. The research team examined the functions of Wnt proteins, which are small, molecular messengers that transmit information between cells and activate signaling via the intracellular molecule β-catenin.

By disrupting Wnt signaling in an animal model using a Wnt pathway inhibitor such as Dkk1 (Dickkopf Wnt Signaling Pathway Inhibitor 1), the team discovered that hair growth was prevented. However, stem cells were still maintained within the dormant hair follicles. When Dkk1 was removed, the Wnt/β-catenin pathway resumed normal function, the stem cells were activated, and hair growth was restored (Cotsarelis & Sang Kwon, 2009).

Despite the future promise of this discovery, more research is still required to improve the understanding of the *Wnt pathway*. However, the study results seem to suggest that developing therapeutic agents capable of decreasing the levels of Wnt/β-catenin signaling in the skin could potentially be used to block the growth of unwanted hair or treat certain skin tumors. Conversely, if delivered in a limited, safe, and controlled way, agents that activate Wnt signaling might also be used to promote hair growth in dormant hair follicles in conditions such as male pattern baldness (Choi et al., 2013).

Notwithstanding these promising discoveries, it is essential to understand that currently, the only efficacious solutions that remain available for the prevention of hair loss are hair-growth stimulants, such as minoxidil, and DHT-conversion inhibitors/blockers, such as finasteride. Again as previously mentioned, the two medications that have FDA approval for growing hair are Rogaine®, a topical vasodilator solution, and Propecia®, an oral, systemic medication. All other claims for growing hair by other companies are not supported by research and hence have not been given the FDA blessing that the medications are efficacious. Therefore, at least for the time being, it is possible to theorize that of the three primary factors responsible for hair loss—*heredity, hormonal stimulation, and aging*—inhibition of testosterone to prevent its conversion to DHT may be the sole factor responsive to medical treatment.

According to Garza et al. (2012), testosterone is necessary for the development of male pattern baldness. However, despite this known fact, the mechanisms for decreased hair growth in this disorder are still unclear. Therefore, the most commonly implicated hormone in hair loss is dihydrotestosterone (DHT), which is a very potent form of testosterone. DHT is estimated to be three to six times powerful than testosterone itself. It is clearly the most potent steroid found naturally in the human body (Newman, 2015).

Testosterone is converted to DHT upon interaction with the 5 alpha-reductase (AR) enzyme. Essentially, enzymes are proteins that speed up biochemical reactions. More specifically, this enzyme removes the C4-5 double bond of the testosterone molecule by the addition of two hydrogen atoms to its structure, hence the name "*di-hydro*" testosterone (Fig. 6.6).

Fig. 6.6: Testosterone-5AR-DHT Conversion Process

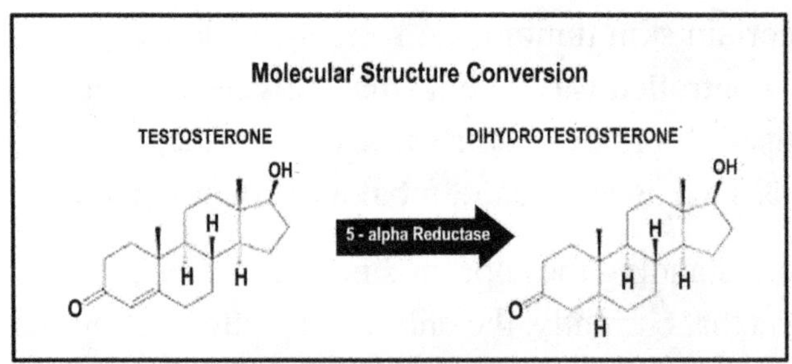

Image Source: By Gustavo J. Gomez Testosterone-5AR-DHT conversion process. Modified image comprised of creative commons public domain images from: Klaus Hoffmeier (Own work) [Public domain], via Wikimedia Commons. https://commons.wikimedia.org/wiki/File%3ATestosterone. PNG; Fvasconcellos (Own work) [Public domain], via Wikimedia Commons https://commons.wikimedia.org/wiki/File% Dihydrotestosterone. Svg

The removal of this bond is important. In this case, it creates a steroid that binds to the androgen receptor much more avidly than does its parent steroid. The enzyme 5-alpha-reductase is present in high amounts in tissues of the prostate, skin, scalp, liver, and various regions of the central nervous system. As such, it represents a mechanism by which the body can increase the potency of testosterone, specifically where a strong androgenetic action is required. However, this localized potentiating mechanism of testosterone is not always a good thing because this stronger androgenetic activity in certain tissues may produce several undesirable side effects. For example, acne is often triggered by dihydrotestosterone activity in the sebaceous glands, and the local formation of DHT in the scalp is the problem that causes AGA.

It would be logical to conclude that if we could decrease the amount of the enzyme 5AR in the blood or in the hair follicles, then less testosterone would be converted to DHT, thus lowering the levels of circulating dihydrotestosterone. Currently, research has been undertaken to develop medications—either systemic or topical—that could block DHT conversion. These drugs contain either topical 5AR inhibitors or androgen receptor blockers. To date, three, chemically distinct forms (isoenzymes) of the 5-alpha-reductase enzyme have been identified (Yamana et al., 2010; Godoy et al., 2011). These are 5-alpha-reductase types 1, 2 and 3 (SRD5A-1, 2, and 3).

The 5AR type 1 is found mainly in the skin's sebocytes and in epidermal and follicular keratinocytes, sweat glands, and dermal papilla cells. The 5AR type 2 is found in the seminal vesicles, prostate, and the inner root sheath of the hair follicle. It is the type 2 that is the most closely linked to male pattern hair loss. The 5AR type 3, according to Yamana et al. (2010) is expressed in the skin, brain, mammary gland, and breast cancer cell lines. The reason each 5AR is given a number is because that is the order they were chronologically discovered.

The only FDA-approved systemic hair-loss drug in the market is Propecia® (finasteride) in one milligram (1-mg) dosage. Propecia® inhibits 5-alpha-reductase types 1 and 2, with greater affinity for type 2. Proscar® is the same drug as Propecia®, but it is available in a 5-mg dosage, which is the dosage indicated for benign prostatic hyperplasia (BPH). The FDA has approved finasteride for the treatment of benign prostatic hyperplasia (BPH) since 1992 and for the treatment of male androgenetic alopecia (AGA) since 1997 (Cather et al., 1999). The drug Avodart® (dutasteride) inhibits all three 5-alpha-reductase isoenzymes—types 1, 2, and 3—and it is only approved by the FDA for benign prostatic hyperplasia (Yamana et al., 2010; Godoy et al., 2011). *Even though Proscar® and Avodart® are strictly designed to treat BPH, they are sometimes used for hair loss off-label by some patients.*

Avodart® has not yet been officially approved to treat hair loss in the United States or the European Union. However, it was approved for that purpose in South Korea in 2009 and has since proven its efficacy, mainly by reducing DHT concentration by 92 % at 24 weeks of treatment. In Japan, Avodart was approved for hair loss in 2015 (Choi et al. 2016). In a study by Olsen et al., (2006), entitled "*The Importance of Dual 5-alpha-Reductase Inhibition in the Treatment of Male Pattern Hair Loss: Results of a Randomized Placebo-Controlled Study of Dutasteride versus Finasteride,*" Olsen discovered that a 2.5 mg dose of dutasteride increased target area hair count versus placebo and demonstrated superiority over finasteride at 12 and 24 weeks period.

Although finasteride has only been FDA-approved for male pattern baldness (MPB), it has been in use off-label for female pattern hair loss (FPHL). At the moment, there is no consensus on the standard treatment options for female pattern androgenetic alopecia (AGA). Therefore, the efficacy of finasteride in women is controversial. In a study by Boersma et al., (2014), entitled *"The effectiveness of finasteride and dutasteride used for three years in women with androgenetic alopecia,"* the *research team concluded that finasteride at 1.25 mg and dutasteride at 0.15 mg given daily for three* years effectively increased hair thickness and arrested further deterioration of FPHL or androgenetic alopecia.

It is important to note that a considerable number of finasteride users have reported numerous sexual dysfunction side effects while on oral finasteride at a dosage of 1-mg per day (Propecia®). These side effects have been classified and reported as *Post-finasteride Syndrome (PFS)* which, seems to persist despite discontinuation of the drug. PFS is a new illness that the medical community has not yet fully recognized. The author will explain the topic of PFS more extensively in the last section of this chapter. The plasma half-life of finasteride is approximately 5 to 6 hours in men aged 18 to 60 and 8 hours in men older than 70. The half-life of dutasteride also increases with age. It is approximately 170 hours or five weeks in men aged 20 to 49 years old, around 260 hours in men aged 50 to 69 years, and about 300 hours in men older than 70. This long-lasting effect of dutasteride poses an even greater risk for libido side effects (Blume-Peytavi, Whiting, & Trüeb, 2008; Blatchley, 2017; Mysore, 2012).

As the result of these potential side effects caused by systemic 5-alpha-reductase inhibitors (5ARIs), there is significant interest in the development of a topical preparation for both finasteride and dutasteride. The objective of a topical formulation is to prevent these side effects from occurring by using a scalp medication that might not penetrate systemically. To date, this topical formulation is not yet available as an FDA-approved medication. However, it is currently available as an off-label pharmacy compounded formulation.

Human Androgen Receptor Binding Theory

Many dermatologists and research scientists specializing in hair loss believe DHT molecules may diffuse into the interior of hair follicle cells—the cytoplasm, or cytosol—and bind with androgen receptors (Fig. 6.7). This complex, both the receptor and the DHT molecule, then enters the nucleus of the cell. In the nucleus of the hair follicle cell, this complex may subsequently alter the rate of protein synthesis in men who are genetically predisposed to baldness (Stewart & Pochi, 1978; Meehan & Sadar, 2003).

Fig. 6.7: Human androgen receptor and androgen binding theory

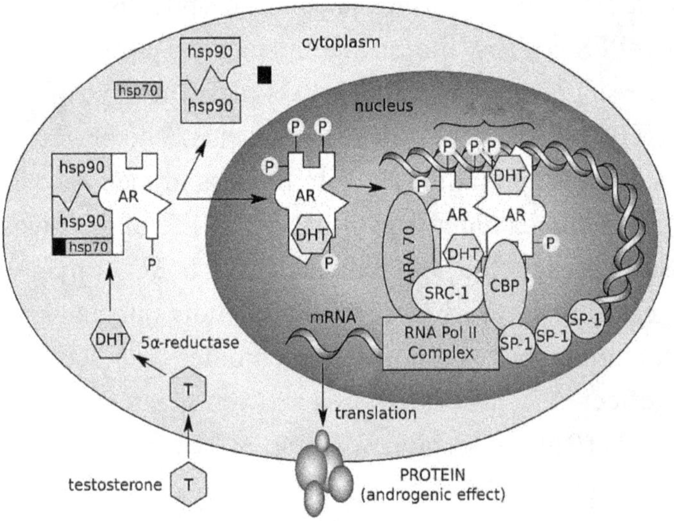

Image Sources: Figure by Jonathan Marcus, based on an original drawing by Dr. Marianne D. Sadar (Meehan, K. L. and Sadar, M. D. Front Biosci. 2003 May 1; 8: d780-800). This file is licensed under the Creative Commons Attribution 3.0 Unported license. https://commons.wikimedia.org/wiki/File%3AHuman_androgen_receptor_and_androgen_binding.svg

As previously mentioned, the only DHT-inhibitor drug for hair loss currently approved by the FDA is Propecia®. Conversely, there are claims that many natural herbs are also considered dihydrotestosterone blockers or inhibitors. For example, saw palmetto, pumpkin seed, pygeum extract, green tea, soy isoflavones, beta-sitosterol, stinging nettle, fenugreek, lycopene, caffeine, and zinc, are considered DHT inhibitors. However, the effectiveness of these natural substances is highly questionable. Regardless of what is available, any drug that is or will be developed will most likely attempt to perform at least one of two things:

- Reduce the amount of testosterone converted to DHT by blocking the effect of the enzyme 5-alpha-reductase.
- Bind DHT to a receptor and thus render it ineffective.

Presently, some investigators are very enthusiastic about the current and future trends of endocrinologic management of androgenetic alopecia (AGA). Famed hair transplant surgeon and researcher the late Dr. Norman Orentreich in 1977 claimed that the era of medical control of premature baldness had begun. Moreover, Dr. Orentreich further raised the hopes of young men with a strong genetic predisposition to balding by stating that hair loss would safely be arrested as more specific endocrine drugs are developed.

However, one big problem in treating androgenetic alopecia or premature baldness by removing the testosterone stimulus from the hair follicle with the use of all these drugs is that the hair follicle that has already been affected by this androgen does not always regain its original hair growth cycle (Hamilton, 1951). According to Dr. Hamilton, this problem implies that in order to treat potentially balding males, treatment would have to be started early enough so that the onset of hair loss could be effectively halted. Hamilton further claimed that, at best, people who are already bald should only expect to keep the hair they presently have. Although, as previously mentioned, the stem cell research undertaken by Garza et al. (2011, 2012) might dispel this theory.

Post-Finasteride Syndrome (PFS)

A word of caution is appropriate at this juncture. Despite the enthusiasm of some investigators, most researchers believe that the clinical use of all these potentially dangerous drugs is premature. For example, Post-Finasteride Syndrome (PFS) is a new illness and is not yet fully recognized by the medical community. PFS is characterized by devastating sexual, neurological, and physical side effects that persist in men who have taken a 5-alpha-reductase type-II enzyme inhibitor, such as Propecia® and Proscar® (finasteride).

The most common and persistent sexual side effects of finasteride are the loss of libido, loss of penis sensitivity, low penile temperature, erectile dysfunction, Peyronie's disease (plaque or scar tissue formation inside the penis), decreased ejaculatory force, penile shrinkage, and gynecomastia.

Moreover, there are numerous non-sexual symptoms associated with the use of finasteride such as depression, suicidal ideation, anxiety, panic attacks, muscle atrophy, cognitive impairment, insomnia, severely dry skin, and tinnitus (Rossi, 2004; Rahimi-Ardabili, Pourandarjani, Habibollahi & Mualeki, 2006; Singh & Avram, 2014). Additionally, a review of 17 randomized controlled trials comprising a study population of more than 17,000 participants demonstrated approximately a twofold increase in sexual, ejaculatory, and orgasmic dysfunction in patients using Propecia® for male pattern hair loss (Marchalik, 2013).

Another study demonstrated changes in the levels of certain steroids in the cerebrospinal fluid of men taking finasteride for hair loss. These steroids have been shown to influence brain function. Their presence may help explain the profound psychological changes observed, such as depression and suicidal ideation, associated with finasteride use. Furthermore, finasteride usage has also been associated with intraoperative floppy iris syndrome (IFIS) and cataract formation (Wong & Mak, 2011).

Unfortunately, PFS is a condition with no known cure and few—if any—effective treatments. As an increasing number of men report persistent side effects to health and regulatory agencies worldwide, medical, and scientific communities are beginning to realize the scope of the problem (PFSFoundation.org, 2013). The continued reporting of these problems has forced the FDA to issue mandated labeling changes for finasteride (FDA.org., 2012).

- A revision to the Propecia® label to include libido disorders, ejaculation disorders, and orgasm disorders that continue after discontinuation of the drug.
- A revision to the Proscar® label to include decreased libido that continues after discontinuation of the drug.
- A revision to both the Propecia® and Proscar® labels to include a description of reports of male infertility and poor semen quality that improved after drug discontinuation.

There are always unintended consequences to every well-meaning intervention. For example, the reason why these 5-alpha-reductase/DHT-inhibitor drugs are administered to patients is because increased levels of DHT have been implicated in androgenetic alopecia (AGA) or male pattern baldness and benign prostatic hypertrophy. In fact, as early as 1986, some authorities suspected that 5-alpha-reductase/DHT conversion might be the primary contributing factor to prostate cancer growth (Petrow, 1986).

Consequently, millions of men worldwide currently take these drugs, as well as natural DHT-inhibiting supplements, to inhibit the 5-alpha-reductase enzyme and decrease 5α-DHT production. However, recent studies have shown correlations between low levels of DHT and reduced survival rate in prostate cancer patients, which is concerning (Nishiyama et al., 2006). In other words, over-inhibiting DHT levels seem to produce more aggressive prostate cancer, resulting in decreased survivability.

Therefore, it appears that over-inhibiting the activity of 5-alpha-reductase can result in unintended negative consequences. While 5α-DHT is considered to be a potential cause of proliferation and growth in the prostate, its metabolite, *3β-Adiol* (5α-androstane-3b,17b-diol), is a differentiating agent that activates estrogen receptor beta (ERβ) and may help prevent cancer. As a result, inhibiting 5-alpha-reductase should be done with caution; without adequate levels of DHT, the production of 3β-Adiol may be over-inhibited as well (Dondi et al., 2010).

Research regarding the benefits of adequate 3β-Adiol is growing. 3β-Adiol is an androgen that stimulates only estrogen receptor beta (ERβ), which has anti-proliferative and re-differentiation activities. Among other functions, ERβ helps regulate prostate growth and differentiation (Weihua et al., 2002). ERβ is also an important modulator of the stress response in the brain (Handa et al., 2008). Over-inhibition of 5-alpha-reductase can result in under-stimulation of ERβ, changing the balance of proliferative/anti-proliferative activity in the prostate and elsewhere.

It would be reckless for individuals afflicted with hair-loss problems to ignore or disregard the potentially dangerous side effects that could result from the use of hair-loss drugs for the sake of growing some hair. The advantages should always be weighed against the disadvantages in any decision made in life. However, the future is definitively brighter than ever before for a possible discovery of a hair-loss cure. Even so, despite the emerging good news about hair-loss research, more data must be gathered regarding the mechanism of the receptors in question. Other drugs with fewer side effects must be developed in order to treat androgenetic alopecia safely and effectively.

7

Effects of Aging on Hair Loss

As previously mentioned, the third factor essential for the progression of baldness is the aging process. It has been observed that there is an increase in the incidence and extent of baldness in normal men and women with advancing age. This hair-loss progression associated with advancing age appears not to be associated with inciting agents like androgens (testosterone). Therefore, the hair, just like the skin, is susceptible to the natural aging process. As a person becomes older, they gradually begin to notice significant differences in their hair's color, texture, thickness, health, and manageability. Hair aging comprises weathering of the hair shaft and aging of the hair follicle. The latter—aging of the hair follicle—manifests as a decrease of melanocyte function, or graying, and a reduction in hair production in androgenetic and senescent alopecia (Trüeb, 2005).

Senescent alopecia, or senile alopecia, was originally thought to affect people who were 50 years of age or older. It is a unique type of alopecia that exhibits a very slow rate of progression with no family history or evidence of male or female pattern baldness. Senile alopecia is described as a diffuse thinning involving the whole scalp due to a steady decrease in thick, terminal hairs but without evidence of increased miniaturization as seen in androgenetic alopecia (Whiting, 2011). Even though this type of alopecia appears to have no direct connection with androgen-mediated signals, it should be noted that senescent (senile) alopecia likely coexists with androgenetic alopecia in many patients. According to the latest study, senile alopecia is associated with changes in alternative splicing (AS), oxidative stress response, and apoptosis (cell death), which are characteristic of aging tissues. According to Dr. Hamilton's theories, hair loss results from independent factors simply connected with the aging process.

Conversely, some investigators believe that other factors, like gonadal (e.g., relating to the testes and ovaries) depression, might account for this loss of hair. The implication is that the gonads of both men and women function less efficiently with advancing age, thereby producing less of the essential androgen responsible for hair growth. On the other hand, it is quite possible that the mere aging process leads to hair loss, just as it affects many other bodily systems and functions. This loss of hair resulting from aging is not only limited to the scalp, but it can also affect the eyebrows, pubic area, legs, and axillary (armpit) hair.

Effects of Scalp Circulation on Hair Loss

The combination of genetic susceptibility and androgenetic inhibition of follicular growth in both male and female pattern baldness is a well-recognized process. However, the role played by the circulatory (vascular) system is not as clear. Even though the position of orthodox (traditional) medicine has always been that circulation has absolutely nothing to do with male and female pattern baldness or androgenetic alopecia, there appears to be sufficient evidence to the contrary. For example, it is recognized that dihydrotestosterone-mediated inflammation damages microcirculation and thus deprives hair follicles of blood and vital nutrients (Kiichiro, Brown, & Detmar, 2001).

Occasionally, it has been postulated that tight scalp muscles, or tight galea aponeurotica, result in hair loss because a tight scalp reduces the amount of circulating blood available to feed the hair follicle. Thus, it deprives it of its vital nutrients (Fig. 7.1).

Fig. 7.1: Galea aponeurotica and scalp muscles associated with a tight scalp

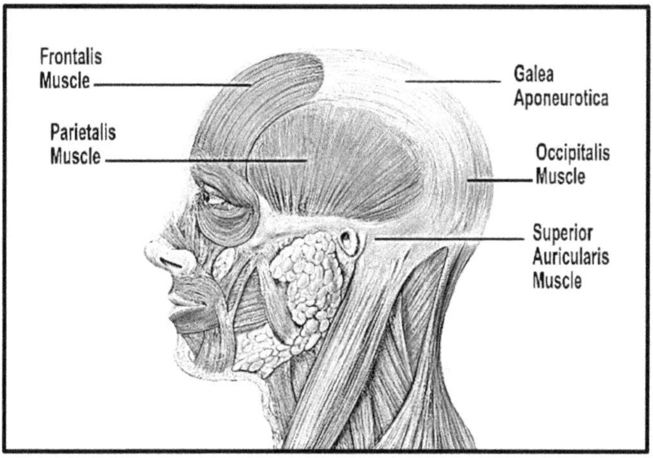

Image Source: By Patrick J. Lynch, medical illustrator. Creative Commons license 2.5. https://commons.wikimedia.org/w/index.php?curid=1498151. Modified image to include muscle classification.

It is a fact that circulatory blood flow is reduced in bald areas, and this diminished blood flow is primarily the result of a decreased demand for the metabolic needs of the area of hair loss. The reason for this reduced demand is that the hair follicles are much smaller and therefore require fewer nutrients. However, while decreased circulatory blood flow to the hair follicle has not been conclusively proven to result in hair loss, it is important to keep an open mind regarding this theory. This could be a theory that becomes invalidated with time since there appears to be some evidence suggesting that improving scalp circulation can indeed lead to hair growth.

For example, a Japanese study found that blood flow to the scalp of a young man diagnosed with androgenetic alopecia was 2.6 times lower than in the normal control group. A research team at Inneov—a subsidiary of L'Oréal—identified diminished circulation as a critical element of the balding process that needs to be addressed in the treatment process if the objective is to attain a cosmetically significant result (Kiichiro et al., 2001).

Furthermore, researchers at Massachusetts General Hospital (MGH) have succeeded in growing hair faster and thicker in mice, which they have attributed to a protein that promotes *angiogenesis* (blood vessel growth) in their skin. The mouse protein-treated hair follicles—while no greater in number than those of normal mice—were individually bigger. In this study, the researchers were able to increase the total volume (thickness) of the hair by 70%. If this protein has the same effect in humans, it could lead to the first *angiogenic therapy* for male pattern baldness.

The results of this study identified vascular endothelial growth factor (VEGF) as a significant mediator of hair follicle growth and cycling. It also provided the first direct evidence that improved follicle vascularization (improved scalp circulation) promotes hair growth and increases the hair follicle size (Kiichiro et al., 2001). VEGF is an endothelial cell mitogen and permeability factor that is potently angiogenic *in vivo*. In-vivo experiments are conducted in living organisms. A mitogen is a chemical substance— usually a form of protein— that encourages a cell to commence cell division, triggering mitosis (cell division).

Additionally, this study provides evidence that diminished microcirculation is implicated in the cause of male and female pattern baldness. It also suggests that the formation of new blood vessels (angiogenesis) causes hair growth in animal models. This new evidence dismisses the traditional medical view that scalp circulation has nothing to do with hair loss. Prior to this study from MGH, no researchers had actually measured how closely blood vessel growth is correlated with hair growth or what might cause scalp blood vessels to grow in the first place (Kiichiro et al., 2001).

Freund and Schwartz (2010) conducted another interesting research study that addressed scalp circulatory blood flow and oxygenation entitled, "*Treatment of Male Pattern Baldness with Botulinum Toxin: A Pilot Study.*" This study is considered important because it demonstrated that testosterone conversion to dihydrotestosterone (DHT) occurs in a hypoxic environment. A hypoxic environment is one where there is inadequate oxygenation of the blood. Moreover, the muscles, or anything that constricts (decreases) blood flow, will also reduce oxygen availability in the scalp and dermal papilla.

According to Freund and Schwartz (2010), the scalp behaves like a drum skin mechanistically, with tensioning muscles around the periphery. These muscle groups include the frontalis, occipitals, superior auricularis muscles, and to a minor degree, the temporalis can create a tight scalp when chronically active (Fig.7.1). Because the blood supply to the scalp enters through the periphery, a reduction in blood flow would be most apparent at the distal ends of the vessels, specifically, the *vertex* and *frontal peaks*. Consequently, these areas of the scalp have manifested the following conditions:

- Sparse hair growth.
- Shown to be relatively hypoxic (inadequate oxygenation of the blood).
- Slow capillary refill.
- High levels of DHT.

Conceptually, Botox® loosens (relax) the scalp muscles, which reduces the pressure on the perforating vasculature, thereby increasing both blood flow and oxygen supply. These researchers contend that the enzymatic (5AR) conversion of testosterone to DHT is *oxygen-dependent.* Thus, in a low-oxygen environment, the conversion of testosterone to DHT is favored. Conversely, more testosterone is converted to estradiol in a high-oxygen environment, which reduces DHT levels (Freund & Schwartz, 2010).

None of the 40 participants who completed the Freund and Schwarz study demonstrated any adverse side effects to the botulinum toxin. Consequently, the study resulted in a treatment response rate of 75%. This investigation also demonstrates that blood flow may indeed be a primary determinant factor in follicular health.

Moreover, strategically placed Botox® injections appear to indirectly modify this variable by improving circulatory blood flow, which results in reduced hair loss and new hair growth in some men with androgenetic alopecia (Freund & Schwartz, 2010).

Yet another study linking reduced scalp circulation to hair loss was conducted in 2008 by Paul J. Taylor entitled *"Big Head? Bald Head! Skull expansion: Alternative Model for the Primary Mechanism of AGA."* Taylor's contention was that steroid hormones such as DHT promote facial and body hair growth. According to Taylor, this premise suggests that DHT should stimulate hair growth within the male pattern balding (MPB) region and not hair loss.

Thus, Taylor postulated that the follicular miniaturization observed in androgenetic alopecia (AGA) might result from an exaggeration of the bone remodeling (expansion) process, causing a reduction in the blood supply to the capillary network within the region or area of hair loss. According to this hypothesis, the adult cranial bones, especially the *frontal* and *parietal* bones, continue to grow in size, even in adulthood, under the influence of DHT, which has an anabolic effect on the skull's bone formation (Fig. 7.2).

7.2: Frontal and Parietal Scalp Bones

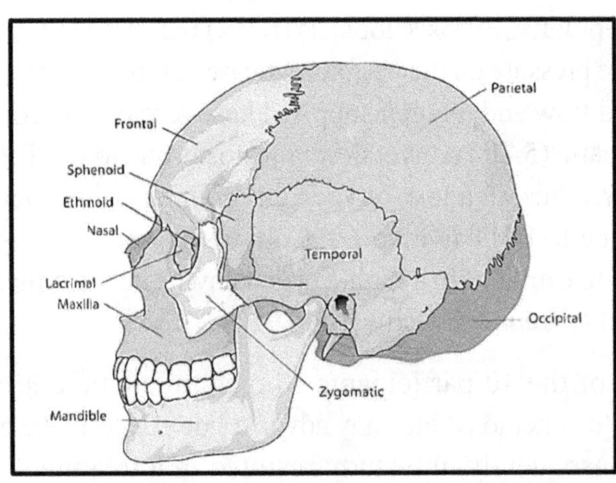

Image Source: By Lady of Hats Mariana Ruiz Villarreal (Own work) Public Domain. https://commons.wikimedia.org/w/index.php?curid=1524860

It is hypothesized that this stimulation of bone growth will overwhelm the hair growth-promoting effects of DHT, which will result in bone expansion and remodeling. This, in turn, would compromise the blood flow through the scalp capillary network in the frontal and parietal areas, thus initiating miniaturization of the hair follicles in these affected areas (Fig. 7.3). Validation of this hypothesis would imply that DHT is primarily involved with androgenetic alopecia (AGA) through its stimulation of the skull expansion process rather than through interaction with the individual hair follicles (Taylor, 2008).

7.3: Hair-loss pattern postulated to occur from expansion of scalp bones in the frontal and parietal areas

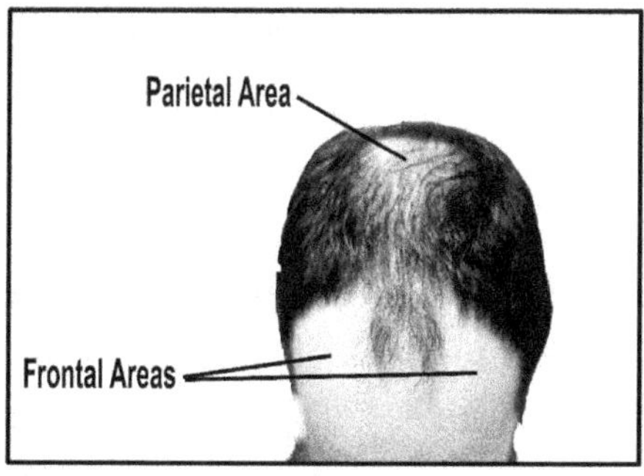

Image Source: http://claytransformations.info/imagehdb-hair-transplant-before-and-after-5000-grafts.html attribution

Furthermore, researchers have demonstrated that the follicles of vigorously growing hair are embedded in a layer of brown adipose (fat) tissue. However, in people with androgenetic alopecia, there is a decrease in the amount of this type of fat around dormant follicles. In fact, it has been observed that there is a depletion of fat tissue in bald areas of the scalp. Conversely, in the occipital region (lower rear area), where hair loss does not occur, a thick layer of adipose tissue is present. Moreover, it appears that the loss of this layer of fat occurs before follicle miniaturization and hair loss begin. Researchers also believe that the skull expansion process might also erode brown adipose tissue, or brown fat, within the skin's dermis. This brown fat promotes new blood vessel formation or angiogenesis, as it is medically called. This brown fat is vital for each new hair-growth cycle if a follicle is to successfully grow hair. Thus, if there is a reduction in brown fat, this could also be a contributing factor to hair loss (Taylor, 2008).

At this juncture, it is important to state that there are always contradictions between research studies. For example, Hamilton's 1951 research study showed conclusively that once the hair follicle has been affected by androgen stimulation—specifically, DHT—there is nothing that can be done to stimulate its regrowth to a terminal hair. This long-standing theory by Dr. Hamilton appears to have been invalidated by the more recent discovery in 2011 by Garza and Cotsarelis' research team from the University of Pennsylvania, and the research team of Bou-Abboud, Nemec, and Toffel in 1990 from the University of Nevada.

Contrary to Hamilton's theory, Garza and Cotsarelis showed that stem cells play an unexpected role in explaining what happens in the bald scalp. Their study uncovered that a balding scalp still possesses the intact hair follicle stem cells. However, certain progenitor cells become depleted in the follicles of the bald scalp. In other words, the follicular stem cells are present, but the activity to initiate growth is not. From this observation, the researchers surmised that balding might arise from a problem with stem-cell activation rather than the number of stem cells in the follicles.

The Bou-Abboud research team studied a 73-year-old white male who had been bald since the age of 28. He had developed Non-A (nonalcoholic) and Non-B-induced liver cirrhosis and had been treated with spironolactone for six years. Because of the exposure to spironolactone, his hair had started to regrow over his bald scalp. The research team postulated that the hair growth might be related to the anti-androgenetic effect of spironolactone. Spironolactone (Aldactone®) is not an FDA-approved hair-loss medication, but it is used off-label as a hair-loss treatment, especially by women. Spironolactone is claimed to stop hair loss, reduce women's body hair (hirsutism), reduce acne, help women with polycystic ovary syndrome (PCOS), and improve seborrheic dermatitis.

Essentially, spironolactone is a potassium-sparing diuretic medication that possesses anti-androgen activity. The drug causes the adrenal glands and ovaries to slow down their production of androgens and blocks the action of the androgens that are produced. One way it does that is by essentially inhibiting dihydrotestosterone (DHT)—the form of testosterone that causes hair loss—from binding to its androgenetic receptor and affecting the hair follicle.

Other Theories Addressing Hair Loss

As previously mentioned, in androgenetic alopecia, what happens is that the hair follicles actually shrink or become miniaturized; they do not disappear. The hairs are essentially microscopic, vellus-type hairs on the bald areas of the scalp in contrast to other areas. The implication of this finding is that there is a problem or defect in the activation of stem cells converting to progenitor cells in balding areas of the scalp. In fact, this is precisely what Garza and Cotsarelis discovered that the hair follicles of bald men contained just as many immature stem cells as healthy hair follicles. However, these stem cells, because of some unknown defect, do not produce as many mature progenitor cells, which essentially are the cells that produce hair (Fig. 7.4).

Fig. 7.4: Stem cells unable to convert to progenitor cells

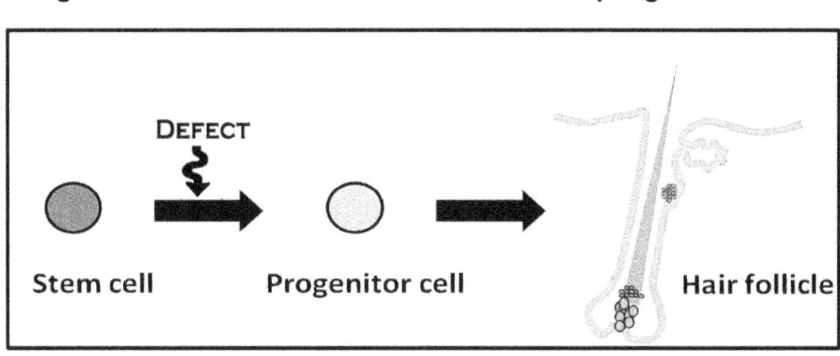

Image Sources: https://www.hairtransplantdubai.com/which-hair-replacement-gives-more-natural-results/

This discovery by researchers Garza and Cotsarelis does not invalidate the significance of DHT's effect on androgenetic alopecia. In fact, it seems that DHT is what keeps the hair follicle stem cells from growing up and becoming progenitor cells that activate hair growth. In other words, it is not so much that the hair follicle itself has a genetic hypersensitivity to DHT, but rather it is the stem cell in the hair follicle that is hypersensitive.

Moreover, in another study, Garza et al. (2012) showed that the enzyme prostaglandin D2 synthase (PTGDS) was elevated in the bald scalp compared to the haired scalp of men with androgenetic alopecia (AGA). The product of PTGDS enzyme activity, prostaglandin D2 (PGD_2), is similarly elevated in the bald scalp. The study showed that PGD_2 inhibits hair growth in explanted human hair follicles and when applied topically to mice. Therefore, the study demonstrates that elevated levels of PGD_2 in the skin develop alopecia, follicular miniaturization, and sebaceous gland hyperplasia, which are all hallmarks of human AGA. These results define PGD_2 as an inhibitor of hair growth in AGA and suggest the PGD_2-GPR44 pathway as a potential target for hair-loss treatment. This research study postulates that if PGD_2 is blocked, it might allow the stem cells to make or facilitate the conversion to progenitor cells again, which should result in hair growth (Nieves & Garza, 2015).

The serendipitous findings from a research study conducted by Dr. Sivan Harel of Columbia University Medical Center addressing the effectiveness of Janus kinase inhibitor drugs in alopecia areata (AA) are also promising. Janus kinase inhibitors—also known as JAK-inhibitors or jakinibs— are types of drugs that inhibit the functionality of JAK enzymes within the body. JAK is a family of intracellular, non-receptor tyrosine kinases that transduce cytokine-mediated signals via the JAK-STAT pathway. The JAK family is composed of JAK1, JAK2, JAK3, and tyrosine kinase 2 (TYK2).

While this topic is a complicated subject, it is important for hair-loss sufferers to understand that these enzymes can cause hair loss, among other things. A research study using mouse and human hair follicles entitled *"Pharmacologic Inhibition of JAK-STAT Signaling Promotes Hair Growth"* conducted by Harel et al. (2015) found that drugs that inhibit or block the JAK family of enzymes promote rapid and robust hair growth when applied to the skin. Although Harel's study focused on alopecia areata (AA), an autoimmune type of hair loss, his study raised the possibility that using JAK-inhibitor drugs could possibly restore hair growth in these types of hair loss. These types of hair loss are induced by male androgenetic alopecia and other forms of hair loss that occur when hair follicles are trapped in a resting (telogen) stage. In 2016, only two JAK-inhibitor drugs were approved by the FDA. Ruxolitinib, and Tofacitinib, neither with a direct dermatologic indication. Ruxolitinib was approved to treat blood diseases, and Tofacitinib was approved for the treatment of rheumatoid arthritis. Both drugs are being tested in clinical trials for the treatment of alopecia areata and plaque psoriasis.

The importance of the Harel et al. (2015) study regarding androgenetic alopecia is that during those experiments, they observed that mice grew more hair when the drug was applied to the skin than when the drug was given systemically. This observation suggested that JAK-inhibitors might be doing something to the hair follicles in addition to stopping the immune system attack from alopecia areata. Moreover, when the researchers observed normal mouse hair follicles more closely, they found that JAK-inhibitors rapidly awakened resting follicles from dormancy, or inactivity.

These researchers observed that JAK inhibitors triggered the hair follicle's normal reawakening process. Mice treated for five days with one of two JAK-inhibitors sprouted new hair within ten days, greatly accelerating the onset of hair growth. However, no hair growth was observed on the untreated control mice in the same period of time. Thus, the contention by Harel et al. (2015) is that it is likely that JAK-inhibitor drugs act on the same pathways in human follicles as they do in mice, suggesting that they may induce new hair growth and extend the anagen (growth) phase of existing hair in humans.

However, whether JAK inhibitors can reawaken hair follicles that have been frozen in a telogen (resting) state because of androgenetic alopecia—which causes male and female pattern baldness—or other forms of hair loss is still unknown. So far, all experiments have been performed on normal mice and human hair follicles. However, research addressing hair follicles affected by other types of hair-loss disorders is in the pipeline.

It has been approximately six and a half years since the first case report showed successful treatment of alopecia areata regrowing hair with tofacitinib on a patient. Since 2015, the interest in the research and development of JAK-inhibitors drugs has increased substantially. As of 2021, not only are their newer options, but there is also a second generation of more selective JAK-inhibitors ready to enter the market. Some of these newer generation JAK-inhibitors are abrocitinib, upadacitinib, and baricitinib, which offer new promising options to treat various dermatologic conditions. Some of these conditions include psoriasis, atopic dermatitis, alopecia areata, and vitiligo. As research has demonstrated, JAK inhibitors are effective across a broad spectrum of autoimmune and inflammatory conditions (Evans, 2021). The future looks bright!!

Hair Restoration Clinics

One of the primary reasons that may explain the popularity and proliferation of today's many hair restoration programs is the belief that improving scalp circulation can regrow hair. Scalp circulation is essentially improved with efforts such as scalp massage combined with the application of numerous topical solutions. It is a well-known fact that just about anything that irritates the scalp can initiate a limited amount of sporadic hair growth (Giacometti, 1982). According to Giacometti, this is the fundamental reason that virtually any hair-loss restorer can cite some positive testimony to back up their claim that they can grow hair.

The majority of these hair restoration clinics employ various methods for treating their clients, such as physiotherapeutic massage of the scalp, either by hand or using vibrators and ultraviolet rays. They also apply stimulating oils, biotin ointments, herbal solutions, vasodilators, and amino acids. McCarthy (1940) advocated these treatment modalities to treat seborrheic alopecia.

Hair restoration clinics utilize these techniques to either improve scalp circulatory blood flow or clean/dislodge debris they claim is blocking or impeding the hair follicle from coming out. Most of these clinics treat hair loss as if all baldness is caused by the same condition, which the scientific evidence proves is not valid. Moreover, these clinics disregard all the other theories that influence hair loss, such as heredity (genetics), androgenic stimulation, and senescence. They continue to operate on the premise that hair will grow again by stimulating the scalp and improving circulation.

Most of the technical personnel working in these hair clinics are not sufficiently trained or knowledgeable about the physiology of hair loss. Their job is to massage the scalp with the topical solutions they claim will regrow hair and provide vague answers to the questions being asked by their clients. Hair restoration clinics have existed for many years and will continue to operate for many more, as long as the public remains uninformed about what can or cannot grow hair. It is the absolute responsibility of consumers to be informed and become educated consumers to avoid being deceived by dishonest hair-restorers. These hair restoration establishments thrive on misinformation and the gullibility of the uninformed public who are just trying to find a solution to their hair loss problems.

It is worth remembering Hamilton's 1951 investigation. He claimed that if the hair follicle had become atrophic, there is no stimulation, hair pills, hair vitamins, hair concoctions, biotin creams, mysterious herbal solutions, vasodilators, or special shampoos that will regenerate the normal function of the hair follicle. The best that can be expected from an effective hair treatment is to retard hair loss and retain some of the remaining hair. Legally, these hair clinic operators are protected because they customarily make clients sign an affidavit stating that they have observed some hair growth. They sign this affidavit within the first month of treatment, a time of excitement and positive expectancy on the client's part. The consumer should be aware that the contract law principle of caveat emptor—let the buyer beware—is applicable in this type of service. That is why it is essential to become an informed consumer before committing to a specific course of action.

While it is true that most of these therapeutic hair treatments are not very effective, one modality— although not a panacea— can regrow hair with a certain degree of satisfaction and effectiveness. This restorative hair treatment solution is hair transplantation. Currently, it is the only effective solution that can regrow hair with any degree of certainty. This surgical hair restoration treatment will be described in more detail in a subsequent chapter. However, although hair research has not yet developed a definitive solution to the problem of hair loss, the discoveries made show a promising future. For example, the testosterone/DHT conversion theory and the stem cell research undertaken by Garza and Cotsarelis (2011) provide valuable information that could potentially resolve the hair-loss enigma within the next decade.

8

Scalp Conditions Resulting in Hair Loss

This chapter aims to educate the reader about the existence of other types of hair-loss conditions besides common male pattern baldness or androgenetic alopecia (AGA). Unlike AGA, these other types of hair loss conditions are the result of an underlying local or systemic disease process, such as inflammation or infection of the hair follicle.

As previously mentioned, most non-surgical hair-restoration programs are dispensed to clients based on the premise that the cause of their hair loss is attributed to inadequate scalp circulation. Other hair restoration programs contend that the cause of hair loss is debris that obstructs the hair follicle, which is the consequence of years of exposure to things such as sebum, hairsprays, dirt, and air pollution. These hypothetical causes are based on the idea that poor scalp circulatory blood flow or exposure to obstructive substances create a sand-like fragment that blocks the exit of the hair shafts.

The goal of these hair-loss restoration establishments is to either improve scalp circulation or remove the debris blocking the hair follicle. They try to accomplish these objectives by massaging the scalp with herbal solutions, vasodilators, or any other topical cleansing concoctions. After the scalp has been cleaned, some of these clinics go so far as to dye the vellus hair on the scalp so that the client can better visualize their new hair growth. The individuals who operate these hair-loss restoration establishments disregard other hair-loss theories with more valid scientific foundations as well as ignoring types of hair loss attributed to local or systemic disease processes that should only be treated by specialized licensed physicians.

Evaluating the Area of Hair Loss

The evaluation of an area of baldness should include the following observations:

1) The pattern of hair loss.

- Bi-temporal.
- Frontovertical (involving the frontal area and the vertex).
- Marginal or patchy.

2) The state of the involved area.

- Presence of scarring.
- Absence of scarring.

3) The presence of any abnormality of the hair loss itself.

Classification of the Various Types of Alopecia

Alopecia is a general medical term used for all types of hair loss. It can be localized or diffuse, and the hair loss can be from the scalp or any part of the body. Alopecia is a disorder that affects the hair growth cycle, usually in two ways. The first way is when hair follicles get damaged, which affects the growth of the hair. The second way is when the hair cycle is disturbed and either the growing period (anagen stage) is shortened or the resting period (telogen stage) is lengthened. Alopecias are generally divided into two categories as follows:

- Non-Scarring (Non-Cicatricial) Alopecia.
- Scarring (Cicatricial) Alopecia.

Non-Scarring (Non-Cicatricial) Alopecia.

This type of alopecia is more common than scarring alopecia. Non-scarring alopecia includes male and female pattern hair loss, diffuse pattern alopecia, diffuse unpatterned alopecia, toxic alopecia, myxedema, hypopituitarism, secondary stage syphilis, following pregnancy (postpartum), anagen effluvium (drug intoxication), alopecia areata, trichotillomania, traction alopecia, and telogen effluvium, as well as other less common conditions such as Demodex mite infestations. Sometimes diseases such as secondary syphilis, thyroid disease, and systemic lupus erythematosus can also lead to non-scarring hair loss (see Table 8.1).

Non-scarring hair thinning can also occur with natural aging, which is known as *senescent or senile alopecia.* Senescent alopecia is a unique type of hair loss that displays a very slow rate of progression. The afflicted group is usually older people— those in their seventies and eighties—and is characterized by diffuse thinning of the scalp hair. It is not clear whether senescent alopecia involves androgen hormones. However, it is generally regarded as a form of hair loss that is distinct from common androgenetic alopecia (AGA).

Non-scarring alopecia refers to a situation where the hair shafts fall out, but the hair follicles are still alive. In other words, it refers to hair loss without permanent destruction of the hair follicle. In this category of baldness, we find the following types of hair loss:

- Male pattern hair loss.
- Female pattern hair loss.
- Diffuse pattern alopecia.
- Diffuse unpatterned alopecia.
- Toxic alopecia.
- Myxedema.
- Hypopituitarism.

- Secondary stage syphilis.
- Post-pregnancy (postpartum).
- Anagen effluvium (drug Intoxication).
- Alopecia areata.
- Hypotrichosis simplex of the scalp (HSS).
- Trichotillomania.
- Traction alopecia.
- Telogen effluvium.
- Demodex mite infestation.

Male Pattern Hair Loss.

This type of hair loss is described as common baldness, common pattern baldness, premature baldness, male pattern hair loss (MPHL), and androgenic or androgenetic alopecia (AGA). As previously discussed, the development of common baldness is dependent primarily on hereditary factors, the influence of androgen (hormonal) stimulation, and the normal aging process (senescence). Many researchers contend that the balding process is multifactorial, with scientific evidence suggesting that there is a genetic (hereditary) tendency or predisposition for acquiring the condition.

Dihydrotestosterone (DHT), a metabolite of the male hormone testosterone, is considered destructive to the hair follicles on the scalp. The simple conversion action of testosterone to DHT is a well-accepted theory believed to be at the root of many kinds of hair loss. Androgenetic alopecia, commonly called male or female pattern baldness, was only partially understood up until the last few decades. In fact, for many years, scientists believed that AGA was caused by a predominance of the male sex hormone testosterone that women also have in trace amounts under normal conditions.

While testosterone is at the core of the hair-loss process, the conversion of testosterone to DHT is believed to be the primary causative factor or culprit for balding. Testosterone converts to DHT with the aid of the isoenzyme 5-alpha-reductase (5AR), which is held in the sebaceous (oil) glands of the hair follicle. Currently, at least three variants of 5AR have been identified: types 1, 2, and 3. These isoenzymes produce DHT that can circulate throughout the body where they can exert their effects in organs other than those where the DHT was produced.

The isoenzyme 5AR type 2 is considered the most active type in hair loss. 5AR type 2 can potentially decrease mean serum levels of total DHT by 71%. Similarly, 5AR type 3, discovered in 2007, has been shown in vitro to inhibit DHT conversion at the same potency as 5AR type 2. Conversely, 5AR type 1 is less effective at decreasing DHT levels by a potency of approximately 30% (Uemura et al., 2007). Drugs such as finasteride, which is sold under the brand names Propecia® and Proscar®, and dutasteride, sold under the brand name Avodart®, are all 5-alpha-reductase inhibitors (5ARIs).

These 5AR drugs are clinically used in the treatment of benign prostatic hyperplasia (BPH), which is a condition exacerbated by dihydrotestosterone (Rossi et al., 2011). Finasteride inhibits the function of the isoenzyme types 2 and 3, whereas dutasteride inhibits all three isoenzymes. This makes dutasteride a stronger and more effective 5ARI. Therefore, Avodart® has a more complete suppression of all three of the 5AR isoenzymes. In fact, as previously mentioned, it inhibits isoenzyme types 1 and 2 better than finasteride, resulting in a reduction of DHT levels by 94.7% compared to 70.8% for the older drug, Proscar® (Clark et al., 2004).

Female Pattern Hair Loss.

Currently, it is not clear if androgens (male sex hormones) play a role in female pattern hair loss (FPHL), although they definitively do play a role in male pattern hair loss (MPH). Most women with

FPHL have normal levels of androgen in their bloodstream. Because of this uncertain androgenic relationship, the term FPHL has emerged as the preferred term for androgenetic alopecia in females (Olsen, 2001).

On average, testosterone levels in the adult male are approximately seven to eight times greater than in the adult female. While female ovaries also produce testosterone, the level of testosterone in the females is only 5%-10% of the level in men (Torjessen & Sandnes, 2004). Scientists now believe that the level of DHT binding to receptors in scalp follicles is the problem, not the amount of circulating testosterone.

DHT shrinks hair follicles, making it impossible for healthy hair to survive. The hormonal process of testosterone converting to DHT, which harms hair follicles, occurs in both men and women. Under normal conditions, women have a minute fraction of the testosterone that men have, but even a lower level can cause DHT-triggered hair loss in women. In fact, this last idea was validated by a study undertaken by Urysiak-Czubatka et al. (2014) entitled *"Assessment of the Usefulness of Dihydrotestosterone in the Diagnostics of Patients with Androgenetic Alopecia."* The research team that conducted this study concluded that the most important factors appeared to be the genetically determined sensitivity of the follicles to DHT and their different reactions to androgen concentration.

The majority of women with androgenetic alopecia manifest a diffuse thinning in all areas of the scalp, except it seems that they do not lose the hairline, according to Ludwig and Savin (Figs. 3.1 and 3.3). Conversely, according to Ebling and Rook's female pattern baldness classification, women can also lose their hairline (Fig. 3.2).

Men, on the other hand, rarely have diffuse thinning. Instead, they have more distinct patterns of baldness. Conversely, as mentioned before, androgenetic alopecia in women is due to the action of androgen that is typically present only in small amounts. In women, androgenetic alopecia (AGA) can be caused by a variety of factors tied to the actions of hormones, including ovarian cysts, taking high-androgen indexed birth control pills, pregnancy, and menopause.

Diffuse Pattern Alopecia.

This type of hair loss does not progress to the point of complete hair loss in any particular scalp area. With diffuse pattern alopecia (DPA), the hairline does not recede. However, diffuse thinning will be visible everywhere else except for the safe donor zone, which is the strip of hair on the occipital (back) scalp that is resistant to dihydrotestosterone (DHT). Since DPA has a clear hair-loss pattern and an intact donor area, it is considered safe for surgical hair restoration. While DPA is similar to MPHL, the difference is that the hair is not lost, but rather it thins enough that the underlying scalp becomes visible.

Diffuse Unpatterned Alopecia.

In general, diffuse unpatterned alopecia (DUPA) tends to advance quicker than DPA. It is a type of diffuse hair loss that permeates the entire scalp and is considered untreatable by hair transplantation surgery. The thinning process in DUPA is so extensive that it progresses into the traditional safe donor zone, thereby rendering the hairs in the safe area unreliable for transplantation. DUPA will usually end up in a horseshoe pattern resembling Norwood stage VII; however, this type of hair loss differs from common pattern balding because the horseshoe fringe on the low back and sides of the head will appear thinner.

Toxic Alopecia.

This type of alopecia is usually of a temporary nature and may follow a severe, often febrile illness, such as scarlet fever. Moreover, certain medications, especially thallium, high doses of vitamin A, retinoids, and cancer medications, may also result in hair loss.

Furthermore, toxic alopecia may result from all of the medical conditions described below.

Myxedema.

Myxedema is a condition resulting from hypothyroidism, which is a clinical syndrome characterized by a deficiency or absence of thyroid hormone that slows the body's metabolic processes. It can occur at any age but typically occurs in older children and adults. This condition can be caused by iodine deficiency in the diet, atrophy of the thyroid gland, or excessive use of anti-thyroid drugs. The term "myxedema" refers to the thickened, non-pitting, edematous changes to patients' soft tissue in a markedly hypothyroid state. This condition may result secondary to hypofunction of the anterior pituitary gland and is further complicated by adrenal and gonadal deficiencies.

Hypopituitarism.

Hypopituitarism is a condition characterized by a deficiency of any of the *trophic* hormones secreted by the adenohypophysis, which is another name for the anterior lobe of the pituitary gland. *Trophic* hormones are hormones that stimulate the growth of tissue and organs. In other words, it produces hyperplasia or hypertrophy of the tissue it is stimulating. The term "*trophic*" originates from the ancient Greek word *trophikós,* meaning *"pertaining to food or nourishment."* The adenohypophysis secretes seven different hormones:

- Follicle-stimulating hormone (FSH).
- Luteinizing hormone (LH).
- Prolactin.
- Adrenocorticotropic hormone (ACTH).
- Thyroid-stimulating hormone (TSH).

- Growth-stimulating hormone (GH).
- Melanocyte-stimulating hormone (MSH).

Hypopituitarism can be difficult to detect and may actually be experienced for years before a diagnosis is made. Some of the symptoms and signs of hypopituitarism include hair loss, loss of body hair, fatigue, weight loss, and anemia, to name a few. Since the hair loss is caused by a hormone deficiency or multiple hormone deficiencies, the use of hormone-replacement therapy can promote hair regrowth as the body's hormone levels normalize. Hair restoration surgery, such as follicular unit extraction (FUE) or follicular unit transplant (FUT), might be unnecessary, and the same goes for non-surgical treatment with medications such as Rogaine® or Propecia® (True & Dorin, 2014).

Secondary Stage Syphilis.

Secondary stage syphilis is a venereal disease caused by the microorganism treponema pallidum. This disease has a three-stage infectious process that results in generalized eruption, mucous membrane lesions, and generalized lymphadenopathy, which is a condition characterized by improper function of the lymphatic system. Balding may result from this disease if the infection infiltrates the hair follicle or if the cervical sympathetic nerves become involved in the infectious process.

Post-Pregnancy (postpartum).

During pregnancy, the hair follicles tend to stay within *their* growth phase (*anagen phase*) longer *than* usual. The pregnancy hormones keep those hairs from shedding, which is why pregnant women›s hair looks as lush and thick as the hair of supermodels. Conversely, postpartum (parturition) precipitates the telogen and exogen stages of the hair-growth cycle, which results in a greater amount of hair shedding for approximately three months following the pregnancy.

Therefore, the abnormal hair loss seen after pregnancy is merely a reflection of the altered physiology of the hair-growth cycle that occurred during pregnancy. After normalcy is restored, regeneration of hair growth should return to normal.

Anagen Effluvium (drug intoxication).

Anagen effluvium, or drug intoxication, is extensive hair loss caused by sudden, profound disturbances to the matrix cells of the hair follicles. The matrix is the part of the hair follicle where matrix keratinocytes proliferate to form the hair shaft of growing hair. Melanocytes are also mixed amongst the matrix cells to provide the hair shaft with pigmentation (color).

Rather than shedding, in anagen effluvium, hair loss occurs from the fracturing of the hair shafts at the level of the scalp. Anagen effluvium occurs after any injury to the hair follicle that impairs its mitotic (replication) or metabolic activity (Schwartz, 2015). This type of hair loss is the result of drug intoxication, usually due to the administration of antineoplastic agents (anticancer drugs), such as cisplatinum, cytosine arabinoside, epirubicin amsacrine, cyclophosphamide (Cytoxan®), etoposide (Taxol®), and ifosfamide, among others. All these chemotherapeutic agents are cytotoxic (toxic to the body cells) in nature, causing cessation of the mitotic process (replication of epithelial cells) in the hair bulb, with consequent loss of anagen (growing) hairs. It can also occur from a deficiency or overdose of vitamin A.

Because chemotherapy targets the body's rapidly dividing cancer cells, the body's other rapidly dividing cells, such as hair follicles in the growing (anagen) phase, are also greatly affected. Soon after chemotherapy begins, approximately 90% or more of the hair can fall out while still in the anagen phase. The characteristic finding in anagen effluvium is the tapered fracture of the hair shafts. The hair shaft narrows as a result of damage to the matrix. Eventually, the shaft fractures at the site of narrowing and causes hair loss (Schwartz, 2015; McAndrews-AHLA, 2004).

Radiation therapy is the other major cause of anagen effluvium. The effect of radiotherapy on hair follicles is dose-dependent, similar to the dose-effect relationship with chemotherapy. Topical minoxidil has been shown to shorten the duration of hair loss due to chemotherapy or radiation by approximately 50 days. However, it is still unable to prevent hair loss due to cancer chemotherapy or radiation therapy (Lee, 2016).

Alopecia Areata.

This type of alopecia is characterized by sudden hair loss occurring in individuals who have no apparent skin disorder or systemic disease. According to the National Alopecia Areata Foundation, alopecia areata is considered an autoimmune skin disease resulting in the loss of hair on the scalp and elsewhere on the body (NAAF. org, 2015). It usually starts with one or more small, round, smooth patches on the scalp or beard. Alopecia areata can further be classified as monolocularis, which means just one circular bald patch, or multilocularis, which means more than one round bald patch (Figs. 8.1 and 8.2).

This disorder is highly unpredictable, cyclical in nature, and often manifests itself in childhood, usually before age 20, and can affect both sexes equally. Severity may differ between individuals. For example, some people may experience many small patches of hair loss while others just experience one big round patch. These patches of alopecia may resolve themselves on their own, or the hair loss may never regrow, even with treatment. The etiology (cause) of this disorder remains unknown, but as previously mentioned, current evidence suggests that the cause is an abnormality in the immune system.

Fig. 8.1: Alopecia Areata

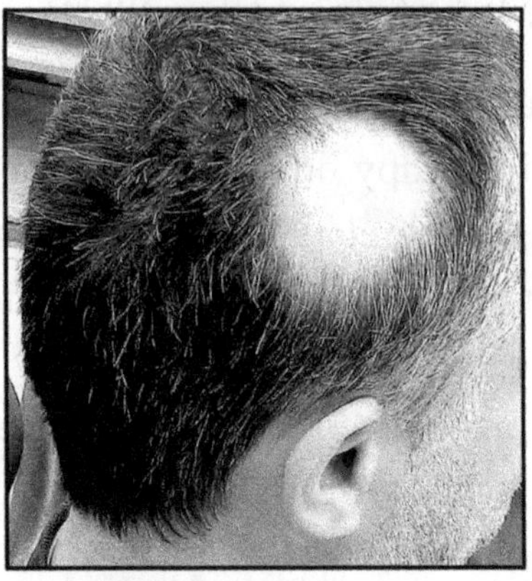

Image Source: Thirunavukkarasye-Raveendran, CC BY 4.0 <https://creativecommons.org/licenses/by/4.0>, via Wikimedia Commons https://commons.wikimedia.org/wiki/File:Alopecia_areata_1.jpg

Fig. 8.2: Alopecia Areata Barbae (Beard)

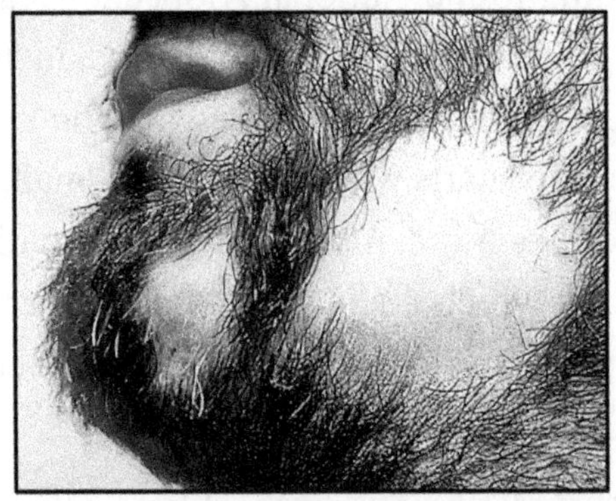

Image Source: http://www.edoj.org.eg/vol009/0901/006/01.htm. An open-access, publication intending to enhance communication between Egyptian dermatologists and the world.

Alopecia areata can progress to include total scalp hair loss, which is called *alopecia totalis,* or it can cause complete body hair loss, which is called *alopecia universalis*. Alopecia totalis is an extreme version of alopecia areata and is one of the worst types of hair loss an individual can contract. The subtypes of alopecia areata are based on the body parts affected and the severity of the hair loss. For example, *alopecia totalis* is the loss of all the hair on the face, scalp, eyebrows, and eyelashes, while *alopecia universalis* is hair loss everywhere on the body.

Fortunately, the good news is that it only affects about one or two individuals per thousand (Fig.8.3). This is an aggressive and frightening form of hair loss:

- A person with alopecia totalis can lose all their scalp hair within a week.
- Alopecia totalis can occur at any time.
- It can be permanent.
- Many different things can trigger it.
- It can run in the family and affect children as well as adults.
- Alopecia totalis is an idiopathic condition, therefore no one knows what causes it.

Fig. 8.3: Alopecia Areata Totalis

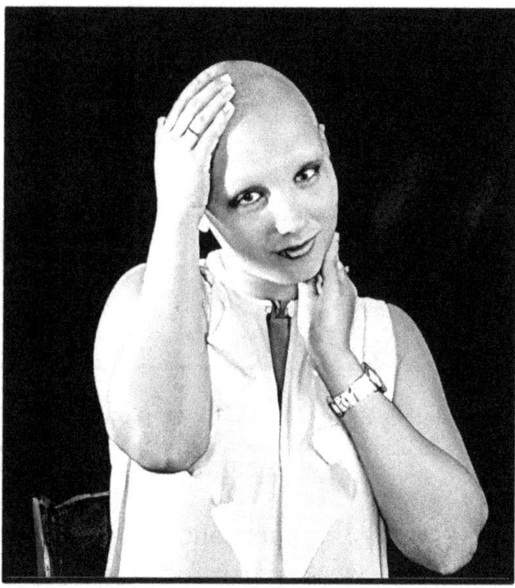

Image Source: http://www.istockphoto.com/photo/female-with-alopecia-gm539334066-96121433

Alopecia universalis is the most extreme and probably the worst version of alopecia areata that an individual can contract. It is considered the most aggressive form of hair loss. As its name implies, it is total hair loss from everywhere on the body, not just the scalp (Fig.8.4). Hair loss can be experienced by the afflicted from nose to toes; in essence, complete baldness develops across the entire body, including the arms, legs, chest, and pubic hair. In fact, losing the hair from the nose and ears can make the afflicted person more susceptible to germs, bugs, and dust, which can then enter the body more easily. In alopecia universalis, just like in alopecia areata and alopecia totalis, the hair can be lost very quickly, causing total loss of scalp hair within a week. Twenty percent of individuals who contract alopecia areata go on to develop the more aggressive form of alopecia universalis.

Fig. 8.4: Alopecia Areata Universalis

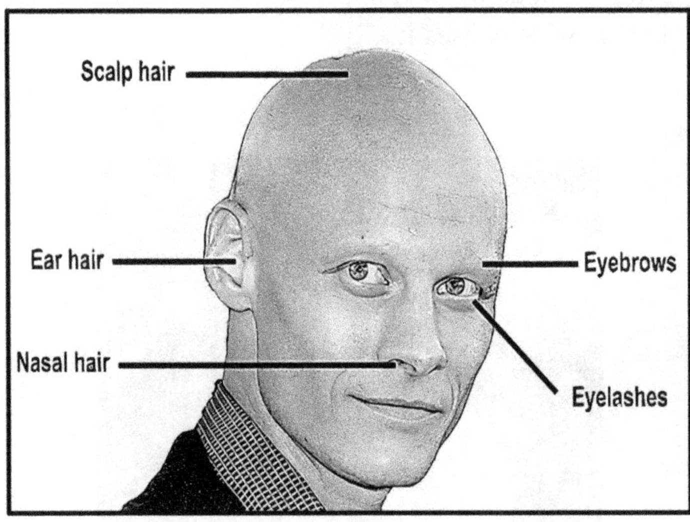

Image Source: Georges Biard [CC BY-SA 3.0 (http://creativecommons.org/licenses/by-sa/3.0)], via Wikimedia Commons https://commons.wikimedia.org/wiki/File%3ATomas_Lemarquis_Deauville_2013.jpg

The good news regarding this condition is that no matter how widespread the hair loss is, most hair follicles remain alive and are ready to resume normal hair production whenever they receive the appropriate signal (naaf.org, 2015). In fact, as stated above, in all cases, hair regrowth may occur even without treatment and even after existing for many years. However, the prognosis of alopecia areata is considered poor if the hair loss is extensive or begins in childhood. If it appears in adulthood and is confined only to a few areas of the scalp, it is often reversible within a few months, though the condition may recur.

Hypotrichosis Simplex of the Scalp (HSS).

Hypotrichosis simplex of the Scalp (HSS) is a rare form of hereditary hair loss without other abnormalities. It is an autosomal dominant form of isolated alopecia, causing almost complete scalp hair loss, with onset in childhood. In hypotrichosis, sparse hair results from a hair regeneration defect caused by impairment in hair cycling and anchoring of the hair shaft in the skin (Ahmed, Almohanna, Griggs, and Tosti, 2019). Toribio and Quinones first described hypotrichosis simplex of the scalp (HSS) in 1974. Affected individuals typically show normal hair at birth but experience hair loss and thinning of the hair shaft that starts during early childhood and progresses with age. Hypotrichosis simplex can be divided into two forms:

- Scalp-limited in which only the scalp hair is affected.
- Generalized in which all body hair is affected.

HSS can be inherited either as an autosomal dominant or autosomal recessive trait. Autosomal dominant means that a single copy of the disease-associated mutation is enough to cause the disease. A child of a person affected by an autosomal dominant condition has a 50% chance of being affected by that condition by inheriting a dominant allele. An allele is one of two or more versions of DNA sequence at a given genomic location (Genome.gov, 2022). If it is a 50/50 ratio between men and women, the disorder is autosomal, which means that one of the parents must have the disorder. Conversely, in a recessive disorder, two copies of the mutated gene are required (one from each parent) to cause the disorder. The available treatment for this type of alopecia, unfortunately, is unsatisfactory. However, topical minoxidil can improve the hair density and texture. But for most patients wearing a wig is the best option (Ahmed, Almohanna, Griggs, and Tosti, 2019).

Although the manifestation of hair loss in alopecia universalis (AU) and alopecia totalis (AT) appears to have similarities to the hair loss caused by hypotrichosis simplex of the scalp (HSS), there is no connection between these conditions. Alopecia universalis and alopecia totalis are a heterogeneous group of disorders with complete or almost complete loss of scalp and body hair. The most frequent cause of AU and AT is alopecia areata (AA), an autoimmune condition. Notwithstanding Alopecia Universalis and Alopecia Totalis autoimmune connection, genetic disorders must be considered, especially in pediatric cases (Zlotogorski, Panteleyev, Aita, and Christiano, 2002).

Anterolateral Leg Alopecia (loss of leg hair).

A concern to many men and women is the unexplained loss of hair from the legs and other body areas. It is not only the scalp that men and women can expect to experience hair loss issues. Other areas, such as hair loss from the arms, chest, pubic area, and armpits, can also be affected. These conditions are more common than people think and can happen for many reasons. This type of hair loss can be independent of any connection to the autoimmune alopecia's areata. It could simply be caused by senescence (aging process). Hair loss in the legs should not be disregarded by the afflicted since it can be a warning sign of a more significant issue, and it is crucial to get to the root of the problem.

Loss of leg hair or Anterolateral leg alopecia, as medically called, was first described in the 1920s, yet the cause of this hair loss pattern remains to be elucidated or explained. Some of the reasons attributed to leg hair loss are leg crossing, tight trouser rubbing, and friction have all been suggested as contributing to this condition. However, a causal relationship has yet to be confirmed by any studies (Siah

& Harries, 2014). Some of the potential contributing conditions causing leg anterolateral hair loss could be due to a more serious underlying condition like the following:

- Peripheral artery disease (PAD).
- Diabetes, which is a risk factor for PAD.
- Chronic rashes from eczema, psoriasis, or other skin conditions.
- Thyroid conditions, especially hypothyroidism.
- Fungal infections.
- Hair follicle infections.
- Severe folliculitis.
- Hormone changes, such as those during pregnancy and menopause.
- Pituitary gland disorders.
- Nutrition deficiencies, such as iron, zinc, and vitamin D.
- Steroid use.
- High levels of stress.
- Wearing tight pants or socks.
- Prescription medications, such as blood thinners.
- A recent illness or major surgery.

Anterolateral leg alopecia is very common in middle-aged and older men but may also occur in women. A previous study estimates the prevalence of anterolateral leg alopecia among males to be as high as 35% (Siah & Harries, 2014). It often presents as symmetrical, sharply demarcated hair loss confined to the anterior and lateral aspects of both legs. This pattern of hair loss is widespread yet hardly described in the medical literature.

Anterolateral leg alopecia is frequently referred to as *peroneal alopecia* as the hair loss occurs in the distribution of the superficial branch of the common peroneal nerve. This distinctive pattern of hair loss is confined to the lower legs and predominantly occurs in male patients. As previously mentioned, the condition is a common, under-recognized hair loss condition with surprisingly limited available information on cause, pathogenesis, course, and treatment.

Trichotillomania.

Another hair-loss condition that may be hard to differentiate from alopecia Areata is the impulse control disorder of trichotillomania, also known as *trichotillosis or hair-pulling disorder.* This condition is a compulsive urge to pull out one's own hair, leading to noticeable hair loss, distress, and social or functional impairment (Fig.8.5). Trichotillomania is one of a group of behaviors known as *"body-focused repetitive behaviors"* (BFRBs), which are self-grooming behaviors in which individuals pull, pick, scrape, or bite their own hair, skin, or nails, resulting in damage to the body.

Fig. 8.5: Result of Trichotillomania

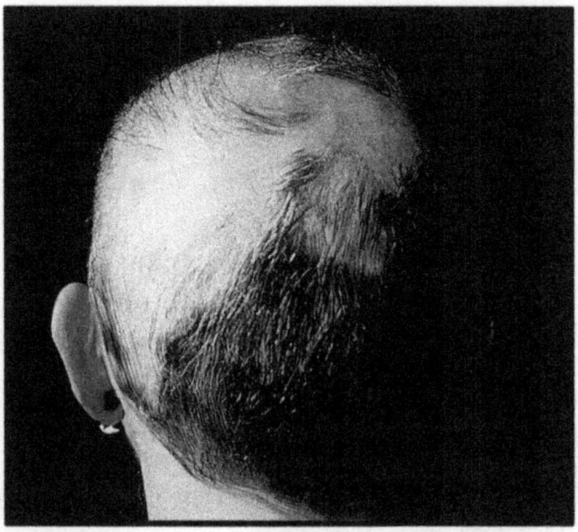

Image Source: By Robodoc (original uploader) (de. wikimedia) [Public domain], via Wikimedia Commons https://commons.wikimedia.org/wiki/File%3ATrichotillomania_1.jpg

If the compulsion to pull out hair also leads to eating one's own hair, the condition is called *trichophagia, or trichotillomania* with gastric trichobezoar. *Bezoars* are collections or concretions of indigestible foreign material in the gastrointestinal tract. T*richophagia*, also called Rapunzel syndrome, is a very dangerous condition that needs to be treated with some urgency. According to Oana-Marginean et al. (2021), Rapunzel syndrome is a rare condition seen in adolescents or young females with psychiatric disorders consisting of a gastric trichobezoar. The delays in diagnosing this condition are common because it is usually asymptomatic in its early stages.

Hair is not digestible in the stomach; thus, it can build up into a hairball (trichobezoar). This hairball can severely irritate the stomach lining, leading to severe ulceration. It is possible to die from trichophagia. Treating trichotillomania is difficult, and therapists can probably help more than dermatologists (Shetty et al., 2013; O'Sullivan et al., 1998; AHLA.org, n.d.).

Trichotillomania is classified as an impulse-control disorder by the *Diagnostic and Statistical Manual of Mental Disorders (DSM)*, published by the American Psychiatric Association. This impulse-control disorder is often chronic and difficult to treat. Trichotillomania is usually confined to one or two sites but can involve multiple locations. The scalp is the most common pulling site, followed by the eyebrows, eyelashes, face, arms, and legs. Some less common areas include the pubic area, underarms, beard, and chest.

Traction Alopecia.

Traction alopecia and trichotillomania are the same disorders in terms of the mechanical action that causes hair loss. In both conditions, the hair is plucked out of the skin, leaving clear, bald patches or diffuse areas of thinning hair. However, traction alopecia is a form of acquired hair loss that results from prolonged or repetitive tension on the scalp hair. Traction alopecia was first described in 1907 in subjects from Greenland who developed hair loss along the hairline due to prolonged wearing of tight ponytails (Dermnetnz.

org, n.d.). The causes of traction alopecia may include pulling the hair into a tight ponytail, wearing tight headbands, wearing certain hairstyles (e.g., braids, cornrow, pigtails, using tight-hair rollers), and anything else that pulls on the roots of the hair (Figs. 8.6 and 8.7).

Fig. 8.6: Results of Traction Alopecia (photo 1)

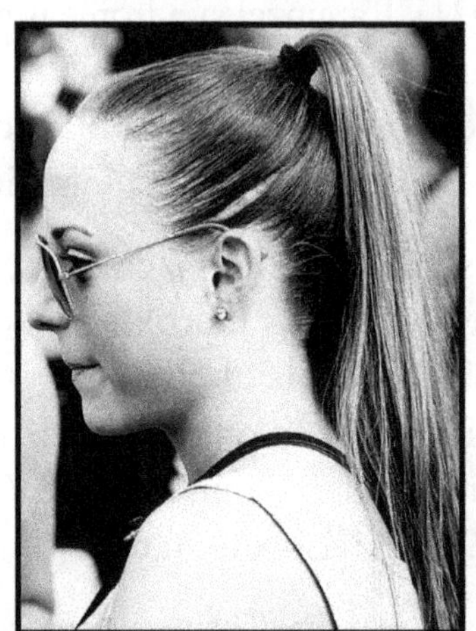

Image Source: By Deortiz from Schweiz, CC BY 2.0 <https://creativecommons.org/licenses/by/2.0>, via Wikimedia Commons https://upload.wikimedia.org/wikipedia/commons/thumb/c/c0/Gnome-emblem-web.svg/100px-Gnome-emblem-

Fig. 8.7: Results of Traction Alopecia (photo 2)

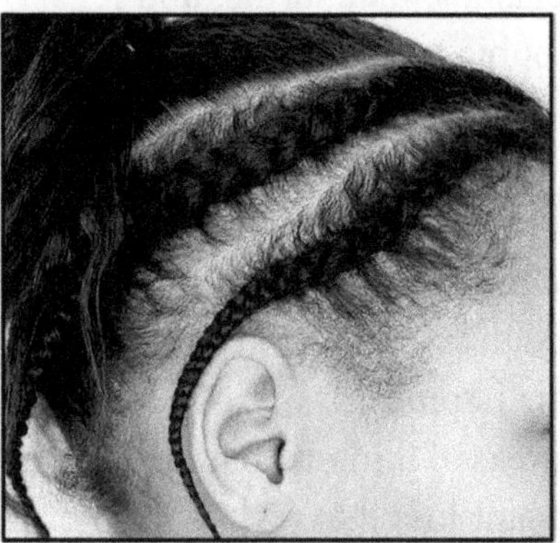

Image Source: http://www.independent.co.uk/life-style/health-and-families/features/traction-alopecia-the-hairstyles-which-can-cause-hair-loss-10516418.html

If the hair traction continues for a prolonged period and the same hair is repeatedly pulled out, then the hair follicles in the area continually subjected to the mechanical pulling action can become so damaged that they stop growing hair permanently.

Telogen Effluvium.

Telogen effluvium is another condition leading to hair loss that results from exposure to different kinds of stressful situations. This hair loss condition was observed by Lynfield (1960) and Kligman (1961), who reported that this type of alopecia occurs following exposure to various kinds of stress, such as:

- Fever.
- Drastic weight loss.
- Surgical operation.
- Pregnancy.
- Emotional disturbances.

It appears that following exposure to some degree of stress, a large number of hair follicles are precipitated into the telogen stage (Fig. 8.8). It is known that approximately 10%-15% of the hair on a person's scalp is in this telogen (resting) stage; however, once a person is exposed to stress, this figure can increase to 30%-50%. Hair loss occurs approximately within 6-16 weeks following exposure to stress. This condition is temporary, and regrowth of the lost hair is usually complete within six weeks (American Academy of Dermatology, n.d.).

Fig. 8.8: A patient stricken by telogen effluvium (TE)

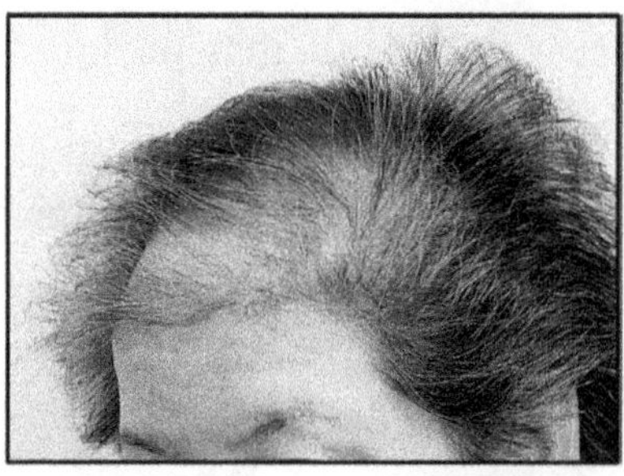

Image Source: By Aisclinic-http://aisclinic.in-tellogen-effluvium_1.jpg. (Use with Permission).

Therefore, telogen effluvium (TE) is a phenomenon in which a person sheds large amounts of hair daily. TE can occur following pregnancy, major surgery, drastic weight loss, fever, or when subjected to any form of extreme stress. This excessive hair loss can usually be experienced when shampooing, styling, or brushing the hair. Telogen effluvium can also be a side effect of a large number of medications (drug-induced hair loss), including antidepressants, beta-blockers, anticoagulants, retinol (vitamin A) and its derivatives, interferons, non-steroidal anti-inflammatory drugs, and antihyperlipidemic drugs (Tosi, Misciali, Piraccini, Peluso & Bardazzi, 1994).

During telogen effluvium, hair shifts faster than normal from the growing (anagen) phase to the resting (telogen) phase before moving quickly into the shedding (exogen) phase. The shed hairs can be recognized as telogen hairs by visualizing a small bulb of keratin on the root end (Fig.8.9).

Fig. 8.9: Telogen Hair Image

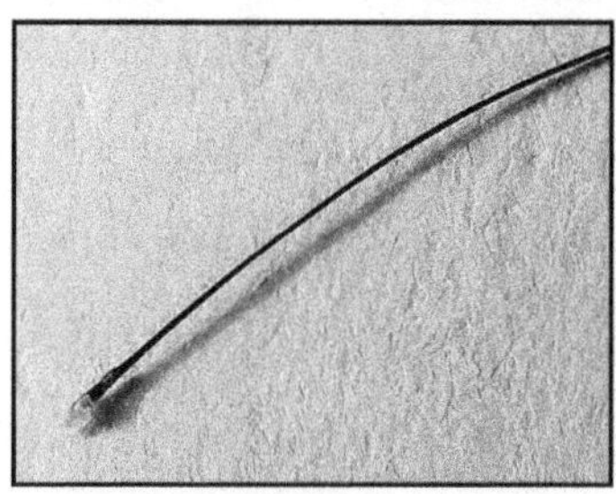

Image Source: My Long Hair Journey by My Long Hair Journey is licensed under a Creative Commons Attribution-NoDerivs 2.0 UK: England & Wales License.

Women with telogen effluvium typically notice hair loss six weeks to three months after a stressful event. At its peak, the individual may lose handfuls of hair. There are no tests for telogen effluvium; however, your physician may ask you about recent life events and look for small, club-shaped bulbs on the roots of the fallen hair (Fig. 8.9). These bulbs indicate that the hair has gone through a complete growth cycle, suggesting that the cycle may have sped up due to stress.

In some cases, such as pregnancy or major surgery, the patient may have to bide their time until the hair loss slows down. If medication is the culprit, then a discussion with the doctor is warranted to possibly lower the dosage of a drug or switch drugs. If the hair loss is stress-related, the patient will have to do their best to relax and reduce the level of anxiety.

The Hair Pull or Tug Test.

It is a well-accepted fact that hair loss is a common phenomenon that results in the shedding of approximately 50 to 150 telogen hairs per day in a healthy adult (Milner et al., 2002; Cheng & Bayliss, 2008; Stenn, 2005). However, if a person experiences a severe increase in telogen hair loss or the presence of anagen hair loss, then this condition is often considered pathological (O'Donnell, Sperling & James, 1992). To diagnose if there is an actual hair loss condition a noninvasive clinical examination, such as a ***hair pull or tug test*** can be used. This simple test measures the severity of hair loss.

To perform a hair pull test, the physician selects 40 to 60 hairs and holds the bundle close to the scalp between the thumb, index finger, and long finger (Fig. 8.10). The clinician then firmly pulls on the bundle of hairs using slow traction as the fingers slide down the hair shaft, avoiding a fast and forceful tug. The hair pulls are performed at the vertex (crown), two parietal areas, and the occipital (back of the head) area of the scalp. Subsequently, the pulled hairs are counted. Any broken hairs that were extracted from the bundle during the pull maneuver are discarded. If more than 10% of the hairs in each bundle are removed from a scalp area, the hair pull test is considered positive. If six or more strands fall out, the patient have what is known as active hair loss. If fewer than 10% are removed, then the hair loss is attributed to normal shedding.

Fig. 8.10: Hair Pull or Tug Test

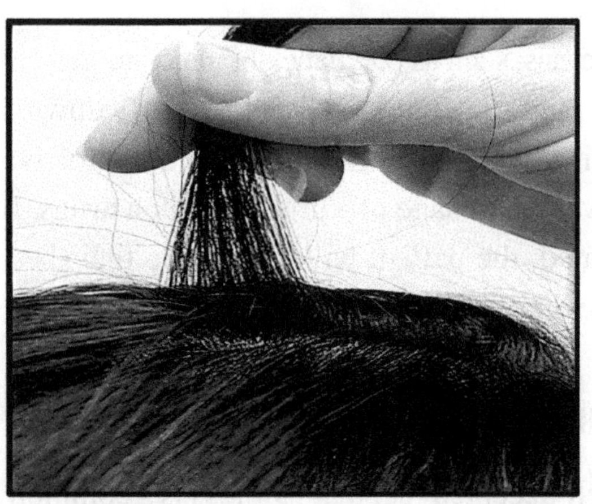

Image Source: https://blabplus.freshdesk.com/support/solutions/articles/14000004450-easy-hair-strength-test

If a pull or tug test is positive in more than one of the evaluated scalp region, the physician can consider the existence of *telogen effluvium* or *anagen* effluvium. In other hair loss disorders such as alopecia areata (AA), the hair pull test might only be positive in the affected area. The hair pull test is ideally used for monitoring the advancing edge of alopecia areata (AA), acute cases of telogen effluvium, anagen effluvium, loose anagen syndrome, androgenetic alopecia (AGA), and scarring alopecia. Patients with scarring alopecia such as Lichen planopilaris, Idiopathic Pseudopelade of Brocq, Discoid Lupus Erythematosus can all trigger increased shedding and thus can also have a positive pull test.

The hair pull test is most effective when the patient has a severe condition and is in the acute phases of hair loss. It is not advisable to use the hair pull test for critical decisions when the patient has a more severe condition (e.g., chronic telogen effluvium) because of the test's low sensitivity and high interobserver variability. Notwithstanding the limitations, the hair pull test is used even though the test lacks validation, strict pretest guidelines, and hair texture considerations. Therefore, a positive pull test is not definitive for any given diagnosis but certainly indicates that something is not quite right with how the patient is losing hair (McDonald et al., 2017).

Human Demodex Mite Infestation.

Androgenetic alopecia (AGA) is one of the most common dermatologic disorders with a multifactorial etiology. Inflammatory activators, such as Demodex mite infestation, may play a role in the pathogenesis of some cases of androgenetic alopecia that are unresponsive to standard treatments such as minoxidil and finasteride (Zari et al., 2008). Demodex is the name given to microscopic parasitic mites that are normal inhabitants of human facial skin and hair follicles. In humans, the Demodex mite is primarily found on facial skin, especially on the forehead, cheeks, sides of the nose, eyelashes, external ear canals, and hair follicles; however, Demodex can also be found anywhere on the human body.

Mites are relatives of ticks, spiders, scorpions, and other arachnids. Over 48,000 species have been described, and approximately 65 of them belong to the genus Demodex. However, only two of those live on the human face: *Demodex folliculorum* and Demodex *brevis* (MacKenzie, 2012). D. folliculorum resides in hair follicles, whereas D. brevis survives in the sebaceous glands adjacent to hair follicles. These two species are evolution's special gift to humans; in fact, they strictly live on humans. Demodex mites are acquired shortly after birth and are considered normal skin fauna that increases in number as people age. A 2014 study of Demodex mites found that 100% of people 18 years old and older had mite DNA on their faces, suggesting that the mites are universal inhabitants of adult humans (Thoemmes, 2014).

D. Folliculorum mites are 0.3-0.4 millimeters long, while D. brevis mites are 0.15-0.2 millimeters. Their size and translucency make them invisible to the naked eye; however, their structures are clearly visible under the microscope. Both the D. folliculorum and D. brevis species are sausage-shaped, with eight stubby legs (called paulus) clustered in the front third of their structure (Fig. 8.11). These mites can move at a rate of 8 to16 millimeters per hour, and this movement mainly occurs during the night, as bright light causes the mite to recede back into the follicle (Ngan, 2005).

Fig. 8.11: Image of Demodex brevis and Demodex folliculorum Mites

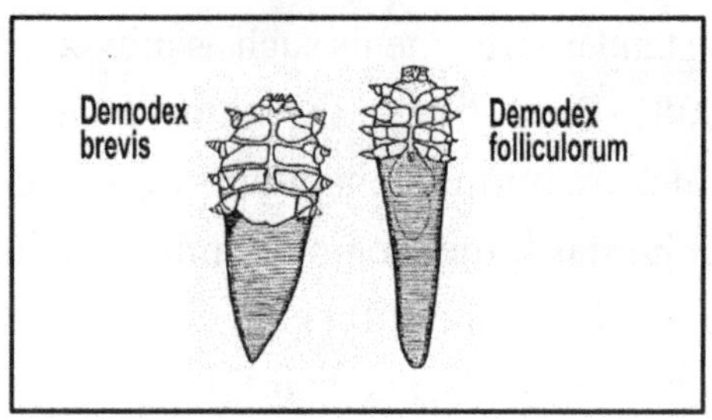

Image Source: By Alan R Walker (talk) 09:16, 28 January 2014 (UTC)] (Own work) [CC BY-SA 3.0 (http://creativecommons.org/licenses/by-sa/3.0)], via Wikimedia Commons

Demodex folliculorum is the bigger of the two species. It was discovered independently in 1841 by two scientists; however, it was only properly described by German dermatologist Dr. Gustav Simon in 1842. While researching acne spots under a microscope, Dr. Simon noticed a *"worm-like animal"* with a head and legs (Fig.8.10). Subsequently, in 1843, English biologist, comparative anatomist, and paleontologist Richard Owen gave the mite the name "Demodex," which is derived from the Greek words *demo,* meaning lard, and *dex,* meaning boring worm. Thus, it is a worm that bores into fat (Young, 2012). Interestingly, Richard Owen was also responsible for coining the term *"dinosaur."*

Demodex mites can occasionally cause a condition called demodicosis, which can have a pathogenic role, but only when there is a high density of mites and when there is an immune system imbalance. However, it is important to be cognizant that even though a Demodex mite infestation usually remains asymptomatic, it could nonetheless be a causative agent for many dermatological conditions, such as acne and rosacea (Rather & Hassan, 2014).

Demodex mites may be best understood in the context of the human microbiome, which essentially describes the ecological community of microorganisms that live within and on the human body. The term microbiome was coined by the late American molecular biologist Professor Joshua Lederberg, who was one of three winners of the Nobel Prize for physiology or medicine in 1958 (Nobelprize.org, N.D.). It is essential to understand that, contrary to popular perception, humans are not biologically self-sufficient organisms whose immune systems must fight off an invasion by microbes and parasites to avoid disease. It is just the opposite; the human body cannot survive without these microorganisms. In fact, it has been common knowledge ever since Antonie Philips van Leeuwenhoek invented the microscope in the seventeenth century that the human body has a population of passengers living on the skin, scalp, and inside the body.

Demodex mites are a natural part of this human microbiome, where they may serve a useful function by feeding on dead skin cells, oils, hormones, and fluids around the follicle to help rid the face of waste (Fig. 8.12). In fact, dead human skin cells are the largest component of household dust, and, just like dust mites, Demodex folliculorum may be part of a natural cleaning system. However, the concern with Demodex mites arises when the infestation is too significant for the body's ability to keep the mites in check. Since the D. folliculorum live in or near the pilosebaceous units, it is quite possible that when something causes the mites to reproduce at a higher rate, they can break out of the hair follicle and may cause acne, hair loss, and other skin conditions.

Fig. 8.12: Demodex folliculorum and Demodex brevis within the Hair Follicle

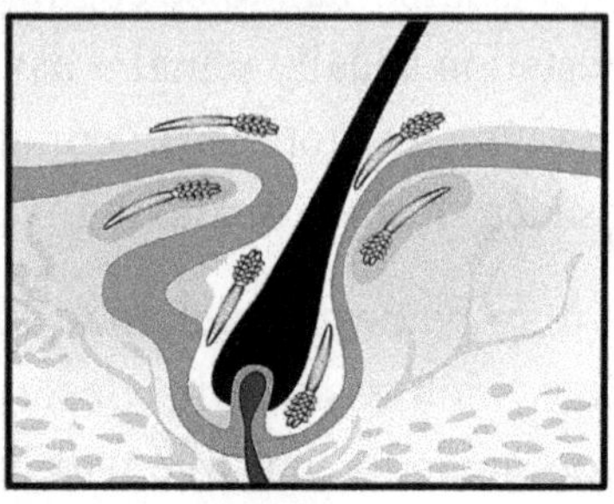

Image Source: http://onliaolah.blogspot.com/2016/12/freerm634.html; https://www.fiuxy.co/informacion/2862900-el-fiel-companero-del-hombre.html. Creative Commons Attribution 4.0 International Public License.

According to Professor Jerry Butler of the University of Florida, under normal conditions, mites produce an antigen when they feed in a hair follicle; subsequently, the human body makes antibodies against the mites, thereby keeping the mites' reproductive ability low and in balance. In fact, Butler further contends that the mites are needed to make the antigen that stimulates the body into making protective antibodies to keep their population under control. Thus, under normal conditions, Demodex mites live harmlessly in the hair and on the skin, feeding on oils, hormones, and dead skin cells. In fact, for most people, Demodex mites live in balance with their human host. However, if there is an overpopulation of mites, they can cause problems like thinning hair, acne, rosacea, and other skin conditions.

Scarring (Cicatricial) Alopecia

Scarring alopecia refers to a diverse group of rare disorders that destroy the hair follicle. It follows scar tissue formation resulting from an infective or inflammatory process and tissue destruction.

The hair follicles are replaced with scar tissue, causing permanent hair loss. Scarring alopecia has two forms. They are classified as either primary or secondary:

- **Primary Scarring Alopecia.**

In primary scarring alopecia, the hair follicle is the affected target of the destructive inflammatory process. Primary scarring alopecia is further classified by the type of inflammatory cells that destroy the hair follicle during the active stage of the disease. For example, the inflammation may predominantly involve lymphocytes, neutrophils, or mixed inflammatory cells, which means that sometimes the process shifts between the two kinds of cells.

- **Secondary Scarring Alopecia.**

In the secondary form of scarring alopecia, the destruction of the hair follicle is incidental to a non-follicle-directed process or external injury. In other words, the hair follicle is an innocent bystander, destroyed by another cause. This cause can be a severe infection, burn, tumor, or radiation.

For injuries, such as burns, physical trauma, and X-ray atrophy (radiation therapy), the cause of scarring is usually apparent. If hair loss results from scar tissue formation resulting from infection, inflammation, or tissue destruction, the prognosis for hair growth is extremely poor.

The cause of the various scarring alopecias is poorly understood. What it is known is that scarring alopecias are not contagious, and they always involve inflammation directed at the upper part of the hair follicle where the stem cells and sebaceous gland (oil gland) are located. However, if the stem cells and sebaceous gland are destroyed, there is no possibility that the hair follicle can be regenerated again, thus resulting in permanent hair loss. Scarring alopecia occurs worldwide in otherwise healthy men and women. It affects all ages but is not common in children (C.A.R.F.org, 2016).

Scarring alopecia usually affects only one family member. However, one exception is central centrifugal cicatricial alopecia (CCCA), which is also referred to as: *hot comb alopecia, follicular degeneration syndrome, pseudopelade in African Americans, and central elliptical pseudopelade in Caucasians.* The cause (etiology) of CCCA appears to be multifactorial, and the condition occurs in all races. Additionally, in this CCCA category, we also find *cicatricial pattern hair loss (CPHL).* CPHL is a CCCA pattern that can be confusing because it can potentially mimic androgenetic alopecia; therefore, it can be difficult to diagnose (Rashid & Thomas, 2010; Blattner et al., 2013).

CCCA is a type of alopecia that commonly occurs in women of African ancestry and may appear in more than one family member. It was first noticed in the 1950s, and subsequently, a study on hot comb alopecia was conducted by LoPresti, Papa, and Kligman in 1968. The occurrence of this type of alopecia was the result of the application of petrolatum, followed by a stove-heated iron comb. The original theory was that the hot petrolatum would travel down to the hair root, burn the follicle, and after repetitive injury, scarring would result (LoPresti et al., 1968; Whiting & Olsen, 2008).

Diagnosing Scarring Alopecia.

The initial step in diagnosing scarring alopecia is to perform a scalp biopsy. The objective of a scalp biopsy is to identify the type of inflammation present, the location and amount of inflammation, and any other pertinent changes in the scalp. Clinical evaluation of the scalp is also essential. For example, symptoms of itching, burning, pain, or tenderness usually signal ongoing activity. Signs of scalp inflammation include redness, scaling, and pustules, which are small bumps on the skin that contain fluid or pus. However, in some cases, there are few symptoms or signs, and only the scalp biopsy demonstrates the active inflammation. A hair pull or tug test could also be helpful to gather additional information. All these findings are necessary to diagnose the type of scarring alopecia, determine the degree of activity, and select the proper kind of therapy.

Other conditions that can result in scarring alopecia are:

- Chronic, deep, bacterial infection.
- Fungal infections.
- Deep factitial (self-induced or artificial) ulcers.
- Granuloma.

Granuloma is a medical condition characterized by a non-cancerous inflammation in the tissue. A granuloma is a tiny cluster of white blood cells and other tissue that can be found in the lungs, head, skin, or other parts of the body. Most granulomas develop as the result of infections, inflammation, irritants, or foreign objects. They seem to trigger a defensive mechanism when the immune system attempts to *"wall off"* substances it perceives as foreign invaders that it cannot eliminate or destroy. Granulomas are often found incidentally on a chest X-ray performed for some other reason.

Some granulomatous conditions are:

- **Sarcoidosis**

  This is a disease of unknown cause that leads to inflammation in any organ in the body, and it does not go away. Instead, some of the immune system cells cluster to form lumps called granulomas in various body organs. These granulomas may change the normal structure and possibly the function of the affected organ(s).

- **Syphilitic Gummas**

  A gumma is a soft, tumor-like growth of the tissues (granuloma) that occurs in people with syphilis. A gumma is caused by the bacteria that cause syphilis. It appears during late-stage tertiary syphilis.

- **Tinea Capitis**

Tinea capitis (TC) is a rash caused by a fungal infection of the scalp. TC usually causes itchy, scaly, bald patches on the scalp. This condition is also called Ringworm because of its circular appearance, although no worm is involved. Ringworm of the scalp is a contagious infection.

Scarring Alopecia Conditions

Table 8.1 shows a variety of systemic and local diseases that can result in varying degrees of alopecia. Furthermore, it describes the onset, course, and nature of the hair loss of all the conditions previously discussed as well as several others. A detailed explanation of all these scarring (cicatricial) diseases that can result in alopecia is beyond the scope and intent of this book. However, sufficient information is provided to the reader to demonstrate the numerous scalp conditions that can result in varying degrees of hair loss other than common pattern hair loss or androgenetic alopecia.

Table 8.1:

Systemic and local diseases that can result in varying degrees of alopecia (hair loss)

Condition	Onset	Course	Nature of Hair Loss
Acrodermatitis Enteropathica Rare childhood disease that is genetically determined, due to zinc deficiency. May be fatal if untreated.	Usually insidious between 3 weeks and 18 months of age.	Intermittent and progressive	Diffuse alopecia of scalp. Eyebrows and eyelashes also involved.

Alopecia Areata Patchy type baldness of unknown cause.	Sudden	Spontaneous recovery usual	Circumscribed. 2 cm to 3 cm patches may enlarge or coalesce. Scalp most commonly involved (occasionally beard or eyebrows). Total loss of scalp or body hair may occur.
Chronic Discoid Lupus Erythematosus A benign skin inflammation characterized by reddish, well-defined scales. Leaves atrophic scars.	Gradual	Variable Can cause permanent Scarring alopecia	Usually patchy involvement of scalp.
Congenital Ectodermal Defect A defect of the outer layer of cell in a developing embryo.	Congenital	Permanent absence of hair in affected areas	Incomplete alopecia. Scalp, eyebrows, beard, and other body hair may be affected.
Dermolytic Bullous Dermatoses A rare, destructive disease of the skin in which inflammation is not necessarily a feature.	Variable. Inherited forms may be present at birth.	Variable with permanent scarring	Cicatricial alopecia in patchy or diffuse pattern.
Drugs Especially anti-cancer drugs that are toxic to cell function.	Variable with drug	Usually reversible	Generalized

Exfoliative Dermatitis Excessive scaling of tissue due to chronic inflammation of the skin.	Variable	Regrowth of hair usual	Mild to moderate. Generalized.
Graves' Disease Exophthalmia Goiter	Usually insidious	Regrowth of hair with treatment.	Diffuse alopecia of the scalp. Temporal hairline recession in some females.
Hypoparathyroidism Insufficient secretion of the parathyroid glands.	Alopecia frequently follows 1 to 3 weeks after titanic episode.	Alopecia usually responds to therapy with secondary forms HPT. Rarely responds with idiopathic forms HPT.	Patchy or complete loss of scalp hair. Scant axillary and pubic hair idiopathic form (idiopathic form).
Hypopituitarism A condition resulting from diminished secretion of pituitary hormones, especially those of the anterior lobe.	Insidious	Partial regrowth with treatment.	Diffuse alopecia of scalp usual. Loss of axillary and pubic hair may occur.
Hypothyroidism A condition due to deficiency of the thyroid secretion resulting in a lowered basal metabolism.	Insidious	Regrowth of hair with treatment.	Patchy alopecia and diffuse thinning of scalp hair. Loss of outer third or eyebrows. Decrease beard and axillary hair.
Iron Deficiency A lack of iron in the Body.	Alopecia may occur with chronic deficiency or following acute blood loss.	Regrowth of hair in 1 to 15 months. May recur with subsequent pregnancies.	Alopecia is most prominent over anterior third of scalp. Diffuse alopecia may occur.

Leprosy (Hansen's Disease) A chronic infectious disease of the skin, tissues, or nerves characterized by ulcers, white scaly scabs, deformity, and wasting of body parts.	Gradual	Hair loss may be reversible with therapy.	Loss of outer third of eyebrows and patchy loss of beard (tuberculoid type). Loss of eyelashes, eyebrows and later, scalp and body hair with (lepromatous type).
Lichen Planus Inflammatory skin disease of many varieties.	Alopecia may precede other lesions.	May be permanent, depending on degree of atrophy.	Irregularly shaped bald patches, with or without scarring (most common with Lichen Planopilaris or atrophic forms of lichen planus).
Mycosis Fungoides A type of lymphoma that is malignant in nature and originates in the reticuloendothelial cells of the skin. It leads to eczematous patches upon scalp.	Usually insidious between 3 weeks and 18 months of age	Intermittent and progressive	Diffuse alopecia of the scalp. Eyebrows and eyelashes also involved.
Myotonic Dystrophy A hereditary disease characterized by muscular wasting, myotonia and cataract.	Early age	Progressive	Frontal alopecia of scalp.
Pregnancy The condition of carrying a developing embryo in the uterus.	Alopecia becomes evident 4 to 20 weeks postpartum.	Regrowth of hair in 1-15 months; may recur with subsequent pregnancies.	Alopecia is most prominent over anterior third of scalp; diffuse alopecia may occur.
Pseudopelade of Brocq It's also known as Alopecia cicatrisata or scarring alopecia.	Usually insidious	Slowly progressive and permanent.	Scarring alopecia in patches up to 1 cm in diameter. Occurs most commonly at vertex of scalp.

Radiation Treatment with a radioactive substance.	Approximately 2 weeks after the radioactive substance application.	Variable with radiation dose.	Hair loss in areas subject to radiation.
Sarcoidosis A chronic granulomatous disease of unknown cause characterized by the formation of tubercle like lesions of the skin, lymph nodes, lungs, and bone marrow.	Gradual	Alopecia is permanent with cutaneous atrophy and scarring.	Patchy alopecia of scalp, often beginning at hair margin.
Secondary Syphilis A chronic infectious venereal disease characterized by lesions, which may involve any organ or tissue.	Alopecia may be first sign of infection.	Hair loss usually not permanent.	Moth-eaten (MEA) alopecia may affect scalp, eyebrows, eyelashes, and body hair.
Systemic Lupus Erythematosus A chronic and usually fatal systemic disease characterized by pathological changes of the body collagen.	Alopecia may precede exacerbation of disease in some.	Regrowth of hair during remission.	Diffuse alopecia of scalp in 20-40%. Patchy alopecia in 3-10%.
Systemic Sclerosis A hardening or induration of an organ or tissue, especially due to excessive growth of fibrous tissue.	Usually insidious	Variable	Partial alopecia or patches of morphea (i.e., localized scleroderma) of the scalp may be present.

Tinea Capitis A fungal skin disease, especially ringworm, affecting the scalp, resulting in dry, brittle hair that is easily extracted with hair shaft.	May occur in epidemic form	Lesions usually resolve at puberty. Occasionally permanent alopecia with Trichophyton infection.	Patchy alopecia of scalp with scaling and broken hairs.
Turner's Syndrome (Gonadal Dysgenesis) A congenital endocrine disorder caused by failure of the ovaries to respond.	Congenital	Chronic	Alopecia of the frontal area of the scalp most common. Occasionally patchy alopecia. Sparse pubic and axillary hairs do to pituitary hormone stimulation.

As previously mentioned, the most common type of hair loss is androgenetic alopecia (AGA) in both genders. AGA is a genetically (inherited) predetermined disorder due to an excessive response to androgens (DHT). This hair loss condition affects 50 million men and 30 million women in the United States. Androgenetic alopecia is characterized by a progressive loss of terminal hair of the scalp following puberty. It follows a characteristic distribution in both males and females. In males, hair loss is most prominent in the vertex (crown) and frontotemporal regions. In women, the frontal hairline is usually unaffected with diffuse hair loss at the crown and the top of the head, with loss often marked by a wider center part. However, as shown in Table 8.1, in some specific cases, other factors like systemic or local disease processes may be the cause of hair loss.

9

Surgical Hair-Loss Restoration Methods: A Historical Perspective

The search for an ideal treatment to correct hair loss has been pursued for a very long time. The constant desire to produce natural-looking results and meet the ever-increasing expectations of patients has driven the evolution of various techniques used to repair or correct hair-loss disorders (Sattur, 2011). Hair transplantation is an increasingly popular surgical procedure for correcting and restoring male and female pattern baldness. In the United States and other western countries, hair-transplant surgeons use a variety of plastic surgery techniques to redistribute the hair available from the patient's donor area (Shiell, 2008). Essentially, there are three broad categories of surgical restoration procedures.

- Scalp flaps (advancement, rotation flaps, and free flaps).
- Surgical scalp reduction.
- Free autograft techniques (punch graft, micro-grafting, mini-grafting, follicular unit transplantation (FUT), and follicular unit extraction (FUE).

The consensus of the hair-transplant industry is that these are the most effective restorative hair-loss techniques that have been developed to date. Although hair transplantation might seem to be a new surgical procedure, the reader will soon discover that it is not. As early as the nineteenth century, surgeons were searching for a solution to cure baldness. They experimented with scalp flaps and free grafts. Among the first written records of such efforts is the published dissertation of medical student Johann Friedrich Dieffenbach in 1822 in Wurzburg, Germany. In his dissertation study, Dieffenbach reported what some researchers consider the first hair transplant performed on a human being.

Dieffenbach, using a needle, made holes in his own arm, and inserted six scalp hair follicles. Of the six transplanted hairs, two hairs dried up and were shed, two were expelled or rejected due to an inflammatory reaction, and two hairs survived the experiment and continued to grow. By extracting single hairs and then transplanting them, Dieffenbach essentially performed the first recorded follicular unit extraction (FUE) transplant operation. Therefore, the FUE method of hair transplantation is actually a technique that is over 195 years old. In subsequent experiments, Dieffenbach improved his transplantation technique and even began to perform eyelash transplantation.

However, while Dieffenbach—a highly skilled surgeon—could successfully and efficiently perform such procedures with the crude surgical instruments of that period, other surgeons were unfortunately not as successful in replicating his success with the same technique. Consequently, due to the lack of progress made following Dieffenbach's discovery, hair transplantation research did not advance, and no new developments were again seen for 100 years (Schultheiss et al., 1998; keratin.com, 2016). Subsequently, Dieffenbach went on to become a world-renowned plastic surgeon recognized as one of Germany's greatest surgeons and among its most prolific medical writers (Lam & Williams, Jr., 2016). In fact, he is generally known in the medical community as the founder of modern plastic surgery (Schultheiss, Knöner, Kramer, & Jonas, 1998).

Regarding the scalp flaps technique, it appears that this procedure dates back to 1894. In 1984 renowned surgeon Herman Tillman, M.D. devised an operation whereby he transposed four pedicle flaps from the margin of a denuded area of the scalp and then sutured the ends together across the wound in a fashion resembling a wheel spoke

(Figure 9.1). This surgical procedure produced a better distribution of hair-bearing skin over a large scalp defect. The primary application of this procedure was for the treatment of scarring types alopecia.

Fig. 9.1: Image depicting Tillman's 1894 pinwheel pedicle flaps method

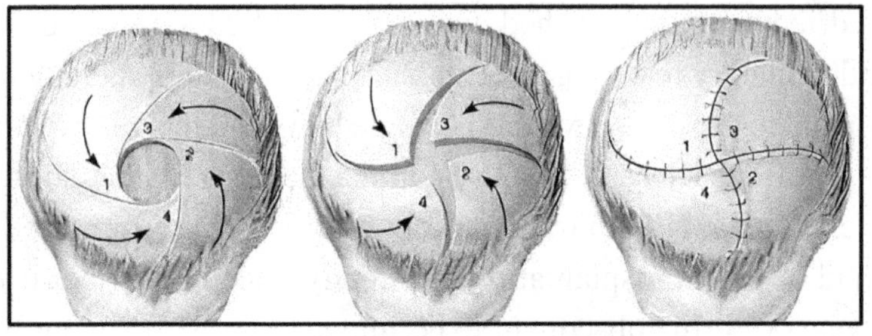

Image Source: https://www.ijhns.com/doi/IJHNS/pdf/10.5005/jp-journals-10001-1098

Other important contributors also paved the way for the acceptance of surgical treatment for male pattern baldness (MPB). For example, Hunt (1926) was the first to propose surgical correction procedures for the treatment of baldness. Passot (1931) proposed the use of transposition flaps for the treatment and correction of alopecia. At the time, his methods were thought to be imaginative and revolutionary, and they are considered the precursors for many of the flap techniques used today.

Tauber (1937) was also considered an important contributor to the scalp flaps method of hair restoration. In his work, Dr. Tauber described the use of local pedicle flaps elevated from the lateral and posterior scalp for the replacement of hair in denuded scalp frontal areas. His technique was essentially a modification of the surgical technique developed by Dr. Passot. Tauber's work was primarily overlooked for two basic reasons: the world was in turmoil at the time because of World War II, and his work was published in an obscure medical journal.

After Tauber's surgical contributions to the scalp flap method, twenty years passed before any significant research was published in any of the medical journals regarding the surgical correction of baldness with the use of the flap technique. In 1957, Dr. Edward S. Lamont published a research paper entitled *"A Plastic Surgical Transformation,"* in which he discussed the surgical treatment of severe fronto-temporal baldness in a 29-year-old male patient using the method of flap transposition as proposed by Passot in 1931.

The flap technique was first performed during the 1930s by Hunt, Passot, and Tauber. However, the procedure never caught on in any significant way until Dr. Jose Juri of Argentina introduced the Juri temporo-parieto-occipital (TPO) flap procedure in 1969. The Juri TPO flap method was the first large, monopedicled flap procedure performed on the scalp for reconstructive and aesthetic purposes (Juri, 1975). The flap method involves removing a large piece of tissue from one area of the scalp and rotating the flap into another site that needs hair. The flap is not entirely removed because it needs to be attached to the major blood vessels that keep the tissue alive (Fig.9.2).

Fig. 9.2: Juri Flap Technique Schematic

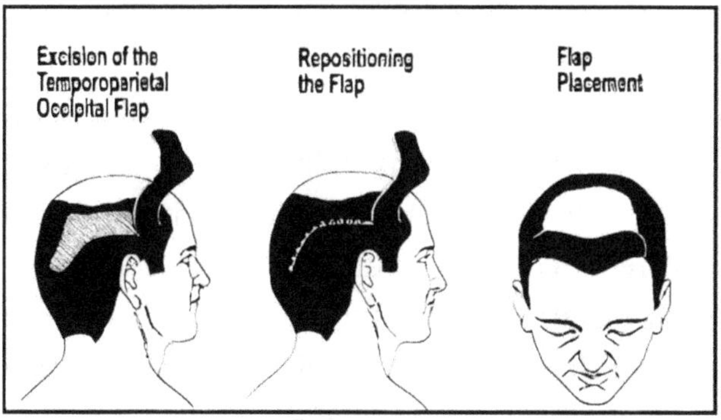

Image Sources: http://kbb.uludag.edu.tr/seminer-fasiyalplastik.htm?ref=SevSevil.Com. Modified image.

The flap method is not always a popular procedure with patients because of the high failure rate associated with the technique. Even when successful, the frontal hair growth is frequently unnatural in density and direction. A scalp flap procedure is a highly invasive operation requiring an exceptional degree of surgical skill to safely and successfully perform the procedure. In current practice, routine use of scalp flaps remains restricted to the hands of a few gifted surgeons, such as the Juri brothers in Argentina, Patrick Frechet in France, and Mayer and Fleming in the United States (Shiell, 2008).

However, it was not until the early 1960s that autograft techniques, such as the punch graft and plug method, were popularized by New York dermatologist Dr. Norman Orentreich. The autograft was the most widely used method until the 1980s. It was also the simplest and least traumatic of all the methods used to correct androgenetic alopecia (AGA) up to that time. Although the punch graft method of hair transplantation was popularized during the early 1960s by Orentreich in the United States, the work of several Japanese dermatologist researchers were unfortunately overlooked, mainly because of World War II and the fact that their research reports were published in Japanese dermatology journals. These Japanese researchers' who contributed extensively to the field of hair loss restoration included Sasakawa, Okuda, and Tamura.

In 1930, Dr. Masao Sasakawa reported on a hair-shaft insertion technique to treat hair loss, probably the first study that intentionally focused on the development of a surgical procedure to treat scalp alopecia. In 1939 another physician named Shoji Okuda also experimented with Sasakawa's technique with highly successful results in 200 reported cases. In these cases, Okuda concentrated on reconstructing cicatricial (scarring) and congenital alopecia that he treated by the punch graft method of hair replacement with satisfactory cosmetic results. He employed small-graft transplantation ranging in size from 1.0 to 5.0 millimeters in diameter. It is important to note that Dr. Okuda was actually a distinguished ophthalmologist, not a dermatologist or plastic surgeon, as previously believed (Hair Transplant Forum International, 2009).

Moreover, Dr. Okuda published a series of five articles in 1939 entitled *"Clinical and Experimental Study of Living Hair Transplantation"* in the *Japanese Journal of Dermatology.* In these articles, Okuda stated that hair transplantation of individual hairs had been performed previously by Dr. Hajime Tamura in 1937. However, Tamura's first 127 hair transplant cases were not successful. Notwithstanding this initial lack of success, Tamura subsequently performed 136 successful procedures in 1939.

Tamura's technique advocated the use of single-hair grafts, which produced an excellent natural appearance. He urged that the donor grafts should be as small as possible. He contended that if the donor grafts were too big, the hair would grow in a very unnatural appearance. In essence, this was the *"doll hair"* look observed in hair-transplants patients in the United States from the 1960s to the 1980s (Fig. 9.3). Furthermore, in 1943, Tamura explained that if the donor punch grafts were too big (6-12 millimeters), they would produce an unacceptably high rate of hair loss in the center of the grafts because of the difficulty oxygen would have diffusing over such large distances. It is important to note that the procedure advocated and described by Tamura was essentially the precursor of the follicular unit transplant (FUT) method still used today.

Fig. 9.3: Round plug hair transplant with the doll hair look

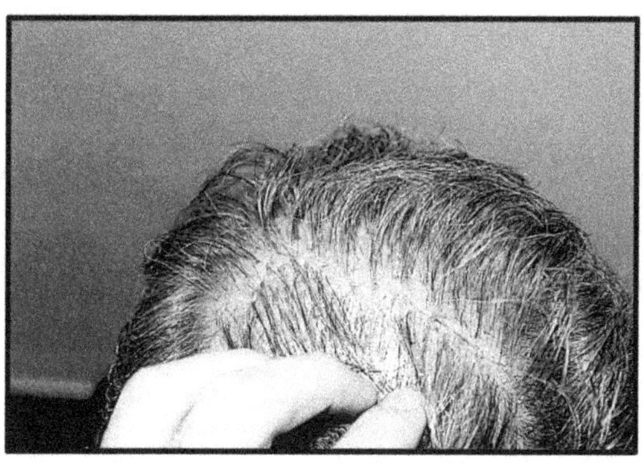

Image Source: https://hairtransplantweb.com/procedures/plugs/

In 1953, another Japanese contributor, Fujita, investigated eyebrow reconstruction via hair graft in leprosy patients. Additionally, Fujita reported on punch hair grafting, a procedure in which a free skin graft containing some hairs was divided into small pieces, each piece containing two, three, or four hairs using a scalpel or a pair of scissors to separate them (keratim.com, 2015). This description sounds quite similar to the strip method and follicular unit extraction (FUE). In the United States, the initial effort to accept a smaller graft size was delayed because of the concern that much smaller grafts may not transplant sufficient hair to make the procedure worthwhile (Bernstein, 2013).

Confirming Tamura's contention regarding the use of smaller grafts, Dr. Robert M. Bernstein (1998) stated that if hair-transplant physicians and surgeons in the United States had recognized and embraced Dr. Hajime Tamura's achievements, the history of hair transplantation in the United States would probably have taken a different direction. It is quite possible that the large punch grafting technique, advocated by Dr. Orentreich, may not have become the standard procedure in the United States for more than 30 years.

Moreover, Okuda's papers contain almost all the information relevant to modern hair transplantation, including the principles of *donor dominance*, which Dr. Orentreich later popularized. Unfortunately, Okuda did not refer to male pattern hair loss (MPHL) as a treatable condition. Therefore, Dr. Orentreich is credited as the first researcher to use these innovative techniques to treat MPHL.

Furthermore, because of World War II, Okuda's work was not known outside Japan. In fact, even in Japan, his writings were unintelligible and difficult to understand because it was written in old kanji, whose origin is pictographs and logographs wherein each character represents an idea. These are often referred to as Chinese characters. Kanji was brought to Japan in the 5th century C.E. because, at the time, Japan had no written language. Japan used the

Kanji language for diplomatic correspondence with China. Therefore, even if his reports had been accessible to western civilization, they were not easy to read (Pathomvanich & Imagawa, 2010).

Fortunately for Okuda, in 1970, German dermatologist Dr. H. C. Friederich discovered Okuda's research papers. He justifiably acknowledged Okuda's significant contributions to the hair-transplantation field and designated the punch graft method as the Okuda/Orentreich technique (Pathomvanich & Imagawa, 2010). Although the Orentreich method of transplanting hair was quite similar to Okuda's, Dr. Orentreich made more far-reaching conclusions from his experimental studies. He started his studies in 1956 and completed them in 1959 when he published his landmark research paper entitled *"Autografts in Alopecia and Other Selected Dermatological Conditions"* in the Annals of the New York Academy of Science. As the result of his study, Orentreich proposed two terms to describe the pattern of hair growth. These terms are still used to this day; they are:

- Donor Dominance Concept.
- Recipient Dominance Concept.

Donor Dominance Concept

The principle of modern hair restoration is predicated on the concept of *donor dominance*. This term addresses the fact that the transposed punch grafts of skin maintain their integrity and characteristics independent of the recipient site. Donor dominance means that transplanted hair will continue to display the exact characteristics of the hair from the location it was extracted. Therefore, donor-dominant transplants continue to show the hair-growing characteristics of hair from the donor site after transplantation to the recipient site. In other words, healthy hair harvested from the back and sides of the scalp that is transplanted to a balding area will continue to grow as if it were still in its original location.

Recipient Dominance Concept

The term recipient dominance addresses the fact that the transposed punch graft of skin takes on the characteristics of the recipient site. Recipient dominance implies the exact opposite of donor dominance, meaning that the recipient area has an influence to some degree over the transplanted hair. *Recipient dominance* expresses itself in unique and subtle ways. For example, in eyebrow hair transplants, eyebrow-region hair that otherwise grows very fast when transplanted can be influenced by the native skin in the eyebrow region so that over time the hair starts to grow more slowly and finer than the original transplant.

Similarly, hair transplanted from the body (e.g., from the chest), can start to grow faster and finer when moved from the body to the scalp (Lam, 2012). In his research to validate the concepts of donor and recipient dominance, Dr. Orentreich studied four different conditions that manifested in different hair-growth problems. These four conditions were:

1. Alopecia Prematura (Androgenetic Alopecia).

2. Alopecia Cicatrisata (Scarring Alopecia).

3. Alopecia Areata.

4. Vitiligo.

Vitiligo is an acquired condition characterized by the absence of melanocytes (i.e., melanin-producing cells), causing low pigmentation areas. Melanin is the substance that pigments or colors the hair and skin. The hair in vitiliginous areas is usually white, and the lesions in the skin are white under a Wood's lamp. Thus, vitiligo is a common, often inherited disorder characterized by well-defined areas of milky white skin and hair (Fig. 9.4). Donor dominance was observed in the following conditions:

- Alopecia Prematura.
- Alopecia Cicatrisata (Scarring).

The Orentreich study was performed by multiple transposition experiments, meaning that punch grafts were relocated or rearrange in the following manner:

1. Hair to hair (which grew hair).
2. Hair to a bald area (which grew hair).
3. Bald area to bald area (which remained bald).
4. Bald area to hair area (which remained bald).

Fig. 9.4: Vitiligo of the hair and skin

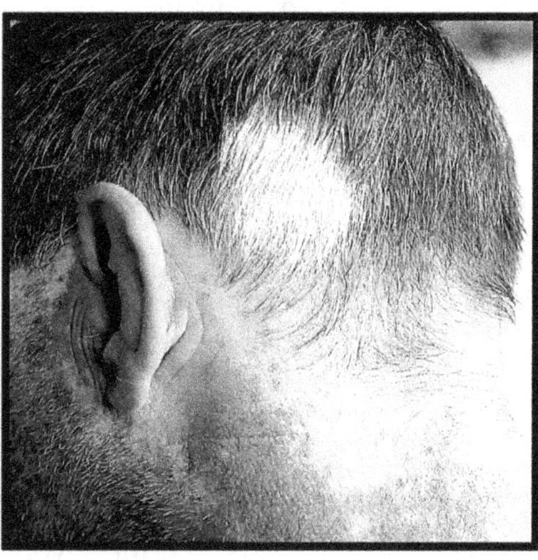

Image Source: By Klaus D. Peter, Gummersbach, Germany (Own work) [CC BY 3.0 de (http://creativecommons.org/licenses/by/3.0/de/deed.en)], via Wikimedia Commons https://commons.wikimedia.org/wiki/File%3AVitiligo_and_Poliosis.jpg

In alopecia areata, hair growth was observed under the experiment's first two conditions (1 & 2), but the hair growth was sparse and weak. No hair growth was evident under the experiment's last two conditions (3 & 4). *Recipient dominance* was observed in the vitiliginous condition when transposition of pigmented skin to pigmented skin remained pigmented. In transposition of pigmented skin to the vitiligo-affected area, the skin became vitiliginous. In transposition of vitiliginous skin to vitiliginous skin, the skin remained vitiliginous, and in transposition of vitiliginous skin to normally pigmented skin, the skin became pigmented.

Two observations can be made from this study. The first has already been mentioned, but this study seems to confirm Hamilton's conclusion that in common pattern baldness, the capacity for the development of hair loss appears to be controlled by factors resident in localized areas of the scalp. Orentreich articulated the second observation, which is that in cases indicating recipient dominance— as in the condition of vitiligo— there seem to be systemic factors or deeper-seated structures and tissues determining the local reaction. Following the publication of Dr. Orentreich's study, many surgically oriented dermatologists began using his technique to treat male pattern hair loss (MPHL). Orentreich's hair-restoration technique was further popularized during the 1960s by some celebrities who were willing to talk about it in magazines and television talk shows.

However, after hair transplantation received its impetus during the late 1950s and early1960s, it created an enormous market potential for unscrupulous opportunists and charlatans wanting to cash in on the human concern for hair regrowth. Hair clinics sprang up all over the country, promising their clients that they would regrow their lost hair with herbal concoctions, vasodilators, scalp massages with and without electric vibrators, ultraviolet rays, biotin creams, and proprietary hair-loss solutions. Not only did corrupt hair-restoration clinics proliferate quickly, but many untrained physicians also began using these hair transplantation techniques as well. The results produced by these unskilled physicians included disastrous disfigurement of the scalp and personal lawsuits.

Inherently, any time there is a scientific discovery that promises to resolve an undesirable human condition, someone will rise to meet the need. This situation usually leads to a proliferation of unprincipled merchants coming to the marketplace to separate the uninformed consumer from their hard-earned money. The only solution to combat such corrupt business practices is by educating the consumer. The consumer should always seek the counsel of a competent and well-trained specialist regardless of the cost. In this situation, the consumer should seek advice from a dermatologist or plastic surgeon. The crucial issue with this kind of surgery is achieving an aesthetically acceptable outcome, and searching for an economical hair transplant can result in unintended consequences.

The hair transplant punch graft method, as described by Drs. Okuda and Orentreich have been used for more than twenty years and remained essentially unchanged until the mid-1970s (Shiell, 2008). During this period, many renowned physicians were responsible for the widespread use of the Orentreich-Okuda hair transplantation method. These prominent physicians included *Ayres, Unger, Jamra, Pierce, Febrier, Norwood, Pirotta, Ponteaux, Smith, Cheikh, Stough, Lebon, Burks, and Kirschbaum.*

Punch Graft Method Refinements

There were numerous practicing physicians during the punch-graft era of hair transplantation that also advocated certain refinements of the punch graft method:

- Kaye and Unger.

- Adamson and Hoston.
- Monell and Berman.
- Seltzer.
- Wilkinson and Iglesias.
- Arouete.

Kaye and Unger.

These researchers advocated the use of the upright position for hair transplantation. However, after proposing the upright position, Kaye ultimately dispensed with this idea and placed his patients in the supine position. The upright position was supposed to offer the advantages of simplifying and speeding up the procedure. For example, the patient could remain in one position throughout the entire operation, the surgical area was prepared as a single field, and the hair grafts were trimmed to a correct level as they were removed from their donor sites and were immediately implanted into their recipient site. Therefore, the surgeon could minimize the time the hair grafts were exposed to the external environment. Additionally, two medical personnel could work on the scalp simultaneously.

Dr. Walter P. Unger further advanced the theory of donor dominance by defining the parameters of what it is called the *"safe donor zone"* from which the most permanent (i.e., DHT-resistance) hair follicles could be extracted for the hair transplant. To determine the safe zone for harvesting or extracting hair, Dr. Unger conducted a research study in 1994 entitled *"Delineating the Safe Donor Area for Hair Transplanting"* (Figs.9.5, 9.6, and 9.7). In this study, Unger examined the scalps of 328 randomly selected men over the age of 65 with varying degrees of MPHL.

Fig. 9.5: Unger's safe donor zone parameters for hair extraction (lateral view)

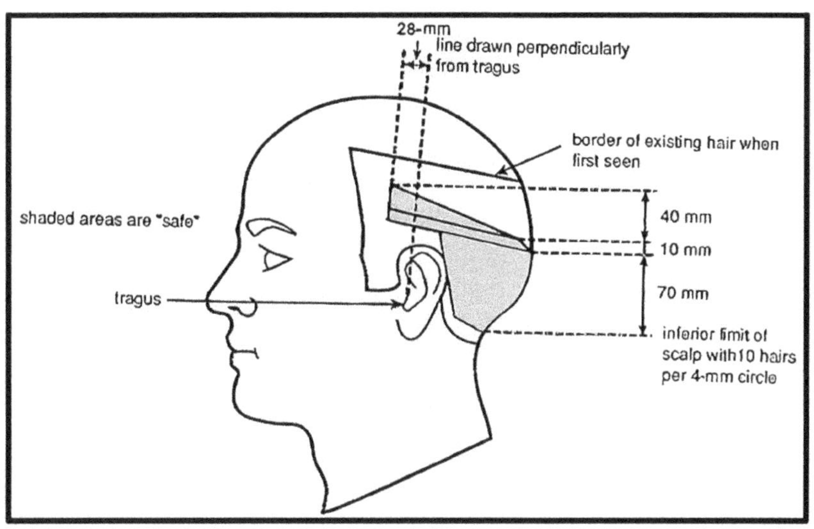

Image Source: By Walter P. Unger, M.D. [CC BY-SA 3.0 (http://creativecommons.org/license/by-sa/3.0) or GFDL (http://www.gnu.org/copyleft/fdl.html)], via Wikimedia Commons. From textbook by Unger, W., ed. Hair Transplantation. 3rd ed. New York: Marcel Dekker, 1995. Pg. 184.

To determine the viability of the hairs to be extracted, Unger looked for areas where there was a minimum of eight healthy-looking hairs in a four-millimeter diameter circle within the remaining or existing hair-bearing fringe. The hairs within this potential donor area are considered the most immune or resistant to dihydrotestosterone (DHT), which is considered the primary causative factor involved in developing MPHL. Although hair continues to be lost throughout the entire hair-bearing fringe of balding men during their lifetime, Dr. Unger was able to outline a zone containing the hair follicles that were most likely to have relative permanence in approximately 80% of patients less than 80 years of age (Kaminer, Dover, & Arndt, 2002).

Fig. 9.6: Unger's safe donor zone parameters for hair extraction (back view)

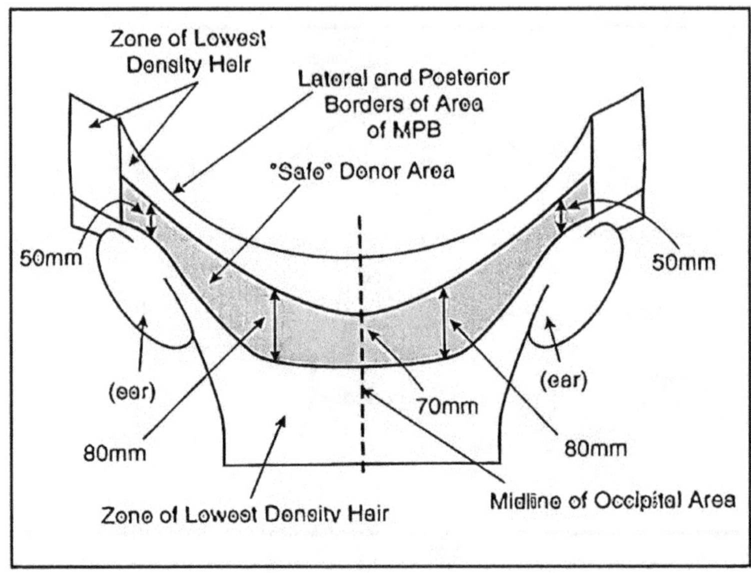

Image Source: Unger WP. "Delineating the 'Safe' Donor Area for Hair Transplanting" The American Journal of Cosmetic Surgery, 1994. https://en.wikipedia.org/wiki/Safe_Donor_Zone. Available under the Creative Commons Attribution-Share Alike 3.0 License. https://en.wikipedia.org/wiki/Safe_Donor_Zone

Fig. 9.7: Marking the safe donor area for hair extraction

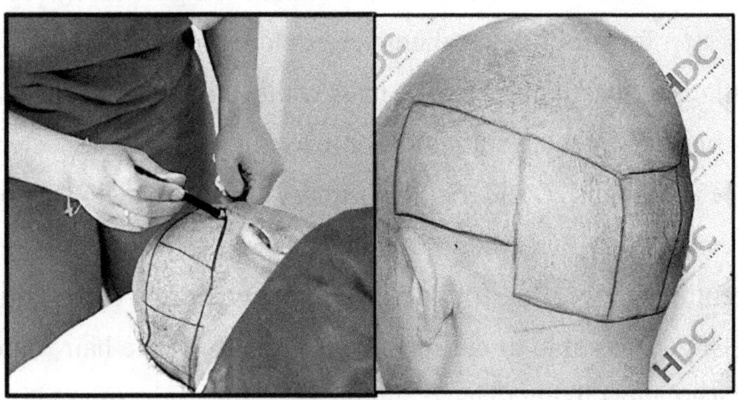

Image Source: http://www.istockphoto.com/photo/hair-transplant-gm496818461-41687298. http://www.hairtransplants-hdc.com/blog/item/state-of-the-art-hair-transplants-in-cyprus (Owner) Used with Permission.

Because the objective of hair transplantation is to use only hairs that are destined to remain permanently in their original site, this quantitative model of a safe donor zone has been and should continue to be the fundamental foundation in hair-follicle harvesting for both the FUT and FUE procedure (Wolff et al., 2002). However, one warning is that the safe donor zone represents a generality that cannot be reliably depended upon for any particular individual (Unger,1994). Unger's concept of the safe donor zone is an important contribution because transplanted hairs will only grow in their new recipient site for as long as they would have grown in their original donor location.

Adamson and Hoston.

Adamson and Hoston advocated using a revolving handpiece run by an electric motor for taking the punch grafts in the donor site. The reason for this refinement was that the proposed device was supposed to shorten the surgery time substantially.

Monell and Berman.

These investigators also advocated using a simple power device motor for removing the punch graft from the donor area since they were extremely concerned about preventing the grafts from drying out. For this reason, they also advocated that grafts be immersed entirely in a chilled (4.4°C), sterile, saline solution.

Seltzer.

Dr. Seltzer advocated using a motorized drill for removing the graft from the donor area. Moreover, Seltzer preferred to perform the procedure under general anesthesia since he could transplant more than 100 plugs in one operative session. He further believed that the motorized drill would reduce bleeding to a minimum.

Wilkinson and Iglesias.

Wilkinson and Iglesias proposed the use of nontoxic tissue adhesive (i.e., isobutyl 2-cyanoacrylate) to prevent the plugs and strips from slipping during the procedure. This team further believed that the tissue adhesive helped prevent the elevation of the hair plugs during the post-operative phase and made bandaging less complicated.

Arouete.

Dr. Jean Arouete advocated using occipital and frontal tourniquets to control the excessive bleeding that could occur during the punch graft technique.

Besides the refinements described above, other physicians such as Lessa and Carreirao advocated new techniques relating to the suturing of the donor site wound so that the patient could have a better cosmetic appearance. Although the round punch graft or plug method of hair transplantation advocated by Orentreich marked the beginning of the era of modern hair transplantation in the United States and was the most popular and widely used technique of its time, other procedures deserve mention from a historical perspective.

Square Graft Method.

Originally, the standard practice for performing hair transplantation surgery was limited to using the round plugs or grafts advocated by Orentreich. However, in the early 1970s, Dr. Felipe Coiffman of the National University of Colombia in South America promoted the use of the square graft (Fig. 9.8). Dr. Coiffman felt that the square graft had certain advantages over the simpler round punch grafts. Coiffman contended that the square graft method minimized the damage to the hair follicle because each graft was handled under direct, magnifying vision using microsurgical techniques. Additionally, Coiffman argued that the donor site of a square-graft hair transplant left a more aesthetically acceptable, straight-line scar after the wound had been sutured.

Fig. 9.8: Square Graft Image

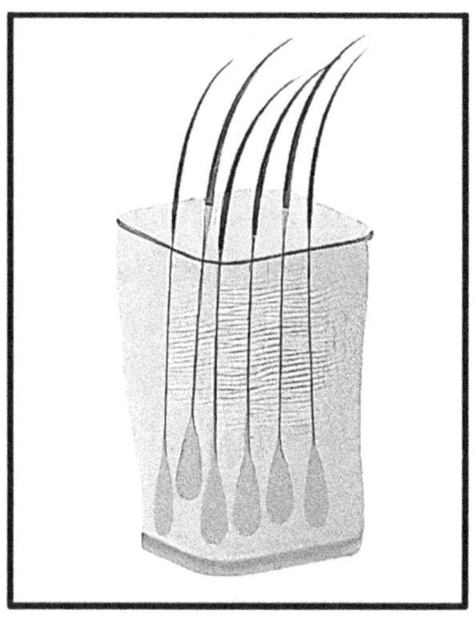

Image Source: By Angela Lehman (Owner). Use with Permission.
https://www.alopecia-hair-transplant.com/hair-loss/hair-transplantation/

Dr. Coiffman further contended that the square graft covered the recipient area more precisely and that each square graft contained approximately 25% more hair than the simpler round punch graft of the same diameter. Coiffman claimed that it was also possible to use the square grafts in combination with the strip graft (FUT) or skin flaps methods. As with any surgical technique, there were also some disadvantages:

- The Coiffman square graft technique was a more involved and complicated procedure than the round plug or punch graft technique.

- It required the use of more specialized instruments and the careful sectioning of the square graft in the donor site under microsurgical techniques.

Hair-replacement surgery appears to date back to Japan in the 1930s with hair transplant pioneers such as Masao Sasakawa, Hajime

Tamura, and Shoji Okuda. However, it was not until 1959, when Dr. Orentreich published his landmark study entitled *"Autografts in Alopecias and Other Selected Dermatologic Conditions,"* that the field of hair restoration evolved significantly from the introduction of his crude, punch graft hair transplants.

In concluding this chapter, it is important to state that hair loss is a pervasive problem that affects both men and women, and it can have profound psychological effects on the afflicted. It is a problem in need of a solution. Therefore, it is not surprising that a solution it is aggressively being sought by the best minds in hair-loss research. However, while we wait for a better solution, hair transplant surgery is still an effective and increasingly popular solution to correct hair loss. The results that hair transplant specialists can attain today are remarkable. In fact, hair transplants can provide an aesthetically natural appearance when the procedure is performed by a skillful and competent surgeon (Rose, 2015). The advances that have occurred within the field of hair restoration have launched a new era of hair transplantation methods. The author will address these advances in the next chapter.

10

New Era of Hair Restoration and Transplantation Methods

While the Okuda-Orentreich hair-transplantation method was a well-accepted procedure for many decades, scientific and technical advances have helped hair-restoration surgeons create *a new era of consistent, safe, effective, and natural-looking results.* The obvious-looking, plug-type transplants (i.e., punch graft) of the past have been replaced with newer procedures that create aesthetic results that defy detection. Microsurgical techniques and new instrumentation, as well as an artistic appreciation of how hair naturally grows, has led to these advances. Some of these new methods are:

- The Strip/FUT Graft Method (also known as follicular unit transplant (FUT).
- Follicular Unit Extraction (FUE).
    - NeoGraft® Automated FUE.
    - ARTAS® Robotic FUE.
    - HARRTS™ i-Brain Robotic FUE.
- Direct Hair Implantation (DHI).
- Hair Stem Cell Transplantation (HST Method).

The Strip/FUT Graft Method

In the 1980s, hair restoration surgery evolved dramatically as the large, round punch grafts were gradually replaced with a more refined combination of minigrafts and micrografts. This combination of minigraft and micrograft hair-transplantation procedures no longer used the punch graft instrument to extract the bald resistant grafts. Typically, a minigraft comprises four to five hairs, and the micrograft is composed of one to two hairs. The strip surgery method is known in the United States by several names, including follicular unit transplant (FUT) or follicular unit grafting (FUG). However, some hair-transplant surgeons feel that a more appropriate term to reference strip surgery is follicular unit strip surgery (FUSS), as described initially by Dr. Alvi Armani in the late 1990s (Abimelec, 2016).

The strip method became the new standard in the field of hair transplantation in the early to mid-1990s. Many hair-transplant surgeons considered it the ***gold standard,*** but with the emergence of the FUE method, it might not be any longer. Notwithstanding the emergent popularity of FUE, FUT still remains, by an overwhelming majority, the most common procedure used to correct pattern baldness (Sutter, 2011).

The strip technique is a method of treating hair loss in which hair grafts are extracted or harvested and then implanted into the patient's balding areas (recipient site). This technique uses a blade to cut out a strip of scalp tissue from the back and sides of the head. Subsequently, this strip of scalp is carefully slivered into small pieces, which are further divided using a microscope (to aid with visualization) into the individual follicular units (FUs), which are the naturally occurring groupings of hair (Figs. 10.1, 10.2, and 10.3).

Fig. 10.1: Strip/FUT Graft Method Steps (schematic)

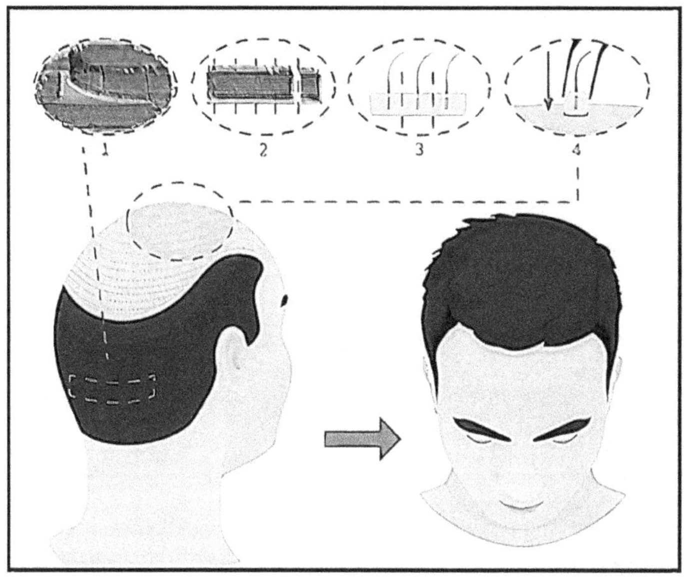

Image Source: http://www.istockphoto.com/vector/fut-hair-loss-treatment-gm639598442-11537173

Fig. 10.2: Strip/FUT Graft Method Steps (photo)

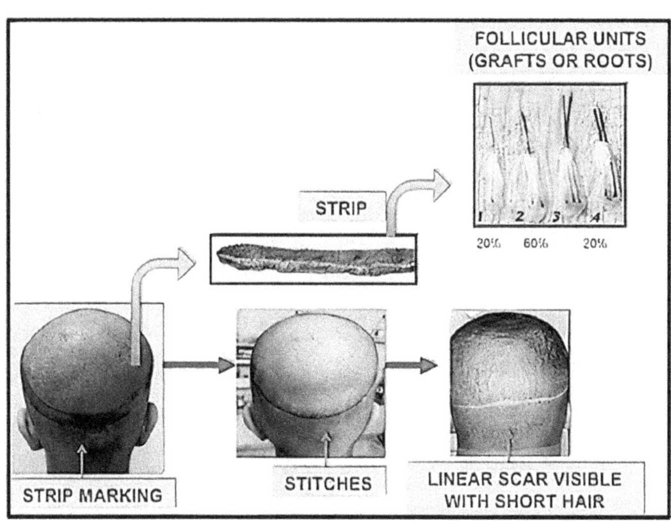

Image Source: By Bishan Mahadevia, M.D. (Owner) http://goodbyehairloss.blogspot.com/2010/03/hair-cloning-hair-multiplication-hm.html/Modified Use with Permission

Fig. 10.3: Photo of the naturally occurring grouping of 1-4 follicular units (FUs)

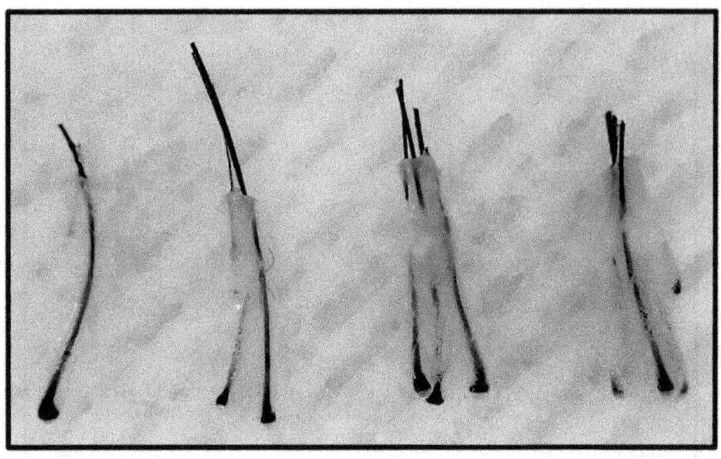

Image Source: By Nicole Rogers, M.D., FAAD (Owner). https://www.hairrestorationofthesouth.com/hair_transplant/fue-hair-transplant/ Use with Permission

Like any other surgical procedure, the strip/FUT hair transplant procedure has some advantages and disadvantages compared to other hair transplantation methods, such as FUE. Some of the advantages and disadvantages of the strip/FUT procedure are listed below.

Advantages of the Strip/FUT Method.

- The strip method is typically less expensive than FUE because it is a less time-consuming procedure.
- A physician can transplant more hair grafts in a single session using FUT compared to FUE. Typically, a physician can transplant 4,000 follicular units or more in a single session with FUT.
- The strip/FUT yields a greater percentage of hair regrowth, typically in the 90% range or higher, depending on the surgeon's competence.

Disadvantages of the Strip/FUT Method.

- The strip/FUT procedure produces a long, linear scar where the strip of the donor's hair has been removed. Although the scar is usually very thin and nearly undetectable when fully healed, it is still visible.
- It is difficult to predict the eventual width of the scar, though skilled physicians can generally keep them to half a centimeter or less.
- It can also result in stretching of the scalp.

Trichophytic Donor Closure Technique.

The problem of unsightly scarring can be minimized if the surgeon is trained in the *trichophytic donor closure technique.* The trichophytic donor closure technique is an advanced surgical procedure that allows patients to have a nearly undetectable, linear donor scar after a strip/FUT hair transplant. Before the trichophytic donor closures existed, patients were expected to have a donor area scar that would range anywhere from zero to two millimeters in width.

While the size of this scar may not be a problem for patients who have long hair that may be utilized to cover the scar, the donor scar would be visible for those who have short hair. The trichophytic donor closure is an overlapping technique that allows hair to grow directly through the donor area scar, making the scar nearly invisible. The *tricho closure technique*, as it is sometimes called, provides a better cosmetic outcome for patients, especially when they choose to cut their hair short after the procedure. Therefore, patients who want to wear their hair very short and are contemplating a strip hair transplant with a surgeon who does not use the tricho closure technique might want to reconsider their decision. Additionally, because the strip method is a more invasive procedure, the donor area requires a longer time to heal, depending on the healing characteristics of the patient. Typically, healing takes approximately ten to15 days.

The strip/FUT method of hair restoration is considered appropriate for patients who have been identified as having Norwood's hair-loss classification levels III-VII. As previously mentioned, one of the advantages of this procedure is that it permits the harvesting of a large number of grafts, typically 4,000 or more follicular units (FUs) per surgery. However, customarily only 1500-2500 FUs are harvested per session. The strip procedure is worth considering if the patient's goal is to quickly treat hair loss with a large number of grafts in a short period of time (Mohebi, 2016).

The creation of natural-looking follicular unit grafts, which mimic the way hair grows naturally, typically requires the use of high-powered magnification. Such magnification enables the surgical technicians to properly visualize the FUs in the donor tissue. They can then isolate the FUs and cut them into one, two, three, and sometimes four hair follicular unit grafts (Fig. 10.3).

Dr. Robert Bernstein proposed the concept of performing the entire hair-restoration procedure using FUs exclusively. This procedure is described in a study entitled *"Follicular Transplantation: Patient Evaluation and Surgical Planning,"* published in 1997 by Drs. Robert Bernstein and William Rassman. Critical to the success of the follicular unit (FU) hair transplant procedure was the introduction of the binocular microscope by Dr. Robert Limmer of San Antonio, Texas, in the late 1980s. Dr. Limmer discovered that by using the binocular microscope to examine the donor tissue, he and his staff could successfully isolate and trim the naturally occurring follicular units into individual grafts (Fig. 10.4). Moreover, doctors could harvest 30% more hair from the donor strip using this new technology.

These new microscopes also allowed finer grafts to be created, which meant that much smaller incisions were required, thereby reducing the possibility of inflicting scalp trauma. The use of the microscope also increased the potential to achieve a more natural and aesthetically pleasing look with greater hair density. Dr. Limmer shared his techniques and findings with his colleagues

Drs. Bernstein, Rassman, and Seager. These surgeons subsequently became persuasive advocates for the follicular unit hair transplant procedure (Hair Transplant Network.com, 2016).

Fig. 10.4: Hair transplant technicians harvesting FUs

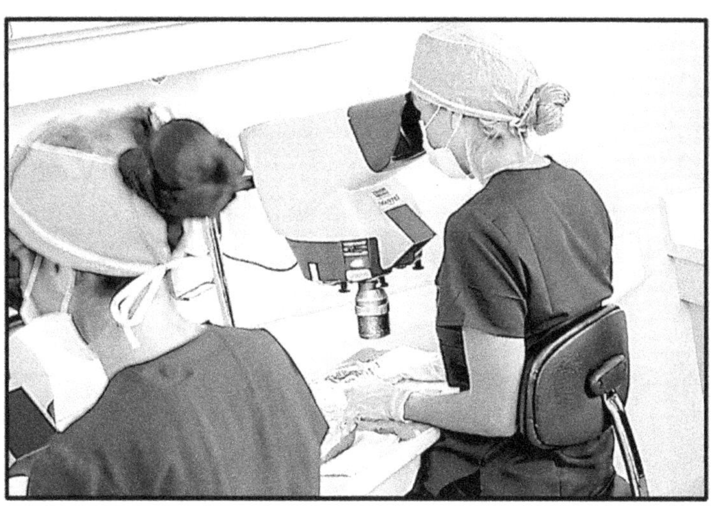

Image Source: http://hairmd.com/traditional-fut/

Follicular Unit Extraction (FUE)

In 1988, Masumi Inaba introduced the use of a one-millimeter punch for extracting individual follicular units (Pathomvanich & Imagawa, 2010). Dr. Ray Woods, the inventor of the FUE technique— also known as follicular transfer— performed the first successful transfer on patients in Australia in 1989. Applying the FUE method, Dr. Woods also performed body hair transplantation (BHT), another procedure he developed where donor follicles are taken from the chest, arms, and other areas and transplanted to thinning or balding areas on the scalp. This procedure was first described in the medical literature in 2002 by Drs. Rassman and Bernstein, in their publication entitled *"Follicular Unit Extraction: Minimally Invasive Surgery for Hair Transplantation"* (Pathomvanich & Imagawa, 2010). Subsequently, Dr. James Harris of Denver developed the patented Harris S.A.F.E.™ (Surgically Advanced Follicular Excision) System and the S.A.F.E

Hex dissection tip, which is an innovative, proprietary technology that improved the existing methodology for FUE (Fig. 10.5).

This breakthrough technology enables the surgeon to perform precise follicular excision without unnecessary follicular damage and the resulting loss that is often associated with the traditional FUE method. It significantly increases the number of grafts that can be transplanted in a single day. Studies show that inexperienced surgeons using the standard FUE technique may damage more than 20-30% of the hair follicles they remove. The comprehensive S.A.F.E™ System developed by Dr. Harris has been proven to help reduce follicle damage to as low as 2.8% or less.

Fig. 10.5: Harris S.A.F.E. System Instrument

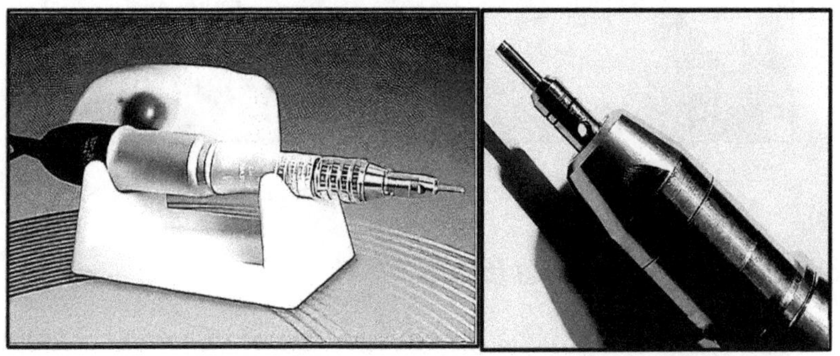

Image Source: http://www.medicalhair.com/hair-restoration
https://www.chaddasurgicals.com/index.php?route=product/product&product_id=175

Follicular unit extraction is a technique that allows hair-follicle harvesting without the use of a scalpel or stitches. Because no scalp strip is removed, this technique does not leave any linear scar, as seen with the strip/FUT method. This method of harvesting follicular unit grafts by removing them directly from the donor area gained popularity in the United States with the publication of "*Follicular Unit Extraction (FUE)*" by Drs. Rassman and Bernstein in 2002. It further gained momentum after the 2005 publication of Dr. James Harris' paper entitled "*The Safe System for Follicular Unit Extraction (FUE).*" Although the FUE method has several limitations, it has proven itself to be useful when strip/FUT harvesting is not indicated.

The main difference between the FUE and the FUT methods lies in how the follicular units (FUs) are extracted/harvested. Using the FUE method, the individual follicular units are extracted directly from the scalp. Essentially, the dominant feature of both techniques is the extraction of the smallest natural hair groups or follicular units. These anatomical follicular units generally consist of one to four hairs and occasionally five hairs (Fig.10.6).

Fig.10.6: One to Five Hair Follicular Units (FUs)

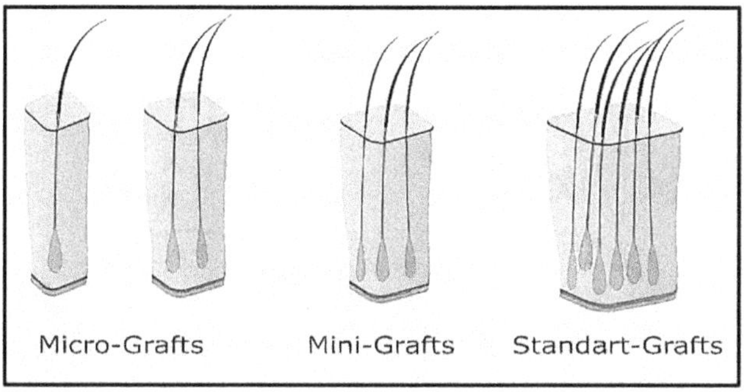

Image Source: By Angela Lehman (Owner) Use with Permission
https://www.alopecia-hair-transplant.com/hair-loss/hair-transplantation/

Both techniques, the FUT and FUE, make use of these natural follicular units. In the FUE extraction method, the size of the punch needles plays a decisive role. Choosing the right size minimizes damage to the donor area. The learning process required to master the FUE method, considered the new state-of-the-art method, is more intensive and time-consuming than when using the strip/FUT extraction method.

The two extraction/harvesting techniques— FUE and FUT— differ regarding the scarring left in the donor area. For example, the strip extraction (FUT) method will leave a narrow linear scar on the back and side of the head; conversely, all that can be seen after a FUE transplant are micro-scars that look like little dots (Fig. 10.7).

However, with the FUE technique, the safe donor zone is exceeded, which means that some of the harvested grafts are extracted from a wide area of the lower scalp. Therefore, this transplanted hair could be lost in the future because the extracted hairs could be from outside the safe donor zone. Notwithstanding this FUE limitation, if the appearance of a scar in the donor area is a patient concern because they want to wear their hair very short, then FUE is the preferred procedure. In contrast, with the strip/FUT method, the hair has to be worn longer to conceal the remaining linear scar.

Fig. 10.7: Extraction difference between the FUE and FUT methods

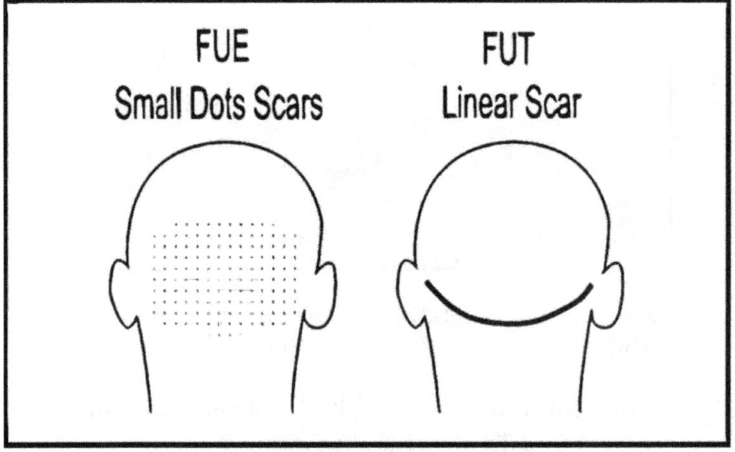

Image Source: https://www.tissuse.com/en/products/regenerative-therapies/.Modified image. (Use with Permission)

New Technologies for the FUE Procedure

The hair transplantation and restoration field have made significant advancements in the past decade. Some of these advancements are technologies developed to perform follicular unit extraction hair-transplantation surgery. All these innovations are aimed at overcoming limitations encountered by previous methods. These technological innovations include:

- NeoGraft® Automated FUE System.
- ARTAS® Robotic FUE System.
- HARRTS™ i-Brain Robotic FUE System.

Neograft® Automated FUE System

The NeoGraft® is the first and only FDA-cleared follicular unit harvesting and implantation system. A NeoGraft® automated system is essentially a machine that performs the extraction process for the FUE procedure (Fig. 10.8). The device helps automate the surgical extraction and collection of individual hair follicles one at a time in a timely manner. Moreover, the Neograft® procedure reduces patient discomfort and recovery time and is more cost-effective for patients.

A point of concern by many hair-transplantation surgeons who have been trained formally through residency is the fact that the NeoGraft® device is marketed to physicians who do not possess formal hair-transplantation training and expertise. These devices are being marketed to physicians with the promise of a simple and lucrative method of increasing the profitability of their practice.

Hair transplantation is not a complicated procedure; however, it is a work-intensive process requiring a surgeon with good surgical and aesthetic skills. Hair transplantation is not a procedure that should be performed by inexperienced surgeons or technicians. It is a well-accepted premise in any field that requires manual dexterity and aesthetic skills that any device or tool in properly trained hands can be a safe and wonderful tool. However, in the wrong hands, it is a disaster waiting to happen. In fact, no matter which device is used to expedite the extraction of intact follicular units, it is important to note that all manual devices are entirely dependent upon the operator's skill. Suffice it to say; these are not skills that can be acquired through a weekend training course.

Fig. 10.8: NeoGraft® 2.0 Automated FUE System

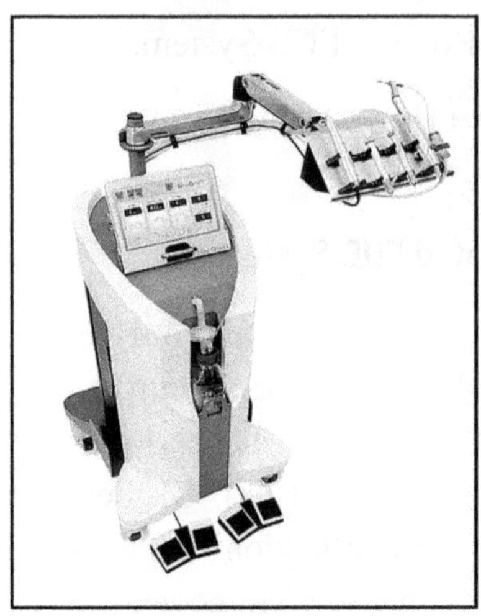

Image Source: https://www.90210surgicalassociates.com/neograft/

ARTAS® Robotic FUE System

The other technological advancement for performing the FUE procedure is the ARTAS® robotic hair restoration platform, which provides multiple advantages over the manual, handheld procedure. The ARTAS® system is a robotic surgical hair-transplantation system developed by *Restoration Robotics, Inc.*, an American, privately-held medical device company founded in 2002 (Fig. 10.9).

ARTAS® was introduced at the annual meeting of the International Society of Hair Restoration Surgeons in 2008. Subsequently, clinical trials were initiated to develop and validate the system's efficacy. The ARTAS® robotic device was approved by the FDA in 2011 for use in harvesting follicular units from brown and black-haired men. However, this limitation of hair coloring can be resolved by dyeing the hair of individuals with blond or white hair. In 2013, the ARTAS® system won the Gold Edison Award in Medicine.

In robotic FUE, the ARTAS® robotic system automates the harvesting of follicular unit grafts, enabling a FUE hair transplant to be performed with unparalleled precision, as claimed by the developers. As previously mentioned, the advantages of the FUE method over traditional hair transplants like the strip method are not having a linear scar in the donor area and eliminating the post-operative limitations on physical activity experienced with the more invasive procedures.

Fig. 10.9: ARTAS® Robotic FUE System

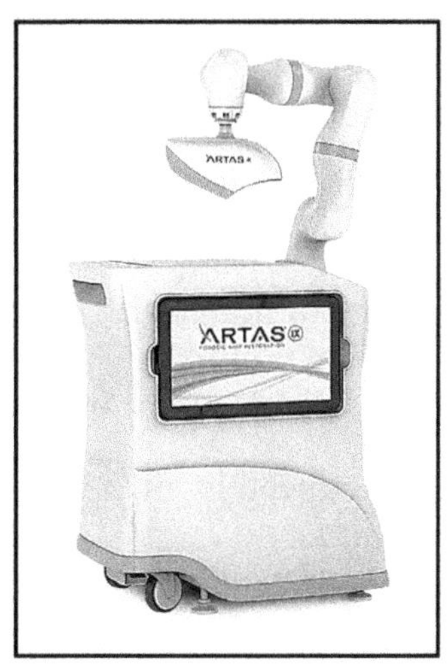

Image Source: https://www.venusconcept.com/en-gl/artas-ix.htm

The ARTAS® robotic system utilizes an advanced optical guidance system to locate and extract the follicular units according to specifications programmed by the physician. It carries out this process hundreds to thousands of times per session with speed and accuracy that is impossible to duplicate with the human hand. The robot can also create recipient sites for the placement of FU grafts according to an aesthetic plan designed by the physician/surgeon. The physician/surgeon uses the ARTAS® system to program these parameters, and the robot executes the plan with greater precision, speed, and consistency than can be accomplished by any manual system. The robot's software allows the physician to specify which size follicular units to harvest, enabling the surgeon to select only those FUs containing the most hair.

A caveat should be reemphasized at this juncture: While machines such as ARTAS® and the NeoGraft® do have value, they cannot replace the expert skill and knowledge of a trained and experienced hair transplant surgeon. It is well-accepted that any type of cosmetic surgery requires a mixture of technical skill and creativity. No one can remove the artistic component of this process if the objective is to achieve natural-looking results (Jones, 2015).

The ARTAS® robotic system possesses many benefits for the patients, but the most important benefits are minimizing donor wounding and making the process more efficient. Some of the potential advantages of this robotic procedure over its manual FUE counterpart are:

- Increased accuracy of graft harvesting.
- Increased survival of harvested follicular units.
- Harvesting time reduced by 50%.
- Computerized selection of follicular units to maximize hair and minimize wounding.
- Easier extraction of grafts from the sides of the scalp.
- Easier extraction of grafts in patients from different racial backgrounds or with atypical.
- hair characteristics.
- Increased speed and accuracy in creating recipient sites.

However, despite all the previously described advantages, the ARTAS® robotic system can only be used on patients with straight, dark hair and is limited to follicle extraction from the back and sides of the head. Patients with lighter-colored hair or with limited hair in the donor area are not suitable candidates for this procedure. Moreover, graft transection (damage) rates are typically 3%-5% with a manual FUE procedure when performed by a skilled and experienced surgeon, while transection rates using the ARTAS® robot are around 8%-10% (Jones, 2015).

HARRTS™ i-Brain Robotic FUE System

The HARRTS™ machine is the world's only robotic hair transplant system that comes with artificial intelligence (AI) and a speech interface. This product was developed by *i-Brain Robotics*, which is a robotics establishment with merchandise ranging from humanoid intelligent android robots to bionic prosthesis and smart medical devices. This same company developed the humanoid robot with artificial intelligence known as Sandy.

According to *i-Brain Robotics,* hair-transplantation technology is evolving rapidly, and with each passing year there is increased demand for the development of less invasive, less time-consuming, and more automated procedures. Consequently, automated FUE is now seen as the preferred choice for hair transplantation, not only for the surgeons but also for the patients themselves. The earlier automated FUE systems that used suction-based harvesting have numerous limitations that have been eliminated with the HARRTS™ robotic FUE (i-Brain Robotics.com, 2016). Some of the limitations that typically accompanied the suction-based systems are as follows:

- Uncontrolled depth while scoring.
- Dehydration of follicular units (FUs) due to the vacuuming effect.
- Trauma to the follicular-unit tissue while traveling through long suction tubes.
- Trauma to the follicular unit while being handled during implantation.
- Trauma to the follicular units during implantation because of pressurized air.
- Buried grafts.

The manufacturer of this hair-transplant machine claims that all the limitations cited above have been addressed and overcome by the HARRTS™ system.

The HARRTS™ robotic system implantation technique uses novel, patented, piston-type implanters with tweezer-free manipulation. The manufacturer claims that this procedure provides the surgeon with more speed and greater depth precision, creating better results. According to i-Brain Robotics, implantation time is approximately 40 grafts per minute, which results in approximately 2,200 grafts per hour when performed by a skilled surgeon. The company also claims that the machine can effectively reduce follicular-unit extraction time by a factor of four. The company further claims that this new hair-transplant system with artificial intelligence (AI) is set to change the landscape of the hair transplant industry globally (Fig. 10.10).

Fig. 10.10: HARRTS™ i-Brain Robotics FUE system

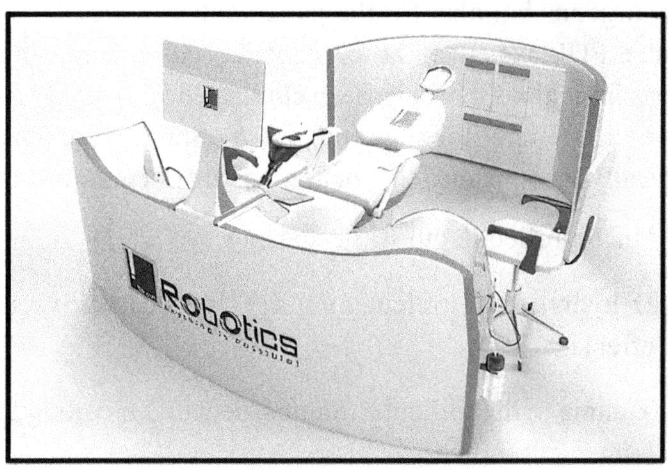

Image Source: http://ibrainrobotics.com/robotic-hair-transplant-system.php

Redefining the "E" in FUE

The term follicular unit extraction (FUE) was coined by Dr. William R. Rassman in 2002. The adoption of the FUE technique began in earnest with the work of several renowned surgeons; Ray

Woods, William R. Rassman, John P. Cole, James A. Harris, and Paul T. Rose. The FUE procedure has undergone various stages of development, from manual to motorized and blunt to sharp, serrated trumpet and flared punches. Presently a robot is also used to perform the FUE procedure with the capability of performing the extraction and incision components.

Since the FUE technique encompasses an extraction and incision component, Dr. Parsa Mohebi, head of the nomenclature committee of the *International Society of Hair Restoration Surgery (ISHRS)*, recommended a name change for the procedure. Dr. Mohebi recommended using the term ***"Follicular Unit Excision"*** to replace *"Follicular Unit Extraction"* as a more appropriate term to describe the FUE technique. Dr. Mohebi and the nomenclature committee contend that this new term explains the two steps of the surgical process: incision and extraction, and the incision component needs to be performed by a physician. FUE is a surgeon-based, time-consuming procedure with a long learning curve (Gang & Gang, 2018).

Direct Hair Implantation (DHI)

Direct Hair Implantation (DHI) is the most recent and costly innovation in the hair restoration field. This procedure is marketed as a pain-free and scar-free procedure, making it perhaps the most sought-after type of treatment for male and female pattern baldness. However, despite these claims, it is important to note that while considered minimally invasive, DHI is still a surgical procedure performed under local anesthetic. Therefore, the patient should expect some minor scarring and a certain degree of pain and discomfort.

DHI is a modified FUE technique. With DHI, hair follicles are implanted one by one directly into the thinning area that needs to be covered. Compared to other hair-transplantation methods, such as FUE and FUT, DHI does not require reception incisions or holes in the recipient area. Hair follicles are implanted directly into the area with a specific angle, depth, and direction using the patented DHI implanter tool (Fig. 10.11). Proponents of this method claim that with DHI, the patient will receive a 100% natural result with maximum hair growth viability. Moreover, with DHI, there is no hair-follicle processing to avoid the risk of necrotic cutting and prevent the negative effects of hair follicles from staying outside their natural environment for too long. Instead, the extracted hair follicles are directly placed and kept at a specific temperature in a solution that enhances their development after placement.

Fig. 10.11: DHI Implanter Tool

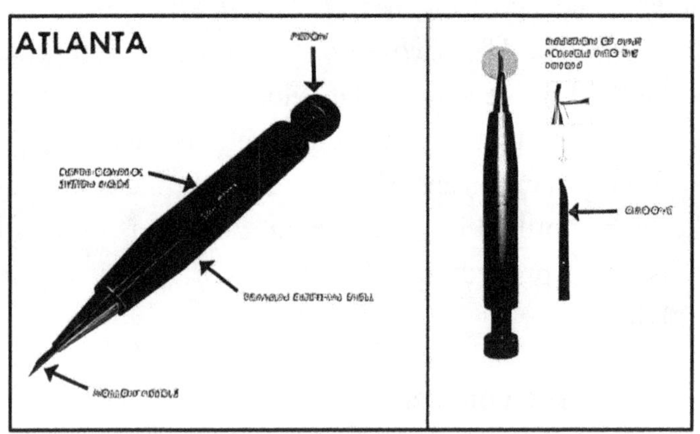

Image Source: http://www.medicaltrain.es/hair-implanter-atlanta-model

Differences Between Hair Transplantation Methods

One of the main differences between FUE and DHI is that patients undergoing the FUE procedure need to shave their scalp before surgery. In contrast, no shaving would be required before undergoing DHI. The DHI technique is a modified FUE innovation that employs a patented implanter tool called the *Choi implanter*. The proponents of DHI claim the technique provides 100% natural results with maximum viability. With the FUE method, hairs are harvested individually or in follicular units of approximately two to four hairs so that roughly 2000-3000 hairs can be extracted and implanted into the bald areas during a single session. During a FUE session, the follicles are often moved using forceps, which can cause damage to the hair follicles and lead to the reduced success of the implanted hair (Fig.10.12).

Fig. 10.12: Follicular Unit Extraction with Forceps

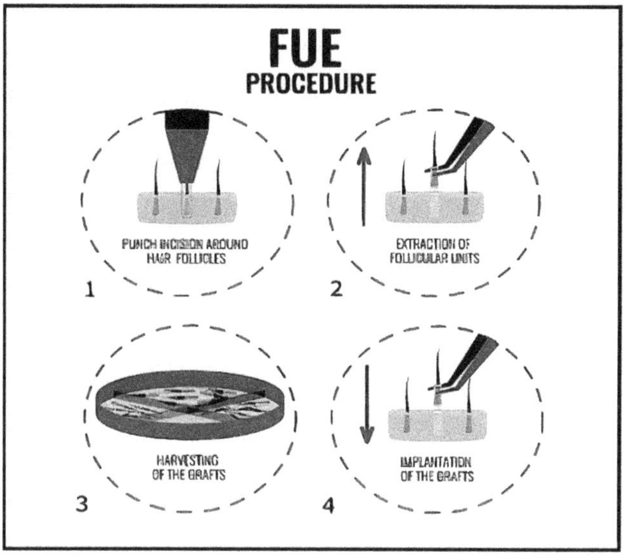

Image Source: http://www.istockphoto.com/vector/fue-stages-treatment-gm643567570-116958313

Conversely, according to proponents of the DHI method, the physician can replace up to a maximum of 6000 hairs in a single session. With DHI, there is no need for reception incisions or holes in the recipient area. Therefore, hair follicles are implanted directly into the recipient site using the patented DHI Choi implanter tool. This implanting tool provides full control of the depth, direction, and angle of placement of each graft, which developers claim diminishes the likelihood of causing damage to the individual hair follicles, thus increasing the procedure's success rate. A prospective patient is more likely to be deemed unsuitable for the FUE procedure compared to DHI because FUE requires a certain type of hair to be successful. In addition, while trained nurses can perform FUE, only specialized doctors can perform DHI.

The Strip/FUT method, as previously mentioned, will leave a scar from where the strip of hair was removed from the back and sides of the head, and the skin must be stitched back together. As with FUE, the hair is implanted using forceps, which can potentially damage the individual hair follicles and introduce human error regarding the direction and angle of the placement of the implanted hair. Furthermore, because the strip/FUT hair-transplantation method is often unsuccessful if the patient has particularly curly hair, there is an increased likelihood that candidates will be unsuitable for this type of procedure when compared to DHI. With the strip/FUT technique, the patient can only hope to receive as many as 5000 implanted hairs in a single session if the patient has a good donor area and excellent scalp elasticity. With a DHI, the claim is that a maximum of 6000 hairs can be implanted (Healthcentre.org, n.d.). Table 10.1 below summarizes the different transplant procedures (methods) and the prices/graft differences in the United States between the strip/FUT, FUE, and the DHI methods.

Table 10.1: Comparison between FUT, FUE, and DHI methods

Compare Surgery	FUT	FUE	DHI
Method	Grafting	Grafting	Immediate implantation
Surgery invasiveness	Moderately Invasive	Minimally Invasive	Minimally Invasive
Donor harvesting	Extracted from strip	Extracted one by one	Extracted one by one
Donor scarring	Long fine linear scar	Tiny circular scars	Tiny circular scars
Donor healing time	14 to 30 days	5 to 7 days	5 to 7 days
Pain-discomfort	Minimum to moderate	Minimum	Minimum

Donor closure type	Sutures	None required	None required
Return to work	2 days	Next day	Same day or next day
Exercise or activities	14 to 30 days	5 to 7 days	5 days
Haircut length	Any length	Shaved donor area	Any length
Graft harvest limits (can vary by physician)	5000 max/ session	3000 max/ session	6000 max/ session
Time hair is out of the body	Up to 10 hours	Up to 6 to 7 hours	Seconds
Procedure time	4 to 7 hours	4 to 7 hours	4 to 7 hours
Cost per graft (approximate cost, can vary)	$3 to $6	$8 to $12	$8 to $12
Results time frame	Permanent	Permanent	Permanent

For many people, the cost of undergoing a hair transplant surgery in the United States is not an affordable option. However, with the advances in technology in other countries, hair transplants have become more accessible, safer, and cost-effective. For most US citizens considering hair transplants in another country, the main deterrent to pursuing the procedure was the lack of reliable information on the prices and the quality of the hair restoration clinics performing the procedures.

The price of a hair transplant in Australia, the United Kingdom, and the United States is substantially higher than in other countries due to the higher operating costs associated with conducting business in those countries. The average price of a 2000 grafts hair transplant in the United States is $16,000, based on an $8.00/graft cost, whereas the average price in Turkey for the same 2000 grafts is $3,000, based on a $1.50/graft cost. The large price differential from country to country is one of the main reasons people choose to get their hair transplant procedure done abroad.

The size of the worldwide medical tourism market reached $11.56 billion in 2020 and $13.98 billion in 2021. It is predicted that the market will continue to grow to $53.51 billion by 2028. Medical tourism has gained immense traction worldwide, especially across developed regions. The Medical Tourism Association (MTA) reports that more than 14 million individuals worldwide travel to other countries for medical treatment each year. This growth in medical tourism poses a significant risk for the hair transplant industry.

For example, some countries offer hair transplants at bargain rates, which are included as a package deal with airfare, luxury hotel accommodations, and transportation. However, the lure of combining an exotic vacation with hair transplant surgery should raise a significant red flag, as *black market hair restoration practices are proliferating unchecked*, leaving patients with disastrous results and no recourse. This medical black market problem has become so serious that the *International Society of Hair Restoration Surgery (ISHRS)* has initiated a worldwide patient awareness campaign to help people recognize fraudulent hair restoration clinics and misleading advertising claims.

Hair Stem Cell Transplantation (HST) Method

The Hair Stem Cell Transplantation (HST) method, also known as the *Partial Longitudinal Follicular Unit Transplantation (PL-FUT)*, is a patented— in the United States and Europe— and sophisticated hair-loss treatment process that attempts to multiply hair follicles. In essence, the HST method utilizes the potential of stem cells to regrow hair. Dutch researcher and hair-restoration expert, Dr.

Coen Gho of the Hair Science Institute developed this technique. Dr. Gho's hair-multiplication method is performed exclusively in their proprietary hair-restoration clinics worldwide in locations like Amsterdam, Maastricht, Cap d'Antibes, London, Vienna, and Jakarta.

The HST method does not remove the entire hair follicle as in most other traditional hair- transplantation procedures. Instead, what is done is to extract several hair stem cells from the donor site, leaving some cells left in the donor area so they can continue to stimulate hair regrowth. Since only a portion of the stem cells and the hair follicle is removed, the remaining stem cells stimulate new hair growth in a matter of weeks, according to Dr. Gho. Furthermore, Gho claims the remaining and transplanted hair stem cells generate the same quality hair as the existing hairs. The results can be observed approximately nine months after a complete hair-growth cycle has passed.

Therefore, the HST method is predicated on the concept that each hair follicle consists of different areas that contain hair stem cells. The scientific studies conducted by Dr. Gho revealed that there was no need to extract the entire hair follicle. According to Dr. Gho, extracting just a small part of the follicle is sufficient to produce new hairs. Under ideal circumstances, this technique can be used to induce hair multiplication, in essence, creating two follicles from a single follicle to generate hair growth (10.13).

Consequently, the donor area can be used for future hair transplants. This method uses a hollow needle of approximately 0.5 to 0.6 millimeters in diameter. The hair shaft is used as a guide for removing part of the hair follicle. By following the hair shaft, the needle automatically reaches the correct location to remove a few stem cells. This technique makes it possible to extract a small portion of the hair follicle, even if the shape is not ideal. The result is a well-preserved donor area that the surgeon can reuse to harvest new hair follicles for future transplants. Some of the purported benefits of the HST method are:

- Multiple transplants can be performed in a single donor area.
- No scarring.
- Painless treatment.

Fig. 10.13: Stem cells left behind to stimulate further hair growth

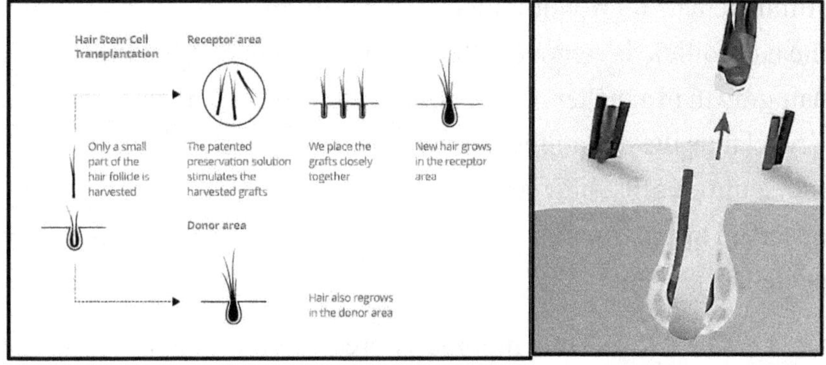

Image Source: Hair Science Institute owner attribution http://www.hasci.com/hair-stem-cell-transplantation/

The reader needs to be aware that the Hair Stem Cell Transplant (HST) method promoted by the *Hair Science Institute (HASCI)* has been the subject of considerable negative debate on Internet hair transplantation forums for quite a while regarding to the donor-area regeneration claims. Some authorities in the hair-transplant community have also criticized it, such as famed hair-transplant surgeon and researcher Dr. William Rassman. The controversy that has arisen regarding this new hair transplant method, which essentially combines elements of hair transplant and hair multiplication, has been fueled mainly by the claim that the developers of the HST method have not presented an independent patient case for verification and analysis.

The literature review conducted on this new hair-regeneration method did not reveal any formal research study addressing this hair-restoration procedure. Therefore, *caveat emptor* and *caveat lector* are applicable principles to be aware of when contemplating this novel hair restoration method. However, despite the lack of documented research on the HST method, it would be safe to say that Dr. Gho's hair transplant advancements at least offer additional hope in the arena of hair restoration. Moreover, it provides the knowledge that fresh approaches and new technologies are being tested and tried with some degree of success.

Innovations and new approaches are always a good thing but, as we all know, not always readily accepted. It is a well-known fact that the success of more traditional hair-transplantation methods is limited by the hair density of the donor area. Dr. Gho's innovative approach promises to circumvent that limitation by creating new possibilities to preserve the donor zone to help men and women afflicted with hair loss. It is appropriate to recall philosopher Arthur Schopenhauer's quote stating that all truths, ideas, or innovations pass through three stages:

- First, it is ridiculed.
- Second, it is violently opposed.
- Third, it is accepted as being self-evident.

As usually occurs, in time, Dr. Gho's innovative approach to preserving the donor zone might prove Schopenhauer's quote correct.

Langer's Lines Concept in Hair-Transplantation Surgery

Langer's lines, cleavage lines, or tension lines are topological lines drawn on a map of the human body. They correspond to the natural orientation of collagen fibers within the dermis (skin) and are generally parallel with the orientation of the underlying muscle fibers. Therefore, Langer's lines is a term used to define the direction within the human skin along which the skin has the least flexibility.

Langer's lines is an important concept relevant to forensic science and crucial to the development of surgical techniques. These cleavage or tension lines are of particular interest to surgeons because an incision made parallel to the lines heals with a fine, linear scar. In contrast, an incision across the lines may set up irregular tensions that result in the development of an unsightly scar (Wolf, 1998). In fact, incisions or wounds against Langer's lines have been described to have a poorer final cosmetic appearance when compared to incisions or wounds along the Langer's lines (Carmichael, 2014). Therefore, Langer's lines are important because they serve as a way to mark the directional growth of the collagen fibers (Fig. 10.14 and 10.15).

Fig. 10.14: Langer's (cleavage) Lines of the Body

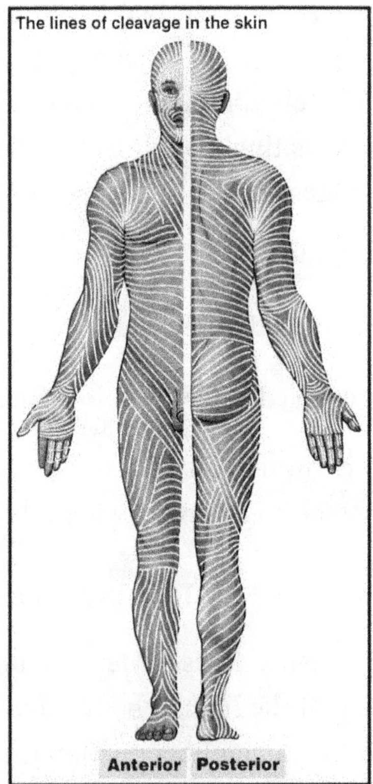

Image Source: http://www.emdocs.net/update-on-the-management-of-skin-abscesses-in-the-emergency-department/. emDocs is licensed under a Creative Commons Attribution 4.0 International License. © 2011 Pearson Education Inc.

Fig. 10.15: Langer's Lines of the Head (frontal and lateral views)

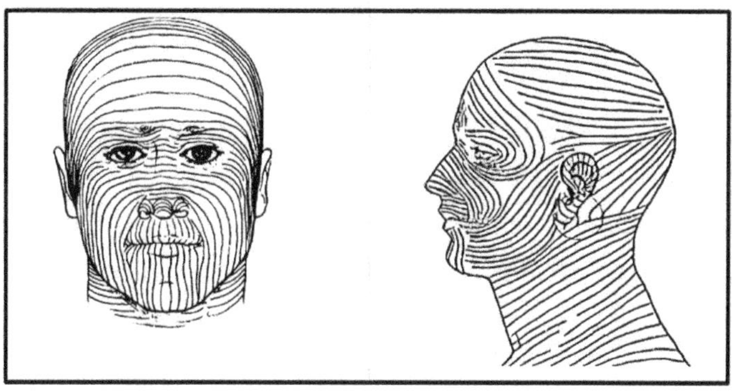

Image Source: Paul SP. Biodynamic Excisional Skin Tension (BEST) Lines: Revisiting Langer's Lines, Skin Biomechanics, Current Concepts in Cutaneous Surgery, and the (lack of) Science behind Skin Lines used for Surgical Excisions. Journal of Dermatological Research 2017; 2(1): 77-87 Available from: URL: http://www.ghrnet.org/index.php/jdr/article/view/1850/2323. Open Access Journal. Licensed under CC attribution (CC BY-NC 4.0)

Understanding the concept of Langer's lines is especially useful for cosmetic procedures, where the ultimate goal is to achieve an aesthetically pleasing outcome with minimal scarring. Austrian anatomist Karl Langer originally discovered the lines in 1861. However, Langer credited the French anatomist and surgeon *Baron Guillaume Dupuytren* as the first surgeon to recognize the cleavage lines phenomenon. Notwithstanding his recognition of Dupuytren's contribution, Langer would decades later propose the concept of the directional growth of connective tissue, which is what determines the size and shape of a wound.

Thus, knowing the direction of Langer's lines within a specific skin area is essential for surgical operations, particularly in cosmetic surgery. If a surgeon chooses where and in what direction to make an incision, they may decide to cut in the direction of Langer's lines. Incisions made parallel to Langer's lines may heal better and produce less scarring than those that cut across the lines. Conversely, incisions perpendicular to Langer's lines has a tendency to pucker the skin and remain visible, although sometimes this is unavoidable. Langer's lines are routinely violated in hair-restoration surgery, and keloids are more common when an incision is made across Langer's lines (Lai Saha & Chintamani, 2014).

Invariably, scars that violate Langer's lines create wider scars when healed. The less parallel the incision is to Langer's lines, the wider the scar. Hair-restoration procedures can afford to violate Langer's lines more frequently than other cosmetic surgeries, primarily because of an abundance of hair that can hopefully camouflage the resulting scar. In fact, certain scalp-expansion procedures regularly violate Langer's lines on principle, as does the circular punch graft device itself. According to Dr. Bradley R. Wolf (2015), hair restoration that can be accomplished with the least amount of scarring will yield the most aesthetically acceptable results.

Besides Karl Langer, other researchers have created their own topological skin maps. For example, Kraissl's lines differ from Langer's lines: Langer's lines were defined from cadavers in rigor mortis, while Kraissl's lines were defined in living individuals, and Langer's lines are defined in terms of collagen orientation, while Kraissl's lines are defined as the lines of maximum skin tension (Bland, Sarr & Csendes, 2008). They are oriented perpendicular to the action of the underlying muscles. Moreover, the method used to identify Kraissl's lines is not a traumatic one (Kraissl, 1951). Later, Borges described relaxed skin-tension lines, which follow furrows formed when the skin is relaxed and are produced by pinching the skin. However, these are only guidelines; there are many contributors to the camouflaging or disguising of scars, including wrinkle and contour lines. Borges' and Kraissl's lines—not Langer's—might be the best guides for elective incisions of the face and body, respectively (Wilhelmi, Blackwell & Phillips, 1999).

In concluding this chapter, it is important to note that the hair-restoration field has had a chequered history. From the days of punch grafting to the present-day follicular unit hair transplantation techniques, the field has experienced numerous beneficial advances.

As with any medical field of practice, innovation continues to drive results. Notwithstanding these innovations, it is essential to understand that in all hair-restoration procedures, the surgeon's expertise and skill are as crucial to the procedure's success as the specific surgical method or technology being used. Moreover, an experienced, well-trained, and skilled surgeon can usually anticipate any cosmetic and psychological problems before they arise and take the necessary steps to mitigate these issues. Therefore, hair-transplantation surgery remains an art form as much as a science, and prospective hair-transplant candidates who ignore this important fact in a rush to use newly available technologies are doomed to disappointment (Shiell, 2008).

11

Alternative Surgical Methods for Correcting Hair Loss

There are two other surgical methods for correcting alopecia, or hair loss, which have nothing to do with punch grafts, strip/FUT, FUE, DHI, HST, scalp reduction, or pedicle flap surgery. These alternative surgical procedures were performed by surgeons to either improve, increase, or reduce scalp circulatory blood flow. Dr. Schein (1909) of Budapest, a dermatologist of high repute, believed that baldness directly resulted from depressed scalp circulation. Schein contended that this reduction in scalp circulation resulted in the improper nourishment of the scalp. In other words, this depressed scalp circulation could lead to an inadequate nourishing influence of the hair papilla, resulting in hair loss.

Surgical Procedure to Increase Scalp Circulation

Dr. Schein further claimed that a degenerative process of the scalp capillaries resulted in baldness because the cranial muscles—the occipitofrontalis and the temporoparietalis— cause a stretching action of the scalp blood vessels and tissues. Consequently, with this tightness of the scalp muscles, the hair bulb receives a reduced capillary blood flow resulting in inadequate nutrition of the hair papilla. Because of Schein's theory, it was believed that baldness was the direct result of diminished or depressed scalp circulation for many years. There have even been surgical procedures developed to relieve the tightness of the scalp in the hope that it would improve scalp circulation and thus its nourishment.

Many investigators advocated for such an operation, intending to reduce the tension of the galea aponeurotica. The galea aponeurotica, also known as the epicranial aponeurosis, is a tough layer of a thick fibrous band that covers the upper part of the cranium in humans and various other animals (Fig.11.1). The surgical procedure developed to reduce the tension of the galea is called a *galeatomy.* It is an operation for dividing the epicranius or the epicranial muscle. A review of the literature indicates that the origin of this surgical procedure dates back to the 1960s. During the 1960s, Dr. Lars Engstrand of Stockholm, Sweden, conducted a study to determine what causes baldness. Engstrand concluded that baldness was caused by the insufficient blood supply to the scalp, which was caused in turn by a thickened scalp membrane, the galea aponeurotica. Moreover, it has been postulated that hormones and stress can make the galea tense and taut, which can further aggravate the condition. Based on the study, Dr. Engstrand surmised that the thickened galea pressured and reduced the blood supply even more as it became enlarged.

Fig 11.1: The Epicranius and Associated Muscles

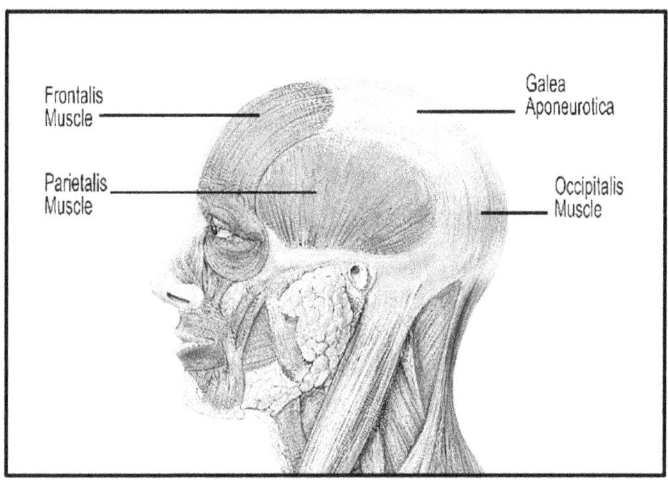

Image Source: By Patrick J. Lynch, medical illustrator- Patrick J. Lynch, medical illustrator, CC BY 2.5. https://commons.wikimedia.org/w/index.php?curid=1498151. Modified image to include muscle classification.

Because of this hypothesis, Dr. Engstrand reasoned that if the galea could be reduced to a normal thickness, the blood supply to the scalp would improve, and the baldness would be stopped, thus facilitating the regrowth of hair. To accomplish this objective, Engstrand developed a surgical procedure called the *"Radical Scalp Operation"* to correct the galea aponeurotica surgically. By performing this operation, the tightness of the scalp would be relieved, which would lead to improvement in scalp circulation and improved nourishment of the hair bulb and dermal papilla. According to a 1964 report, Dr. Engstrand had performed more than 1,000 successful operations, with 70%-80% of the patients experiencing hair regrowth within six months to a year after the operation. Moreover, even in cases of complete baldness, there was supposedly new hair growth in 40%-50% of the cases (Segrave, 1996).

Although the galeatomy operation has been around for more than half a century, it is not presently performed in the United States. However, the procedure is currently performed in Belgium by the Wellness Kliniek and in Thailand by Urban Beauty Thailand Co., Ltd. The Wellness Kliniek claims that they have been successfully performing the surgery for more than ten years, with a patient satisfaction rate of over 98%. Additionally, the clinic claims that the results have been assessed in accordance with the quality standards of ISO 9001(WellnessKliniek, 2016). ISO 9001 is essentially a set of international standards for management and verification of good quality management practices. ISO (International Organization for Standardization) is a worldwide organization that certifies that businesses, government organizations, and social entities meet certain common standards of quality (ISO.org, 2016).

The Urban Beauty Thailand establishment recommends combining conventional hair transplantation with a galeatomy. They contend that the galeatomy is a surgical operation that serves to prevent further hair loss. They further claim is that undergoing the galeatomy procedure significantly decreases the probability of having to readdress hair loss soon after restorative hair-transplantation surgery. Despite the claims of success by the Wellness Kliniek in Belgium and Urban Beauty Thailand Co., Ltd regarding their galeatomy operation, not every authority agrees with these results.

According to present-day, world-renowned hair-transplantation surgeons William R. Rassman and Bishan Mahadevia, the scalp has a clear blood supply coming from the front, sides, and back of the head. These physicians contend that the blood supply lies above the galea aponeurotica; therefore, cutting the galea makes no logical sense. Thus, cutting the galea will not increase the blood supply to the scalp. In fact, Dr. Rassman adamantly contends that competent doctors do not perform this barbaric procedure to treat hair loss, even though Dr. Lars Engstrand reported successes with the procedure during the 1960s. Here we see the ever-present conflicting evidence that can result from research reports.

Some well-known physicians who have used the galeatomy surgical procedure, albeit not always successfully, are renowned surgeons Humplik (1959), Friederich (1959), P.F. Corso (1961), and Ponten (1963). While some of these investigators performed this procedure and reported successful results, in 1961, Dr. Sandler reviewed this subject extensively and concluded that the results were less than impressive. Furthermore, Sandler criticized all operations that were performed to supposedly relieve the alleged abnormal tension of the scalp.

Because of Dr. Schein's theory, hair-restoration establishments have attempted to improve scalp circulatory blood flow in several ways:

- Physiotherapeutic massage of the scalp, either by hand or mechanical vibrators.
- Devices to stand on the head for several minutes a day.

- Massaging proprietary herbal solutions on the scalp.
- Massaging oils, such as rosemary, geranium, lavender, almond, olive, and coconut oil.
- Application of vasodilator drugs, like minoxidil.
- Biotin creams, gels, and other proprietary solutions.

These methods to improve scalp circulation have been used by hair-restoration establishments, most of which have been ineffective in restoring hair loss. The objective of all these treatment modalities is to separate the consumer from their hard-earned money. In fact, confirming the lack of efficacy of these treatments, back in 1980, an advisory panel to the U.S. Food and Drug Administration (FDA) was convened to evaluate many of the substances contained in hair-loss lotions and creams. Some of these substances were amino acids, aminobenzoic acid, ascorbic acid, benzoic acid, B vitamins, hormones, jojoba oil, lanolin, sulphanilamide, tetracaine hydrochloride, urea, wheat germ oil, and polysorbates 20, 40, and 60. Polysorbates are a class of emulsifiers often used in cosmetics to solubilize essential oils into water-based products. Additionally, the FDA evaluated other balding remedies that were considered ineffective in resolving hair loss, such as scalp massage, frequent shampooing, scalp electrical stimulation, Chinese herbal extracts, and dietary modification (Orentreich & Orentreich, 1995).

Following its evaluation, the FDA panel recommended that all these products should be removed from the market (Hecht, 1985). In view of the ineffectiveness of the majority of these topical hair-loss products, it is strongly recommended that individuals experiencing hair-loss problems become informed consumers by seeking the advice of competent healthcare professionals well-versed in the field of alopecic conditions before seeking help from any hair-restoration establishment.

Surgical Procedure to Decrease Scalp Circulation

In 1977, Dr. Raymond E. Marechal proposed another interesting theory for the treatment of seborrheic alopecia. His hair-loss treatment aimed to treat hair loss by inducing a hypoxic (low-oxygen) environment that he believed would inhibit the enzymatic systems and lessen the damaging action of androgen and lipid factors on the pilosebaceous effectors. In essence, what Dr. Marechal was attempting to inactivate was the testosterone/DHT conversion metabolism by inhibiting 5-alpha-reductase (5AR), which is the enzymatic system that facilitates the conversion of testosterone to DHT and is currently believed to be the mechanism responsible for androgenetic alopecia (AGA).

Dr. Marechal's surgical treatment for alopecia was geared at bilaterally ligating the superficial temporal and posterior auricular arteries. His contention was that by performing this ligature procedure, the arterial circulatory hemodynamics of the scalp's ligatured areas would be converted into a slower capillary-type circulation, thereby reducing the speed of the normal circulatory blood flow in the hair-loss-affected areas by what he estimated to be a factor of approximately 200.

Marechal's contention was that the reduction in circulatory blood flow from the procedure would produce a state of hypoxemia (low oxygen level in the blood) by diminishing the partial pressure of oxygen (PaO2) (i.e., a deficiency in the amount of oxygen delivered to the body tissues) in the ligated affected areas. The hypoxemic state produced by the reduction in blood flow would tend to inactivate the conversion of testosterone to DHT, which is the enzymatic system currently believed to be responsible for balding by androgenetic stimulation. By producing this hypoxic state, Dr. Marechal claimed that the action of the androgen testosterone and lipid factors on the pilosebaceous system would be brought under control.

While this theory has not been fully accepted worldwide, Marechal claimed that 57% of the 1,300 cases he performed the procedure on were cured; another 19% showed improvement, and 24% remained unchanged. Moreover, to validate his findings, he presented histological evidence demonstrating a reduction in sebum production, and he showed evidence that the appearance of the hair follicle was distinctly improved. He further believed that the best candidate to undergo the procedure was a young, balding patient because the surgery would halt or stop the evolution of the disease process toward a more severe and extensive type of hair loss.

Furthermore, Marechal also disagreed with the claims that epicraniotomies (galeatomies) increased blood circulation of the scalp. On the contrary, he contended that what this surgical procedure actually did was to reduce the circulation to the scalp. In fact, he claimed that the good results obtained through the incision of the epicranial (galea) aponeurosis were comparable to his own results because the technique produced the same circulatory result, which was restraining transportation of blood to the level of hair. If these claims by Dr. Marechal are valid, they would indicate that— if a galeatomy decreases scalp circulatory blood flow rather than increase it, as Drs. Schein and Engstrand suggested— then the reason for some of the successes of this procedure is because it inactivates the testosterone/DHT conversion system due to the hypoxemic environment created by a reduction of scalp circulation.

An interesting research study conducted by researchers Freund and Schwartz (2010) seems to contradict Dr. Marechal's research conclusions that a low-oxygen (hypoxic) environment inactivates the testosterone/DHT conversion process. The study was entitled "*Treatment of Male Pattern Baldness with Botulinum Toxin: A Pilot Study.*" This study is considered important because it demonstrated that testosterone conversion to dihydrotestosterone (DHT) occurs in a hypoxic environment. Freund and Schwartz contended that the muscles, or anything that constricts (decreases) blood flow, would also reduce the availability of oxygen in the scalp and dermal papilla.

According to Freund and Schwartz (2010), the scalp behaves like a drum skin mechanistically, with tensioning muscles around the periphery. These muscle groups— the frontalis, occipitals, periauricular, and to a minor degree, the temporalis— can create a tight scalp when chronically active (Fig. 11.1). Because the blood supply to the scalp enters through the periphery, a reduction in blood flow would be most apparent at the distal ends of the vessels, specifically, the vertex and frontal peaks. Consequently, these areas of the scalp have manifested the following conditions:

- Sparse hair growth.
- Shown to be relatively hypoxic (inadequate oxygenation of the blood).
- Have slow capillary refill.
- Have high levels of dihydrotestosterone (DHT).

Conceptually, Botox® loosens the scalp muscles, which reduces the pressure on the perforating vasculature, thereby increasing both blood flow and oxygen supply. Freund and Schwartz (2010) contend that the enzymatic conversion of testosterone to DHT is oxygen dependent. Thus, in a hypoxemic (low-oxygen) environment, the conversion of testosterone to DHT is favored, which contradicts Dr. Marechal's theory. Conversely, in a high-oxygen environment, more testosterone is converted to estradiol, which reduces DHT levels (Freund & Schwartz, 2010). In essence, Freund and Schwartz discovered the opposite finding from Dr. Marechal. Here again, we see the conflicting findings that can frequently occur among research studies.

Of the forty subjects who participated in and completed the Freund and Schwarz study, none demonstrated any adverse side effects to the botulinum toxin, and the study resulted in a treatment response rate of 75%. This study concluded that there was a statistically significant increase in hair count of 18% between baseline and week 48 of the study. Furthermore, hair loss was reduced by 39%. Therefore, the researchers concluded that strategically placed Botox® injections appear able to indirectly modify this variable by improving circulatory blood flow, which results in new hair growth and reduced hair loss in some men with androgenetic alopecia (Freund & Schwartz, 2010). The Freund and Schwarz research is another study that also appears to demonstrate that improved scalp blood flow may indeed be a primary determinant factor in follicular health.

12

Scalp Reduction Surgery

An interesting and logical spinoff from scalp-flap surgery was the development of the alopecia reduction (AR) operation around 1977 (Unger & Unger, 1978). Chapter 2 addressed some of the various hair-loss classification systems that have been used to differentiate the different stages, or degrees, of baldness. For example, it emphasized the Hamilton and Norwood classifications since these scales are the most commonly used classifications. The degree of hair loss seen in Hamilton's classifications V, VI, and VII and Norwood's IV, V, and VI are quite extensive. In these advanced hair-loss stages, the results that the hair-transplantation procedure can attain are not satisfactory because of the limited donor area.

Because of the unacceptable results attained by the hair transplant procedure in these advanced degrees of baldness, a surgical procedure was developed to serve as a complement to hair transplantation surgery. This surgical procedure has been called scalp reduction, scalp lifting, alopecia reduction, male pattern reduction (MPR), and galeoplasty (GP). This procedure aims to reduce the amount of existing bald areas by resection. The scalp-reduction procedure reduces the balding areas by removing segments of the bald scalp and stretching the hair-bearing scalp to a higher position (Sattur, 2011).

What this procedure accomplishes is saving hair-bearing grafts that can be used for future transplant surgeries. It also reduces the enormity of the operative task for the surgeon because fewer hair grafts will be required to complete the hair transplant operation. Blanchard and Blanchard (1976, 1978) first initiated this procedure during the early 1970s. It was a new surgical approach to correct androgenetic alopecia (AGA) and complement hair transplantation.

A significant reduction can be performed if the scalp is loose enough. Usually, the surgeon can remove a portion of the scalp, two to five centimeters (3/4″ to 2″) wide in one session. Because the scalp is stretched, this procedure diffusely separates the hair in fringe areas, creating an excellent cosmetic effect. Scalp reductions leave scars within the bald areas of the scalp, which are camouflaged by hairstyling or by hair-grafts transplantation. The scalp reduction procedures can either be performed before starting the hair transplant or after the completion of the hair transplant. In the latter situation, the grafts are inserted in such a pattern that leaves an area of the bald scalp to be removed at a later session.

In some cases, a limited number of hair grafts can be done simultaneously with scalp reductions. However, when combining both the scalp-reduction and hair-transplantation (grafting) procedures in the same operation, dangerous consequences can occur. For example, if the overall scalp experiences too much trauma, blood flow may be interrupted, which could result in scalp shock and tissue necrosis (Sattur, 2011; Brandy, 2002).

Scalp Reduction Techniques

Over the years, several scalp-reduction techniques have been developed. However, no one method is adaptable to all patients. The choice of technique is based upon considerations that may include the degree of hair loss, scalp laxity or mobility, the amount of and quality of the hair in the donor area, and whether hair transplantation will be used as a complementary procedure. The scalp-reduction technique is largely a matter of the scalp incision pattern, such as a midline sagittal ellipse pattern, which is the easiest to perform, a Y-pattern, an S-pattern, a circumferential pattern, a lateral crescent pattern, or a Star pattern. Figure 12.1 below shows a few of these scalp-reduction patterns.

Fig. 12.1: Various patterns of scalp reduction incisions

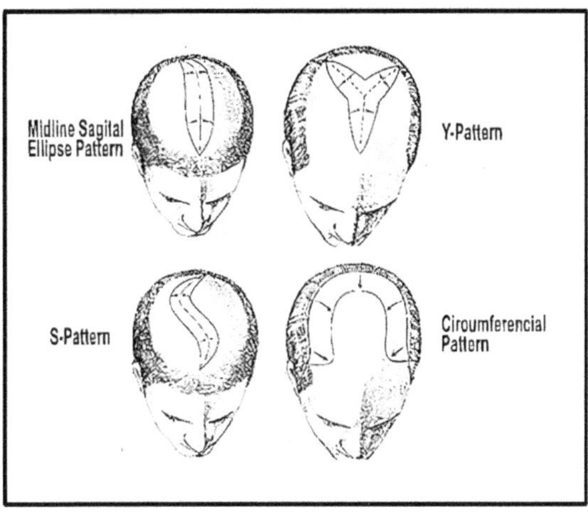

Image Source: https://klinikakolasinski.pl/lysienie-przeszczep-wlosow/odtwarzanie-owlosienia.html

The selection of any particular technique and the rationale for the selection is based on the patient-physician consultation. Any non-emergency surgical procedure must be justified by its applicability and ultimate value to the patient. This is especially true for elective cosmetic procedures such as hair restoration. Therefore, to be considered a good candidate for scalp-reduction surgery, the following criteria should exist:

- The operation recipient must be classified as having Hamilton's baldness classification degree V, VI, or VII or Norwood's IV, V, or VI.
- The recipient should have mobility of the scalp, which essentially means having a loose scalp. This mobility can be estimated or assessed by compressing the parietal area's skin (side of the head) toward the midline.
- The recipient should have a donor area that has sufficiently dense hair on the back and sides of the head to ensure a uniform appearance after surgery.
- The recipient should be a male who is middle-aged or older.

This evaluation is important because the procedure tests the adherence of the skin to the underlying tissue; it does not test the skin's elasticity. Most scalp reductions are performed in several sessions in order to accomplish the final results. The interval between sessions is usually no longer than six weeks.

Potential Complications and Side Effects

Careful planning and expert operative skills are necessary to achieve good scalp reduction results and prevent possible complications and side effects from the procedure. Complications are rare if a skillful and competent surgeon performs the surgical procedure; however, they can and do occasionally occur. The major problems associated with scalp-reduction procedures are typically cosmetic. The following postoperative complications can occasionally occur after a scalp-reduction procedure:

- **Scarring at the Suture Lines.**

  If the procedure is performed improperly, the shape of the residual bald area can become increasingly irregular and more difficult to conceal with each additional reduction procedure.

- **Stretch-Back of Scalp.**

  The scalp has a surprising capacity to stretch, which means that much of the initial baldness, or scalp reduction, can be lost over subsequent months. This phenomenon, called stretch-back, can consume up to 50% of the original gain. In fact, even when all the bald area is removed, the surgeon will still have the problem of future expansion of baldness, which can expose the old scars (Shiell, 2008). Therefore, because of skin elasticity, very often most of the benefit of the resection of the bald scalp is lost over time as the skin stretches back. Due to this inherent skin phenomenon, there is no longer a role for scalp reductions in current hair-transplantation procedures (Dauer, 2014).

- **Slot Deformity Scar.**

  When a scalp-reduction procedure is performed, a large swath, or strip, of bald skin is removed from the crown, and the skin edges are then sewn together. This procedure sometimes left a sizable scar in the midline of the scalp. This type of scar is commonly referred to as a *slot deformity.* That is, the angulation of the hair around the midline scalp scar changes direction and grows out from the scar, looking like a large slit in the middle of the scalp.

Besides the post-operative complications that can result from the scalp reduction procedure, there are some possible side effects:

- Temporary discomfort.
- Swelling.
- Numbness in the surgical area.

Objective of Performing the Scalp Reduction Procedure

It is appropriate to reiterate that scalp or alopecia reduction is a surgical procedure aimed at reducing the size of the area of hair loss by resection. Figure 12.2 below shows a schematic representation of the possible results for a Y-pattern scalp-reduction procedure with its possible visual outcome.

Fig. 12.2: The Y-Scalp Reduction Method

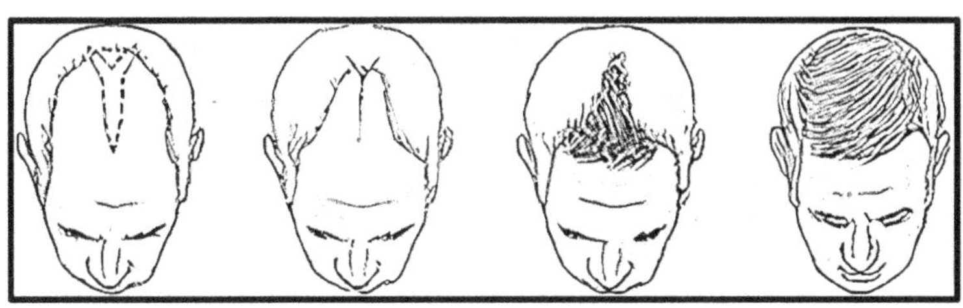

Image Sources: http://www.iranhaircenter.com/english/glossary-e.htm. Modified image.

Visualizing the images above from left to right demonstrates the potential outcome of a Y-pattern scalp-reduction operation:

- In a Y-scalp reduction technique, the skin is removed from within the dotted lines, and the scalp edges are pulled upward and stitched in place.
- Potential results after one or two scalp reductions. Further reduction procedures may be done.
- The bald area has been reduced by scalp reduction. Hair grafts are shown filling in the remaining bald areas.
- An example of hair styling, with the complete result after multiple scalp reductions and hair grafts.

The primary reasons for performing this surgical procedure as an adjunct or complement to hair transplantation are:

- To reduce the number of hair-bearing grafts that will be used during the hair transplantation procedure.
- To reduce the number of sessions required to complete the results of the hair transplant surgery.
- To increase the density of transplanted hair.
- To produce a better cosmetic appearance.

At the time that it was introduced, the scalp reduction procedure appeared to offer great possibilities for a more advantageous, pleasing, and better-looking hair-transplant operation. However, this surgical procedure has fallen out of favor in recent years and is not used very extensively due to the superiority of newer hair-transplantation methods (e.g., follicular unit micrografting, such as FUT and FUE; NeoGraft® automated FUE, ARTAS® and HARRTS™ robotic FUE, DHI, and HST).

13

The Initial Physician-Patient Consultation

It takes a considerable amount of time for a potential hair-transplant candidate to make the final decision to see the hair transplant surgeon. The patient may make several appointments to visit the physician and then cancel them or perhaps not show up at all. Every patient seems to experience an extraordinary amount of fear and anxiety when contemplating the surgical procedure for the very first time. Their fear and anxiety are attributed to their lack of understanding regarding the surgical procedure.

Eventually, out of frustration— because the potential patient has already spent thousands of dollars attempting (unsuccessfully) to find a viable hair-loss solution option— the patient finally decides to visit the physician for consultation. Sometimes the decision to follow through with the appointment is facilitated by seeing and talking with a patient who has had a good hair transplant. This process is probably one of the best ways to select a physician; the patient can view the caliber of work the surgeon is capable of performing.

The initial consultation is the most crucial moment of the patient's association with the physician. During this consultation, some of the fears and anxieties of the patient are alleviated. This consultation allows the patient to ask the surgeon as many questions as necessary regarding the procedure. Conversely, the physician will educate the prospective patient about what hair-transplant surgery is and what it is not. This consultation session is also the time when the physician determines if the patient's donor area makes the potential patient a good candidate for the procedure. Some of the topics that should be discussed during the initial consultation period are:

- Degree of discomfort after surgery.
- Appearance of the final result.
- Cost of hair transplant surgery.
- Age of the patient.
- Long-term results of the hair transplant procedure.

Degree of Discomfort After Surgery

The physician must be very specific when explaining what can be expected from the procedure and the possible resulting discomfort to the potential patient. The patient should be informed that depending on the donor site's health and density, the process could entail a long series of tedious operative procedures that will require considerable patience since hair growth is a slow process.

The patient should also be made aware that the final outcome of the hair transplant procedure depends on how much hair density is available in the safe donor zone. The patient should understand that the original density of hair growth can never be regained, no matter how many operations are performed. Because a hair transplant is essentially a redistribution of hair from a donor site to a recipient site, the quantity of hair is a limiting factor.

The patient should also be made aware that there is a certain degree of pain and discomfort associated with the procedure, both during and after surgery. Usually, the degree of discomfort and pain is minor, especially with the newer, minimally invasive methods such as the NeoGraft® automated FUE, ARTAS® and HARRTS™ robotic FUE, and DHI. Depending on the procedure, most of the pain associated with hair-transplant surgery occurs during the injection of local anesthetic solution into the donor and recipient areas. In fact, to minimize discomfort during the surgical procedure, it is crucial to provide preoperative sedation to reduce patient anxiety, raise the patient's pain threshold, and induce a state of amnesia.

To accomplish this level of comfort for the patient, the physician must consider the following; the choice of local anesthetic agents, the infiltration technique to be used, optimal field and nerve blocks, the timely readministration of anesthesia, maintaining patient hemostasis, and the possible use of analgesics intraoperatively with the goal of keeping the patient comfortable and pain-free. Ensuring the smooth implementation of all these steps is fundamental for a successful hair transplant procedure. Furthermore, to reduce the pain of infiltration, a buffering and warming local anesthetic solution can be administered, as well as employing techniques that decrease sensation or by partially anesthetizing the skin prior to injection (Nusbaum, 2004).

It is essential for the potential hair-transplant candidate to understand that in any hair-restoration procedure, the surgeon's skill is as important as the precise surgical method selected (Shiell, 2008). Consequently, the competence and skill of the surgeon will also directly impact the degree of pain and discomfort the patient will experience.

Appearance of the Final Result

The patient should be aware that, at best, if they cooperate and complete all the transplant sessions that have been suggested, a good and acceptable appearance can be attained. The optimal results in hair transplantation—as they relate to thickness and fullness—are attainable with any well-performed technique, especially in patients with minimal hair loss and an abundant donor site. It is a matter of supply and demand. With male pattern baldness, we are dealing with an increasing demand for a diminishing supply. However, if the loss of hair is slight, then it is possible to achieve an excellent dense growth of hair.

Therefore, if the patient has an ample supply of hair in the donor site and the surgeon is a highly skilled professional, the results can be very natural and satisfactory. It is also important to consider that even with competent surgical technique and no complications, some candidates do not seem to grow transplanted hair as well as others. This is a crucial point that the person contemplating transplant surgery should remember. It is difficult to predict the degree of hair growth that may be attained after hair transplant surgery.

Then again, the patient who understands and accepts the limitations and discomfort of hair-transplant surgery and is still sufficiently motivated to undergo the operation is considered a good candidate. This fact is especially important for the patient who just wants a little more hair and is not expecting a miracle. Any individual planning to follow through with the operation must be patient and motivated since the most common cause of dissatisfaction with the procedure is the failure to complete the required number of hair-transplant sessions suggested by the surgeon.

Cost of Hair Transplant Surgery

It is well documented that most would-be recipients of hair-transplant surgery have not undergone the operation because of the expense associated with the procedure. Currently, the industry-standard regarding pricing is based on a per-graft basis. This pricing model allows each client to pay for only the number of grafts they need, unlike a flat rate that could end up being more expensive.

The per-graft cost of a strip/FUT procedure is generally less expensive than a FUE procedure. However, in response to the rising popularity of the FUE technique, many hair-transplantation clinics have started lowering the cost per graft on FUE procedures so that the cost differentials between the two types of methods are not that significant. The cost of medical procedures always varies by a patient's condition, needs, and objectives; therefore, prices are quite elastic. Moreover, the hair-restoration industry is becoming extremely competitive, and that competition leads to lower prices.

Typically, if hair loss is not that extensive (i.e., requiring under 1,000 hair-transplant grafts to cover the bald area), the cost is usually $3.00 to $5.00 per graft for a FUT hair transplant. However, should the patient desire to have a FUE hair transplant procedure, the cost is approximately $7.00 to $9.00 per graft. If an extensive hair transplant is required— greater than 1000 grafts— the cost per graft could be $5.50 to $7.00 per graft or lower. Therefore, the cost per graft becomes more economical if the hair transplant requires a large number of grafts. In other words, doubling the number of grafts the patient receives will not necessarily double the price of the hair transplantation procedure. The hair- transplantation and restoration industry is a competitive environment subject to the laws of supply and demand. This means that prices could fluctuate from state to state and city to city, and country to country. The reader should be aware that the graft prices described herein are for informational purposes only since the industry is very elastic and costs will vary.

It is crucial at this juncture to issue a warning to anyone who might be contemplating hair-transplant surgery. The potential hair-transplant recipient should not look for bargains or the cheapest transplant available, including in the United States or any other countries abroad. For example, hair transplantation in Turkey has skyrocketed in popularity in recent years, thanks mainly to the growing popularity of this operation and the economical price of the procedure. Hair transplantation has become so popular that, according to market sources, the industry will reach the $40 billion target by 2025. Moreover, with the rise in the popularity of hair transplantation, even hairstylist establishments have risen to the occasion to satisfy the soaring demand for this service (Avi Stern, 2022).

Furthermore, because of the increased demand for hair restoration services worldwide, the ISHRS faces a growing problem of fraudulent, illicit clinics performing hair restoration surgery on unsuspecting consumers. ISHRS members continue to report that they are seeing an increasing number of patients seeking treatment to repair previous hair transplants performed on the black market. Due to this concerning safety issue, the ISHRS recently started a public awareness campaign called "***Fight The FIGHT,***" which stands for ***Fight the Fraudulent, Illicit & Global Hair Transplants,*** to address the alarming problem of non-physicians illegally performing hair restoration surgery around the world.

Looking for the most economical hair transplant is a dangerous selection practice that could lead to disastrous consequences, including disfigurement of the scalp resulting from an improperly performed hair transplant. As with any restorative surgical procedure, looking for a cheap transplant is asking for trouble. Always look for the best, and if you cannot afford it, then do not do it until you can afford it. It might be of interest to the reader that the cost of hair transplant surgery may be covered by insurance in some cases of hair loss resulting from trauma, such as scarring-type alopecia or a disease process.

Age of the Patient

There is some controversy regarding early hair transplantation on individuals who are not yet extensively bald. The controversy arises because hair transplantation on a younger individual before the hair-loss pattern has been fully determined makes it a risky procedure. The risk lies in the fact that for younger individuals, the hair-loss process may continue to occur for many years.

Most conscientious hair-transplant surgeons would prefer first to stabilize the patient's hair loss using available hair-loss medications before contemplating the hair-transplant procedure. The situation is substantially better if the candidate is over 30 years of age since the pattern of baldness in this age group is usually pretty well determined, in contrast to candidates in their early twenties. What the physician is trying to determine here is the progression of the pattern of baldness, which is sometimes hard to decide when the patient is in his twenties.

Most patients who become severely bald lose most of their hair during their twenties, which makes them only average candidates for hair transplant since the progression of their hair loss is unpredictable. Conversely, patients in their 30s usually lose their hair slowly and in a more predictable pattern, making them better candidates than the twenties age group.

Another postulated theory regarding early hair transplantation is that in androgenetic-type alopecia, early transplanting into an area exhibiting progressive baldness might slow down the progression of hair loss. The premise behind this postulated theory is that— as demonstrated in macaque monkeys— the pilosebaceous unit, in areas of active androgenetic baldness, produces increased amounts of dihydrotestosterone (DHT), which results in hair loss (Novak & Meyer, 2009). This increased amount of DHT formed in the hair follicle will not only affect the particular hair follicle but will also have an impact on the surrounding hair. Therefore, the assumption is that if bald grafts are removed during transplantation from the recipient site, which contains high levels of DHT, the circulating tissue level of DHT will be reduced by the removal of the bald grafts. However, while this hypothesis appears to have some merit, the theory has not yet been proven in human beings.

Long-Term Results of Hair-Transplantation Surgery

One crucial question that arises in people's minds regarding hair-transplantation surgery is: How long will the transplanted hair grow after the procedure? According to Dr. Orentreich's observations, hair-bearing grafts continue to grow in their recipient sites as long as the hair on the donor site continues to grow. This is the primary reason why determining the *safe donor zone* of follicular extraction, as proposed by Dr. Unger, is of vital importance for the ultimate success of hair transplantation (Fig. 13.1).

Fig. 13.1: The safe donor zone for follicular unit extraction

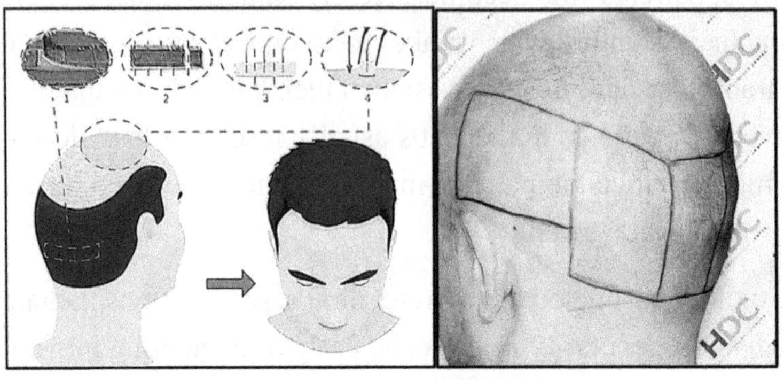

Image Source: http://www.istockphoto.com/vector/fut-hair-loss-treatment-gm639598442-115371733. http://www.hairtransplants-hdc.com/blog/item/state-of-the-art-hair-transplants-in-cyprus. (Use with permission).

Many surveys have been performed to ascertain the longevity of transplanted hair. The results indicate that approximately 90% of people who have undergone hair transplantation surgery are satisfied with their results for many years after their initial surgery. As previously mentioned having realistic expectations of the hair transplant surgery was an essential element in avoiding dissatisfaction with the hair transplant procedure. Every potential patient contemplating surgical hair restoration should recognize that hair-transplantation surgery is not a panacea. However, in the past decade, the hair-restoration industry has made significant strides in creating safer, minimally invasive hair restoration methods with an exceptional aesthetic appearance.

According to results reported from the 2020 practice census survey conducted by the International Society of Hair Restoration Surgery (ISHRS), the number of people seeking proven medical and surgical treatments for hair loss grew by 13% from 2016 to 2019. In 2019, specifically, 735,312 surgical hair restoration procedures were performed worldwide, representing a 16% increase from 2016.

Moreover, there were 1,401,589 nonsurgical patients treated in 2019, a 13% increase from 2016. These figures reflect that more than 2 million patients sought treatment for hair loss in 2019.

This increase represents a continuing trend over the last decade of more men and women of all ages turning to hair restoration surgery to resolve their loss problems. The ISHRS has reported a 157% increase in hair restoration patients from 2008 to 2019. The ISHRS attributes the growing popularity of hair restoration surgical procedures to advances in the field and the countless educational opportunities the Society affords physicians to learn the latest techniques from its own expert physician members. With more people seeking treatment for hair loss in 2019, the estimated worldwide market for surgical hair restoration has increased by 10% since 2016. This increased demand for hair restoration services represents an increase of $ 500 million from $4.1 billion in 2016 to $4.6 billion in 2019 (ishrs.org, 2020).

The hair plugs of the past, with their clustered, doll-hair appearance that was part of older hair transplant procedures, are now considered history (Fig. 9.3). Modern hair-restoration surgical practices utilize new technologies, such as platelet-rich plasma (PRP) therapy, platelet-rich fibrin matrix (PRFM) therapy, and specialized surgical techniques such as the NeoGraft® automated FUE, ARTAS®, and HARRTS™ robotic FUE and direct hair implantation (DHI). With these hair restoration methods, the hair follicles for transplantation can be painlessly extracted from the scalp one hair at a time. The hair to be transplanted can now be relocated to thinning scalp areas without leaving any linear scar whatsoever, as is observed with the strip/FUT method.

Chart 13.1 below shows the growth comparisons between the FUT and FUE procedures performed between 2004 and 2014. The chart indicates that in 2014 the FUT procedure was preferred and accounted for a 51% utilization rate compared to a 48.5% utilization rate for the FUE procedure. In 2019, the latest reported data from the International Society of Hair Restoration Surgery (ISHRS) regarding this metric showed that the FUE procedure has continued to increase in popularity. As of 2019, the latest reported statistics, the FUE procedure was used 66% of the time compared to the FUT procedure, which was used only 29.8%. A substantial decrease from 2014, see Chart 13.2 (ishrs.org, 2020).

The main differences between a hair transplant procedure and any other hair-restoration solution are the permanence and results. A hair transplant procedure provides results that look and feel natural. If a skilled and competent surgeon performs the surgery, no one should be able to detect the surgery. The industry's current state has produced advances in medical technology that have not only made restoring one's hair a reality but have also accomplished the dream of creating a natural-looking appearance.

Chart 13.1: Growth progression of FUT vs. FUE from 2004-2014

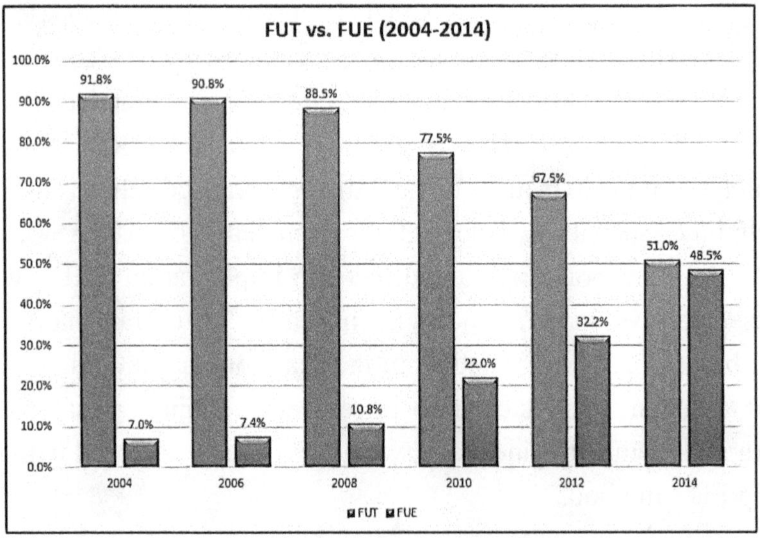

FUT vs. FUE (2004-2014)

	2004	2006	2008	2010	2012	2014
FUT	91.8%	90.8%	88.5%	77.5%	67.5%	51.0%
FUE	7.0%	7.4%	10.8%	22.0%	32.2%	48.5%

Image Source: International Society of Hair Restoration Surgery (ISHRS)

Chart 13.2: Growth Progression of FUE vs. FUT Method 2019

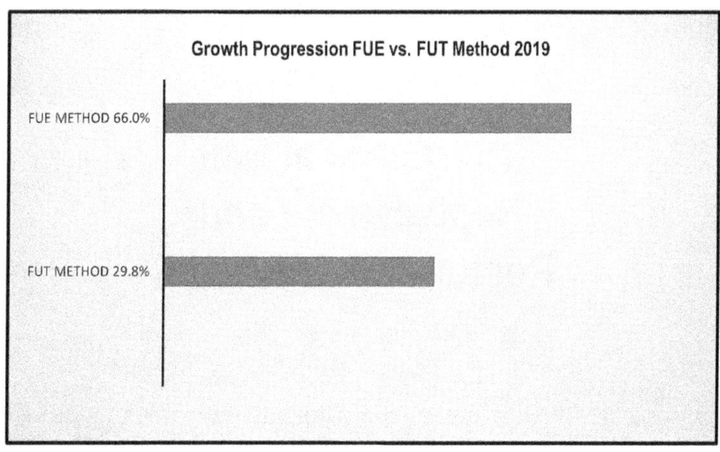

Image Source: International Society of Hair Restoration Surgery (ISHRS)

The hair-transplant surgeon has several different techniques they can use to extract and transplant large numbers of hair follicles. As shown in Chart 13.1, and Chart 13.2 there are essentially two primary techniques used for hair transplantation. These are the FUT and FUE methods, whose primary difference is how the hair follicles are extracted or harvested from the donor area. For more information on these two hair transplant techniques and several others, see Chapter 10.

14

Non-Surgical Hair Replacement and Restoration Methods

This chapter will address the alternative non-surgical of hair restoration methods and replacements available to the consumer. The procedures in this category could either be minimally invasive or non-invasive. This chapter will also address the psychological effects hair loss can have on those afflicted with the condition. The hair-loss restoration industry is full of competing products, such as prescription and over-the-counter (OTC) drugs, shampoos, foams, creams, and lotions that promise the prevention or restoration of the hair. The industry also promotes the use of synthetic hair implantation and the quintessential hair-replacement solutions such as wigs, hairpieces, hair weaves, and toupees. Another non-surgical hair-restoration treatment modality claiming positive results is low-level laser (light) therapy (LLLT).

With the abundance of products and treatment modalities competing for the consumer's dollar, getting objective, reliable information from the mainstream media is quite difficult. Most of the available information provided to the consumer comes directly from either the companies that sell their own hair-loss products or the medical providers offering their therapies. These sources can result in an inherent conflict of interest. They offer plenty of information on their websites; however, getting objective, third-party information not provided by these establishments is difficult to obtain.

In fact, according to a report in the Washington Post, hair-loss sufferers in the United States typically spend well over $3.5 billion per year purchasing hair loss products in an attempt to treat and correct their alopecic affliction. However, the unfortunate truth is that the majority of the products marketed in the ethically challenged hair-loss treatment industry are completely ineffective for most individuals. In reality, according to Spencer Kobren, founder, and president of the American Hair Loss Association (AHLA) and author of *The Bald Truth: The First Complete Guide to Preventing and Treating Hair Loss,* 99% of the hair-loss treatments available today do not work at all.

Moreover, the AHLA— a consumer advocate and non-profit organization— contends that hair loss is an extremely emotionally distressing condition that can make afflicted individuals particularly vulnerable to marketing and advertising scams. For this reason, the AHLA recommends against purchasing any hair-loss product that has not been clinically tested and approved by the FDA or recommended by AHLA.

Some of the minimally invasive and non-surgical methods of hair replacement and restoration described in this chapter are:

- Synthetic Hair Implantation.
- Wigs, Hairpieces, Hair Weaves, and Toupees.
- Low-Level Laser (Light) Therapy (LLLT).

Synthetic Hair Implantation

It is well known in the hair-restoration industry that not every patient is a good candidate for hair transplant surgery. The reason for inadequate candidacy could be that the available hair density in the donor area is insufficient. Moreover, the client might be too young with an undefined baldness pattern that makes it difficult to predict the progression of the hair loss. The physician faced with these dilemmas might recommend one of the non-surgical alternative hair replacement and restoration methods as a better choice. One of these alternatives for hair-replacement methods is the synthetic hair implantation procedure called the dermis inversion process. This hair replacement method utilizes synthetic fibers inserted into the skin with a microscopic anchor that keeps the hair-like fiber embedded in the underlayer (dermis) of the skin. The initial aesthetic results of this method are quite good.

However, the use of artificial hair fibers in hair restoration is controversial. While this alternative product has been marketed as a simple, cosmetically effective remedy, physicians have not widely accepted it because of the lack of proper evidence. The primary problem with this method of fiber implantation is the intense, local reaction that can occur on the scalp resulting from the body's rejection of the synthetic fibers and the anchors used to hold them. This reaction can lead to severe inflammation followed by local infection and necrosis (death) of the skin tissue. Other possible complications include facial swelling, foreign body granulomas, scarring, and permanent hair loss (Mysore, 2010).

Scientific investigation of patients who have undergone synthetic fiber implantation revealed that nearly 100% of the fibers implanted had fallen out by the tenth week following the procedure. In some of these cases, the damage that occurred was so extensive that reconstructive plastic surgery was required to remove the severely scarred and necrotized tissue. The reconstructive procedure required skin grafts and large pedicle flaps.

The potential complications and high monetary expense of hair-fiber implantation make this method an unacceptable type of therapy (Hanke & Bergfeld, 1981; Shiell & Kossard, 1990; Lange-Ionescu & Frosch, 1995; Agrawal, 2008). Because of these unfortunate results, in 1983, the FDA banned this product because of the danger associated with its use. The reasons cited by the FDA for the ban are:

1. The fibers presented risks of illness or injury due to non-biocompatibility of the fibers and non-medical performance of the implant.

2. The fibers presented fraud due to:

- Spreading of misleading information on the efficacy of the results.
- Inadequate information on the risks deriving from the implant method.
- The implant method did not demonstrate any benefit for public health.

The ban on prosthetic hair fibers is regulated by the ***Code of Federal Regulation (CFR) Title 21, Section 895.101, Volume 8,*** which was revised on April 1, 2015. The exact language used by the FDA for the ban reads:

Sec. 895.101 Prosthetic Hair Fibers:

Prosthetic hair fibers are devices intended for implantation into the human scalp to simulate natural hair or conceal baldness. Prosthetic hair fibers may consist of various materials; for example, synthetic fibers, such as modacrylic, polyacrylic, polyester, and natural fibers, such as processed human hair. Excluded from the device banned are natural hair transplants, in which a person's hair and its surrounding tissue are surgically removed from one location on the person's scalp and then grafted onto another area of the person's scalp.

[48 FR 25136, June 3, 1983]

Wigs, Hairpieces, Hair Weaves, and Toupees

The terms "wigs, hairpieces, hair weaves, and toupees" are often erroneously used interchangeably. Therefore, it can be difficult to tell the difference between them and even harder to know which system may be the most appropriate alternative for the user. These alternative hair-replacement options have their aesthetic usefulness in contemporary society. They can be made from either human or synthetic hair. Human hair offers the most natural look and feel. It is also remarkably soft, with shine and movement not easily duplicated with synthetic hair. There are generally four basic types of human hair used to make wigs:

- **Chinese**

Chinese hair has a thicker denier, which results in the hair being extremely straight. Denier is a unit of weight used to indicate the fineness of fiber filaments. This type of hair is more resistant to curling and can, therefore, be harder to style.

- **Indonesian**

Indonesian hair is found in greater supply, and hence it is less expensive. This type of hair can typically be found in ethnic style wigs.

- **Indian**

Indian hair wigs have a thinner denier quite similar to European/Caucasian hair but with a bit more texture. A ***denier*** is a unit of measurement that expresses fiber or hair thickness.

- **European/Caucasian**

European/Caucasian hair is the most sought after for its fine denier. However, due to its increasingly limited supply in the marketplace, it is the most expensive.

The use of human hair is by far the superior choice if the quality is the primary factor being considered. Notwithstanding the quality consideration, it is important to note that human hair's primary shortcoming or deficiency is the amount of maintenance required to retain that quality.

However, synthetic hair has come a long way with new technological advances in recent years. In some cases, it is quite difficult to tell the difference. Even the denier and texture are of such high quality that the fibers feel almost like human hair. In fact, with some of the higher-quality synthetic wigs and hairpieces available today, the consumer would be hard-pressed to differentiate between natural, human-hair products and synthetic hair.

The most appealing aspect of synthetic hair is that it can often be worn right out of the box, requiring little or no styling. However, what synthetic hair offers in ease of use, it lacks in versatility. For example, the product cannot be styled in a variety of different ways like its human hair counterparts. However, the limited versatility of synthetic hair becomes less of a consideration when one factor in affordability (Wigs.com, 2016).

The difference between a wig, hairpiece, and a toupee has to do with the covered portion of the head. A wig is considered one of the oldest hair-replacement systems, dating back several centuries. Wigs can be seen in artifacts recovered from ancient Egypt, Greece, and Rome. A wig is designed to cover the wearer's entire scalp, whether the user is bald or not. Typically, wigs are removed nightly by the wearer upon retiring for the day and are not worn during certain activities, such as bathing. Conversely, a hairpiece is designed to cover part of the scalp or may be added in as a hair extension with the existing hair to make the hair appear fuller or longer or to create highlights within the hair. In contrast to wigs that are used to cover the entire scalp, hairpieces can be worn in more diverse ways.

A toupee is essentially a hairpiece or partial wig worn to cover a limited area of baldness, or in some cases, for theatrical purposes. While toupees and hairpieces are typically associated with male wearers, some women also use hairpieces to lengthen existing hair or cover a partially exposed scalp. Toupees are generally worn to disguise a bald spot on the wearer's head. It is usually attached to the user's head by an adhesive, but the cheaper versions often merely use an elastic band. It is a well-accepted fact that toupee usage is currently on the decline, due in part to better alternative methods of addressing baldness and greater cultural acceptance of alopecia.

This toupee usage decline notwithstanding, it is essential to note that the first patent for a toupee was filed in 1921, and the first patent for a hairpiece was filed in 1956. The toupee and hairpiece industries have constantly been striving to develop better-quality materials and better overall products. These efforts have resulted in the attainment of 60 patents for toupees and over 260 patents for hairpieces (U.S. Patent Database, n.d.).

Hair weaving is another method of hair replacement. A hair weave is essentially a hair-extension technique where human hair is constructed on a weft (woven hairs). They are sewn directly onto a plaited cornrow (braid) base using a hair-weaving needle and thread, thus attaching it securely to the client's scalp. Hair weaving is a technique in which the base of the hairpiece is woven into whatever natural hair the wearer still retains (Fig. 14.1). For this method to work adequately, the client's existing hair must be suitable for this process. This technique requires the natural hair to be healthy and strong enough to withstand the tightness of the braid and the weight of the weave or hairpiece.

Fig. 14.1: The cornrow (braid) base where the hairpiece is attached.

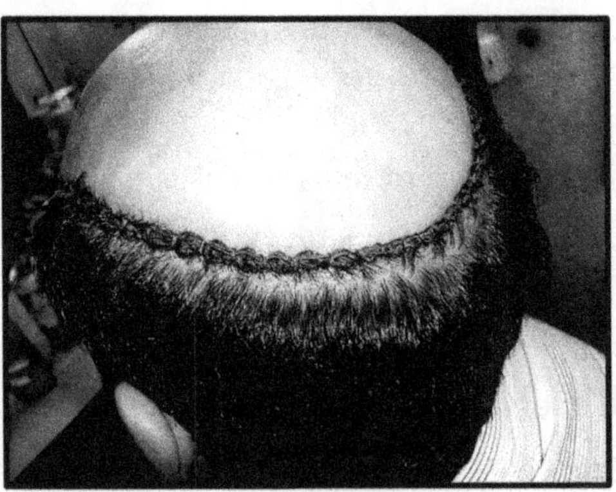

Image Source: http://www.drhaircareclinic.com/drhair/index.php/hair-weaving is licensed under a Creative Commons Attribution-NoDerivs 2.0 UK: England & Wales License.

A professionally done hair weave can last up to three months before the braided hair starts to loosen up. Therefore, this hair replacement method requires periodic readjustments of the hairpiece or toupee since the hair has to be rebraided as it grows. Otherwise, the hairpiece will feel loose and will be mobile on the scalp. Moreover, the hairpiece wearer can experience discomfort and sometimes hair loss (traction alopecia) from frequent retightening of the weave as one's hair grows. Hair-weave methods were very popular during the 1980s and 1990s but are not usually recommended anymore because of the potential for permanent hair damage and hair loss.

Low-Level Laser Therapy (LLLT)

Low-Level Laser Therapy (LLLT) is another alternative hair-loss treatment modality. LLLT, or cold laser therapy, is the application of specific wavelengths of coherent laser light to injuries, skin, cells, and tissue to initiate a healing response. Low-level lasers are referred to as cold lasers because they do not release energy in the form of heat (Acvi et al., 2013). Laser therapy has been heavily debated by reputable hair-restoration physicians and patients for some time. While some physicians reject the use of this treatment modality entirely, others have embraced the therapy and have incorporated it regularly into their medical practice. Moreover, some hair specialists believe that applying LLLT can assist with the post-operative healing process following hair-transplant surgery.

LLLT: A Historical Perspective.

Even though Albert Einstein did not invent the laser, his work laid the foundation for its development. In his 1916 paper entitled *"Zur Quantum Theories der Strahlung,"* which translates to *"The Quantum Theories of Radiation,"* Einstein describes the possible occurrence of stimulated emission of radiation. In fact, the acronym LASER means "Light Amplification by Stimulated Emission of Radiation." Therefore, all it took to eventually invent the laser was for an investigator to find the right kind of atoms and add reflecting mirrors to help the stimulated emission along.

The effects of red light on cellular function have been known since 1880; however, the clinical benefits of red light were discovered serendipitously—as often happens in research—in 1967 during the performance of a laser safety test. A few years after the first working laser was invented, Dr. Endre Mester, a professor of medicine at Semmelweis University in Budapest, Hungary, became interested in determining if laser light could cause cancer.

To test his theory, Dr. Mester shaved a group of mice, trapped half of them in a cage, and exposed them to constant, cold-laser light, leaving the other half unexposed as a control group. To Mester's surprise, exposure to the light did not cause cancer in any of his animal subjects. Instead, what happened was that the mice that were exposed to the laser light therapy grew back their shaved fur much faster than the mice in the control group. Mester's discovery was the first demonstration of what he later termed *"Laser Photo-Biostimulation."*

Mester's contention regarding his study was that the laser light somehow stimulated the hair cells into an accelerated state of hair growth. This discovery led Dr. Mester to become the pioneer of laser medicine, which includes the use of LLLT. Consequently, he is credited as the discoverer of the positive, biological effects of low-power lasers. Subsequently, medical treatment with coherent light sources (lasers) and non-coherent light sources (light-emitting diodes, or LEDs) has evolved as an acceptable treatment modality. Currently, LLLT, also known as cold laser, soft laser, photo-biostimulation, and photo-biomodulation, is used as an effective therapeutic modality in many parts of the world (Hamblin, 2008).

In fact, since the invention of lasers 52 years ago, it has been known that the use of low levels of visible or near-infrared (NIR) light is effective in reducing pain, inflammation, and edema, as well as promoting the healing of wounds, deeper tissue, and nerves.

Originally thought to be a peculiar property of laser light (i.e., soft, or cold lasers), this treatment modality has now broadened to include photo-biomodulation and photo-biostimulation using non-coherent light. Despite many reports citing positive findings from experiments conducted in-vitro, animal models, and randomized, controlled clinical trials, Low-Laser Light Therapy (LLLT) remains a controversial treatment modality. The controversy typically arises for two primary reasons, which are:

- The biochemical mechanisms underlying the positive effects of low-level laser are not completely understood.
- The complexity of rationally choosing from among many illumination parameters such as wavelength, fluence, power density, pulse structure, and treatment timing has led to the publication of many negative and positive studies, leading to increased confusion (Hamblin, 2008).

LLLT as a Hair-Loss Treatment Modality.

In today's society, LLLT is being used as a hair-loss treatment modality. To treat baldness with laser light therapy, the laser rays are directly applied to the scalp by a mechanical device so that red blood cells are stimulated. It is hypothesized that the primary mechanism of LLLT is the stimulation of epidermal stem cells in the hair follicle bulge and shifting the hair follicles into the anagen (growth) phase. Another hypothesis is that lasers work by converting adenosine triphosphate (ATP) to adenosine diphosphate (ADP), releasing energy, and causing cellular metabolic changes (Acvi et al., 2013). During this process, additional nutrients and oxygen are provided to the scalp, assisting the normal chemical processes performed by those cells and increasing overall blood circulation. When applied to the scalp and hair, lasers have been claimed to improve overall hair quality, promote hair growth, and increase the hair shaft's diameter. In several controlled clinical trials, it has been demonstrated that LLLT stimulates hair growth in both men and women (Acvi et al., 2013).

In a recent study by Jimenez et al. (2014) entitled *"Efficacy and Safety of a Low-level Laser Device in the Treatment of Male and Female Pattern Hair Loss: A Multicenter, Randomized, Sham Device-controlled, Double-blind Study,"* the question of whether LLLT is safe and efficacious in the treatment of hair loss was investigated. The objective of this study was to determine if the HairMax LaserComb®— an FDA-cleared, low-level laser device— increases terminal hair density in both men and women with pattern hair loss.

The study by Jimenez comprised 146 males and 188 female subjects with pattern hair loss. A total of 128 males and 141 female subjects were randomized to receive either a laser comb— one of three models— or a sham (dummy) device in concealed, sealed packets. The subjects' entire scalps were treated three times a week for 26 weeks. Subsequently, the terminal hair density of the target area was evaluated at 16-week and 26-week follow-ups. The scalp was analyzed to determine whether the hypothesis formulated prior to data collection— that laser comb treatment would increase terminal hair density— was correct.

This study determined that there was a statistically significant difference in the increase in terminal hair density between laser-comb and sham-treated subjects. Moreover, there were no reported serious adverse events, rendering the device safe. The study results suggest that the application of LLLT may be an effective option to treat hair loss in both men and women. Therefore, since male and female pattern hair loss is a common, chronic, dermatologic disorder with limited therapeutic options, the application of LLLT can now be considered an additional treatment modality in the prevention of hair loss.

In 2009 the research team of Leavitt, Charles, Hayman, and Michaels conducted another 26-weeks double-blind, sham device-controlled, multicenter study specifically to evaluate the effectiveness of the HairMax LaserComb® in restoring hair loss. This study by Dr. Leavitt comprised 110 male-only participants with Norwood-Hamilton classes IIa-V androgenetic alopecia (AGA) who completed the study. The subjects in the HairMax LaserComb® treatment group exhibited a significantly greater increase in mean terminal hair density than subjects in the sham device group. The study results suggest that the HairMax LaserComb® is an effective, well-tolerated, and safe laser phototherapy device for the treatment of AGA on males.

Conversely, another LLLT study entitled *"The Growth of Human Scalp Hair in Females Using Visible Red-light Laser and LED Sources"* conducted by Lanzafame et al. (2014) emphasized the effect of LLLT on female participants only. The study included 47 female participants between the ages of 18 to 60. Moreover, these participants manifested a Fitzpatrick phototyping scale of I–IV, with a Ludwig-Savin baldness scale classification of I-2, I-3, I-4, II-1, and II-2.

Forty-two of the original 47 participants completed the study, which included 24 active and 18 sham participants. There were no adverse events or side effects reported in the study at the diode laser level of 665 ±5 nanometers (nm) and LEDs of 655 ±20 nm. The laser was administered in a bicycle helmet-like apparatus. The study demonstrated a 37% increase in hair growth in the active treatment group compared to the placebo group. Thus, the study concluded that LLLT of the scalp at a wavelength of 655 nm significantly improved hair counts in women with androgenetic alopecia at a rate similar to that observed in male studies using the same LLLT parameters.

Furthermore, well-respected Brazilian dermatologist Dr. Maria A. Muricy (2008) also conducted a HairMax LaserComb® study in Brazil, whose results were subsequently presented at a meeting of the International Society of Hair Restoration Surgery (ISHRS) in Las Vegas. This study evaluated hair growth with the HairMax LaserComb® alone and in combination with minoxidil. The study confirmed an increase in hair shaft diameter, fullness, and overall improvement in hair quality using the laser hair treatment alone.

During the study, biopsies were obtained, and the results of the study demonstrated a reversal of follicular apoptosis (cell death) using B-cell lymphoma 2 (Bcl-2) markers. According to Cleary, Smith, & Sklar (1986), the Bcl-2 gene is the founding member of the Bcl-2 family of regulator proteins that regulate cell death by either inducing (pro-apoptotic) or inhibiting (anti-apoptotic) cell apoptosis. Apoptosis with premature termination of hair follicle growth induces several types of hair loss and is one of the crucial factors of hair loss (Kim, Kim, & Yang, 2014). The Bcl-2 protein is involved in these signals by controlling the intrinsic pathway of apoptosis (Botchkareva, Ahluwalia, & Shander, 2006).

Additionally, Muricy's study demonstrated some statistically significant evidence that LLLT, when combined with 5% minoxidil, provided noticeable cosmetic benefits, especially for women. This finding suggests that LLLT might be a complementary and synergistic hair-loss treatment modality. Some laser treatment devices have a similar appearance to a hood hairdryer, which is placed over the top of the head (Fig. 14.2). The low-level laser will rotate, allowing laser rays—usually red in color— to discharge into the scalp. Handheld devices resembling hairbrushes, such as the HairMax LaserComb® and the Laser Band®, have also been developed (Figs. 14.3 and 14.4).

Fig. 14.2: A Laser Hood Device

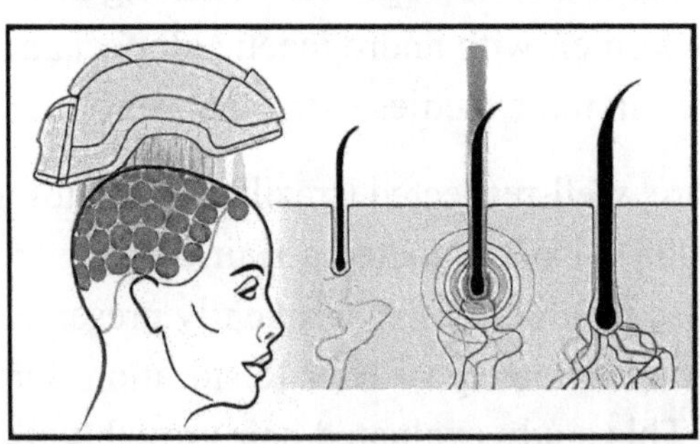

Image Source: http://buytheradome.com/

Fig. 14.3: Low-level laser therapy application with laser brush device

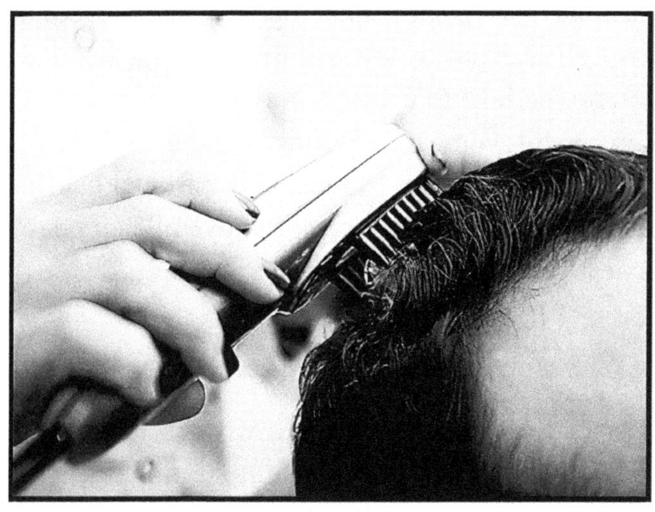

Image Source: http://www.istockphoto.com/photo/hair-therapy-gm171148998-1975600

Fig.14.4: HairMax LaserComb® and LaserBand®

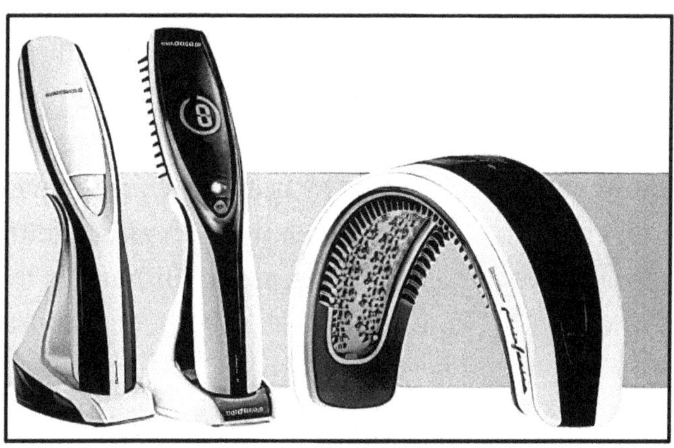

Image Source: https://www.herringtoncatalog.com/products/hairmax-cordless-laserband/?gdffi=dc27bddbbedb44da8220d3b219c6b454&gdfms=DE87DCCAC2934C4FABFB1B126C6E1D1E&gclid=CM6-5N-6rNMCFZm3wAodqWIlew

Physicians have long shared varying views on whether hair laser therapy is a viable treatment modality. While some well-respected physicians reject its use entirely, some believe that LLLT can provide benefits for both men and women suffering from AGA. Furthermore, some physicians believe that laser treatments can assist a hair transplant patient's postoperative wound-healing process as well as expedite new hair growth (Jimenez et al., 2014). Other doctors believe that LLLT may provide similar hair-loss prevention benefits comparable to minoxidil in the mid-vertex and crown areas. However, any benefits to the frontal hairline region are generally attributed to an increase in overall hair quality rather than hair-loss prevention.

Medical Community Opinion on Low-Level Laser Therapy

Most practitioners believe that LLLT works better when combined with other acceptable hair-loss treatment modalities to elicit a synergistic effect. For example, with Propecia® (finasteride) and Rogaine® (minoxidil). As with any treatment modality, LLLT may help some patients more than others, and it has been found to be more efficacious in patients experiencing minimal hair thinning. A growing number of physicians believe that in some patients, LLLT can promote healthy hair growth and increase the hair shaft diameter of miniaturized hair that has been affected by male and female androgenetic alopecia (Muricy, 2010). However, despite the numerous points of view held by healthcare practitioners, it has become apparent that laser hair therapy is an effective treatment modality for hair loss in some patients, as demonstrated in the studies of Jimenez et al. (2014), Leavitt et al. (2009), and Lanzafame et al. (2014).

Despite the emerging positive evidence about laser therapy, some physicians are still skeptical about its effectiveness. In spite of numerous studies to the contrary, these physicians feel that the only thing medical lasers can offer is to deliver energy to target cells. They contend that the only thing that happens when the laser strikes the target cells is that the energy is absorbed and converted to heat, despite the proven fact that cold lasers do not release energy in the form of heat. The consensus among these physicians is that more compelling evidence is required to promote LLLT as a hair-regrowth or hair-loss prevention solution ethically.

Conversely, as previously mentioned, a growing cadre of physicians have embraced laser hair therapy and believe that it works by delivering gentle, nourishing laser light to the hair follicles, stimulating energy production, and creating a healthier environment for hair growth. It is postulated that the boost in laser energy stimulates hair growth by increasing cellular energy through enhanced ATP production and increased blood flow to the follicle, thus supplying more oxygen and nutrients, activating antioxidant defenses, and speeding up the elimination of waste products such as dihydrotestosterone (DHT). Despite the lack of scientific evidence, there have also been claims that LLLT affects and possibly inhibit scalp DHT, the androgen substrate believed to cause the miniaturization process of the hair follicles.

According to the developers of the various FDA-cleared laser hair therapy devices, the creation of a healthier hair-growth environment with improved overall circulatory blood flow can result in the following hair improvements:

- Improved Hair Quality.
- Stimulation of Hair Growth.
- Hair Shaft Diameter Growth.

FDA Clearance of Laser Hair Therapy

The claim by developers of LLLT devices is that the device works by enhancing the natural hair-growth cycle through a process known as *photo-biostimulation*, a term coined by Dr. Mester. The theory is that LLLT devices stimulate the hair follicles to stay in the anagen (growth) stage so that thinning hairs are much more quickly replaced by growing ones. This process helps fight male pattern baldness by shortening the buildup of DHT, which binds to hair follicles, cuts off blood flow and nutrients, and eventually forces the hair to be shed.

Furthermore, as previously mentioned, it is hypothesized that these LLLT devices increase ATP levels, which in turn increase cellular metabolism and cellular activity. Consequently, the hair follicle now has the building blocks and energy to transform from a weakened follicle to a healthy one capable of producing thick terminal hair (Acvi et al., 2013). The claim is that the light delivered by the laser device effectively awakens the individual hair follicle because of the enhanced environment. This improved environment, in turn, invigorates the hair follicle, produces healthier hair, prevents further hair loss, and stimulates the regrowth of hair.

Scientific studies have been performed showing that increases in the amount of the ATP molecule cause the individual cells to increase their activity. ATP is integral to the function of the cell as an energy transporter. The end result is healthier, thicker, and more vibrant hair (Muricy, 2008; Acvi et al., 2013). Figure 14.5 depicts a laser-energized hair follicle.

Fig. 14.5: A Laser-Energized Hair

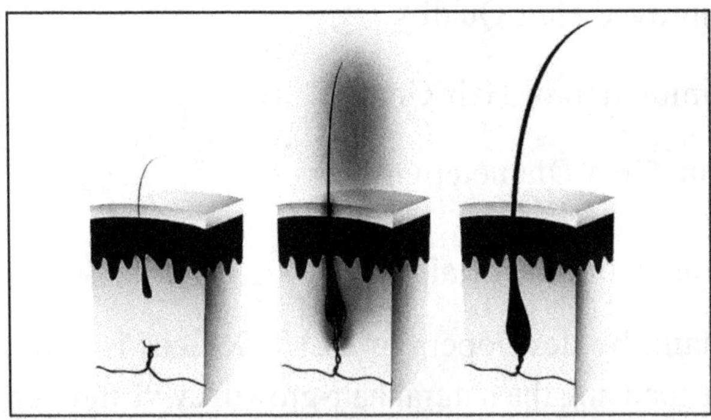

Image Source: http://www.dehaarspecialist.be/186/hairmax-laser-technologies

While many of the LLLT devices evaluated in multicenter clinical studies have been deemed safe for consumers, they are classified as FDA-cleared devices, not FDA-approved. It is not clear to what extent the FDA reviewed or cleared these devices in terms of their effectiveness in treating hair loss. However, it appears that the laser hair therapy industry is promoting their devices as FDA-approved for hair loss as if they are equivalent to the only two FDA-approved hair loss solutions available: Propecia® (finasteride) and Rogaine® (minoxidil). However, until the laser hair treatment industry provides more compelling, non-company-funded studies showing effective hair loss treatment, it is quite possible that some companies will overpromote the effectiveness of LLLT.

It is recommended the reader visit the FDA website (www.fda.gov) to learn more about the FDA standards for approving food and drugs and clearing medical devices. As a convenience to the reader, below is the language used by the FDA on their website clarifying the difference between FDA-approved and FDA-cleared medical devices.

When an FDA review is required prior to the marketing of a medical device, the FDA will either:

- **Clear** the device after reviewing a premarket notification, known as a 510(k)— named for a section in the Food, Drug, and Cosmetic Act— that has been filed with the FDA,
- **Approve** the device after reviewing a premarket approval (PMA) application that has been submitted to the FDA. Whether a 510(k) or a PMA application needs to be filed depends on the classification of the medical device. For example:

To acquire a clearance to market a device using the 510(k) pathways, the submitter of the 510(k) application must show that the medical device is *substantially equivalent* to a device that is already legally marketed for the same use. *To acquire* approval of a device through a PMA application, the PMA applicant must provide reasonable assurance of the device's safety and effectiveness.

In concluding this chapter, it is essential to understand that all the hair replacement and restoration methods described in the book have their own particular limitations in regrowing or restoring hair. However, despite their inherent limitations, they all have a valuable and valid function in contemporary society by alleviating the psychological distress that both men and women can experience when afflicted with any form of alopecia.

Hair loss can be as devastating to men as it is to women. However, short of undergoing hair-transplantation surgery, there is no single effective method available to prevent hair loss or restore the hair if the individual is predisposed to hereditary hair loss complemented by androgenetic stimulation. Notwithstanding these limitations, there are currently many more options to restore and possibly reverse a hair loss condition. Moreover, one thing is clear: Neither men nor women should resign themselves to feeling less attractive than they should because of an alopecic condition, especially with so many useful surgical and non-surgical hair restoration methods available.

15

Topical Hair-Loss Treatment Modalities

At the moment, it is a well-known fact that there are only two FDA-approved hair-loss treatment modalities available in the marketplace. These are Propecia® (finasteride), a systemic treatment modality, and Rogaine® (minoxidil), a topical scalp solution. There is a multitude of non-FDA-approved hair-loss remedies available to consumers. These remedies can be either oral or topical, and they are extensively promoted as efficacious hair-regrowth solutions.

There is no question that effective marketing campaigns often overreach or exaggerate in an attempt to sell a product, whether or not the product is efficacious. Therefore, the safety of the consuming public is constantly at risk. The only defense available that can counteract this inherent, ever-present conflict of interest between the consuming public and the companies attempting to promote their products is to create an informed and educated consumer— one of the objectives of this book.

The hair-loss industry, like any other industry where there is the potential for conflicts of interest, can engage in unethical, self-dealing practices. Conflict of interest refers to any situation where a person's public decisions are improperly influenced by his personal affiliations or interests. In other words, a conflict of interest is a set of circumstances that creates a risk that professional judgment or actions regarding a primary interest will be unduly influenced by a secondary interest (Lo & Field, 2009). Therefore, it cannot be stressed enough that the only way to oppose unethical, corruptive behavior in any industry is by creating an educated consumer.

Today's society has accepted and even embraced hair loss to a certain extent. For example, shaving one's head is an acceptable grooming style. However, hair loss is still an extremely emotionally distressing condition. It makes those affected particularly vulnerable to potential unethical marketing scams. For this reason, the American Hair Loss Association (AHLA) recommends against purchasing any hair-loss product that has not been clinically tested and approved by the FDA or recommended by the AHLA.

The hair-product industry is an enormous, 83 billion-dollar industry that is mostly unregulated. Therefore, when product complaints are launched against a company, not much is done about it. There is no legal requirement for a company to inform the FDA when they receive any type of product complaint. More disturbing still is the fact that the FDA has not updated its policies on personal-care products since 1938 (Duarte, 2016). Furthermore, the FDA has come to rely heavily on the cosmetic industry to regulate itself to ensure consumer safety. Recent criticism alleges that this system of self-regulation is ineffective, inefficient, and inappropriate (Lee-Daum, 2006). Hence, the risks of creating potential conflicts of interest are enormous.

Available Hair Loss Treatment Modalities

There are many topical hair-loss treatment products and restorative solutions available for the consuming public to resolve or alleviate their hair-loss issues. These are generally classified as:

- DHT Blockers and Inhibitors.
- Hair Growth Stimulators.
- Hair Loss Thickening Fibers Concealers.

DHT Blockers and Inhibitors

Dihydrotestosterone (DHT) blockers and inhibitors attempt to treat hair loss at the root. The use of these two terms can create some confusion. Thus, it is essential to clarify their meanings. The proper term for a drug or chemical that slows or prevents the conversion of testosterone to DHT is a 5-alpha-reductase inhibitor (5-ARI). 5-ARIs are a class of drugs with antiandrogen effects used primarily in the treatment of benign prostatic hyperplasia (BPH) and androgenetic alopecia (AGA). Some well-known drugs that are classified as 5-alpha-reductase inhibitors are finasteride, dutasteride, and alfatradiol.

Conversely, a drug or chemical that stops the effects of androgen by binding to the androgen receptor and preventing androgen binding would be classified as an androgen receptor blocker, or simply, antiandrogen. Antiandrogens, or androgen blockers, discovered in the 1960s, prevent androgens— like testosterone and its strong metabolite, DHT— from expressing their biological effects in responsive tissues. Essentially, antiandrogens work by altering the androgen pathway by either blocking the appropriate receptors or by affecting androgen production (Mowszowicz, 1989; Hitner, 2016). Some well-known antiandrogen drugs are spironolactone and cyproterone acetate (CPA).

However, a once-promising antiandrogen compound that is not as well-known to the consumer as the ones mentioned above that the reader should be aware of is RU-58841. RU-58841 (also known as HMR-3841 or PSK-3841) is a non-steroidal, antiandrogen compound research chemical that was previously investigated for use as a topical treatment for acne, androgenetic alopecia (AGA), and hirsutism (Battmann et al., 1994; Münster et al., 2005). The chemical RU-58841 was first synthesized at Roussel-UCLAF pharmaceutical— hence the prefix RU— in Romainville, France, by Battmann et al. (1994) as part of experiments to identify antiandrogen drugs.

The initial studies on RU-58841 reported excellent results in treating hair loss in animal models without any side effects. The lack of side effects was because the medication was explicitly designed to limit its action to the application site. Supposedly, there was no systemic absorption of the chemical. Additionally, De Brouwer et al.'s research team (1997) conducted a study entitled *"A Controlled Study of the Effects of RU58841, a Non-Steroidal Antiandrogen, on Human Hair Production by Balding Scalp Grafts Maintained on Testosterone-Conditioned Nude Mice."* De Brouwer's study demonstrated a positive action for RU-58841 on human hair growth from balding samples grafted onto testosterone-conditioned nude mice. Thus, the study encouraged further clinical trials to evaluate its potential in treating androgen-dependent alopecia.

Unfortunately for RU-58841, Roussel-UCLAF was absorbed in 1995 by a merger with Hoescht, a German pharmaceutical company. Subsequently, Hoescht and Roussel-ACLAF were themselves absorbed in a merger with American company Marion Merrel Dow becoming the HMR Group. Thus, RU-58841 became known as HMR-3841. Following this merger, the rights to RU-58841 or HMR-3841 were acquired by a Scottish pharmaceutical company called ProStrakan, which changed the compound's name to PSK-3841.

ProStrakan performed limited research studies with the chemical PSK-3841, including human trials. For example, in 2002, ProStrakan conducted a study under the direction of Dr. Evelyne Guénolé entitled *"A Double-Blind, Randomized Vehicle-Controlled, Safety and Tolerance Study of Topical PSK 3841 Solution at 5% Administered Twice Daily Over Four Weeks to Healthy Caucasian Males and Females with Androgenetic Alopecia."* As far as the literature review is concerned, it appears that this study was never published.

Although the results from the ProStrakan trials were reported to be encouraging, the company abandoned all future research and development (R & D) of the compound. It is speculated the R & D was discontinued because of a 2005 Morgan Stanley financial analysis that concluded that the market potential for the drug was a modest one, only $100-$200 million. Further speculation for ProStrakan abandoning the drug was that the company believed that the product was no better than minoxidil or finasteride or that the compound was already old with insufficient time left in the patent to justify any more financial investment.

In 2011, ProStrakan was acquired by Tokyo-based Kyowa Hakko Kirin Co., Ltd. Then, on April 18th, 2016, ProStrakan was rebranded as Kyowa Kirin. The Japanese company decided that to portray a consistent image worldwide, all of its western pharmaceutical subsidiaries were to adopt the Kyowa Kirin name.

Some investigators believe that the potential of RU-58841 as a potential baldness cure was lost in the pursuit of profits. However, apparently, these financial decisions are not an uncommon practice in the pharmaceutical industry. In fact, the World Health Organization (WHO) estimates that only 37% of known human diseases are being targeted by pharmaceutical companies, entirely due to perceptions about possible profits.

Officially RU-58841 has never been approved by the FDA for human use. The compound is strictly sold as a research chemical. Notwithstanding the illegalities of the product as a topical hair-loss solution, RU-58841 has found its way into the market. In fact, it is being sold in Indonesia as an over-the-counter topical solution called MezogenRx™ in combination with minoxidil in a 2% and 5% strength solution. It is also sold as a pre-mix formulation by Anagenic, Inc., RegenRx, and VentanexCorp. These products can be purchased from these providers directly or can be purchased through Amazon. Needless to say, again, this is one of those areas where caveat emptor (buyers beware) is applicable. Essentially, caveat emptor is the principle that the buyer alone is responsible for checking the quality and suitability of goods before a purchase is made.

Non-FDA-Approved Topical Hair-Loss Solutions

There are only two FDA-approved hair loss drugs with either DHT-inhibitory or DHT-blocking properties. However, there are many non-FDA-approved topical hair-loss solutions claiming to possess the same effects as these two FDA-approved medications.

Because it is challenging to keep up with the onslaught of these hair loss products, only the most familiar will be addressed here. Some of the topical hair-loss treatments available in this category are:

- Revivogen MD.
- Crinagen.
- Procerin.
- Progesterone creams.
- Azelaic acid.
- Xandrox.

Revivogen MD.

Revivogen is a topical hair-loss formula made from natural ingredients that claim to promote hair regrowth. It is described as a dermatologist-formulated hair-loss product effective for androgenetic alopecia (AGA). The active ingredients of Revivogen include alpha-linolenic acid (ALA), gamma-linolenic acid (GLA), linoleic acid, oleic acid, azelaic acid, zinc, vitamin B6, beta-sitosterol, saw palmetto, and oligomeric proanthocyanidins (OPCs), which is found in grape seed extract.

The manufacturer of this product claims that all these natural ingredients have been proven to reduce DHT production, block the androgen receptors, limit DHT uptake, and initiate the hair follicles' rejuvenation cycle.

Crinagen.

Crinagen is another topical hair-loss formula that can be used or applied as a spray or dropper solution. The product is made from natural ingredients similar to those in Revivogen. Some of the ingredients found in Crinagen are azelaic acid, vitamin B6, zinc acetate, Serenoa repens, niacin, saw palmetto, Ginkgo Biloba, and proanthocyanidins from grape seed extract. The product was developed by Dr. Nasser Razack after he began to experience hair loss as a college student in his mid-twenties. According to Dr. Razack, Crinagen only contains ingredients and compounds that have proven medically effective in treating hair loss.

Crinagen is promoted as a DHT-inhibitor and vasodilator that increases scalp circulatory blood flow to the hair follicles. It also claims to suppress immune system reactions that can cause inflammation of the scalp, which can exacerbate the damage DHT can inflict to the follicles. Furthermore, Dr. Razack also claims that Crinagen has been proven to reduce DHT production in the scalp by up to 98%. Unlike other topical scalp solutions, Crinagen is not sold with the usual, associated combination of shampoos, conditioners, and pills. However, the developer does recommend that an anti-inflammatory shampoo like Nizoral or T-Gel be used with the formulation. Moreover, Crinagen, like other over-the-counter (OTC) hair-loss products, can take a long time to produce results. The claim is that the user must be patient because it takes approximately three months to see results if the product is effective for the user.

Procerin.

Procerin is another popular, natural, OTC hair-loss product available as a supplement in tablet form and as a topical solution. The developers claim that the product works by blocking the metabolite DHT without interacting with testosterone itself. Thus, according to the developers, Procerin targets the specific chemical process that transforms testosterone into the hair-damaging byproduct DHT. It is important to note that, despite the claims that Procerin and most other hair-loss formulations containing similar ingredients can block the effect of DHT, this is not proven science. While some of the natural ingredients in these hair-loss products may possess some anti-DHT properties, none have ever been formally tested as a hair-loss treatment.

Some of the ingredients contained in the Procerin formulation are saw palmetto, nettles, zinc sulfate, vitamin B6, Gotu kola, magnesium, and azelaic acid. The product was designed for men to use twice daily, once in the morning and once at night. Although the product claims to be side-effect-free, Procerin can cause mild stomach discomfort, which can be remedied by taking the tablet with a meal. Moreover, the manufacturer also advises that men with sensitive skin should only use the solution once per day for the first week to prevent skin irritation.

Progesterone creams.

Progesterone is a hormone found in men, women, and children. Everyone needs a small amount of progesterone for good health and longevity. Progesterone is crucial to the health of everyone regardless of sex or age. Contrary to popular belief, progesterone is not a feminizing type of hormone. That distinction actually belongs to estrogen. Progesterone is a natural antagonist (enemy) to estrogen. In fact, progesterone helps balance and neutralize the powerful effects of excess estrogen in both men and women. Without sufficient progesterone in the body, estrogen dominance may result, which can be harmful to the individual.

In the presence of low progesterone levels, the body responds by increasing its production of adrenal cortical hormones, such as aldosterone and cortisol. These hormones have a variety of roles that are crucial for the body's response to stress. However, they can also convey androgenetic (male-like) properties, such as male pattern baldness. When the progesterone hormone levels are raised through supplementation, the adrenal cortical hormones levels will gradually stabilize, and normal hair growth will eventually resume within four to six months (Jockers, 2011).

The progesterone hormone is an effective therapeutic modality in treating hair loss in both men and women with androgenetic alopecia. Progesterone is a natural 5-alpha-reductase inhibitor and can bind to androgen receptors. Thus, the application of topical progesterone has been shown to arrest the progression of female and male pattern baldness. *However, it does not promote the regrowth of the hair; it just slows the progression.*

Azelaic acid.

Azelaic acid is a naturally occurring, saturated, dicarboxylic acid found in wheat, rye, and barley. It is produced by *Malassezia Furfur*, a harmless fungus (yeast) present on the skin of most adults. It is a weak acid with antimicrobial activity that affects keratin production and reduces inflammation. Azelaic acid was first approved as a new molecular entity by the FDA in 1995 as a topical 20% cream produced by Allergan. In the form of a cream, azelaic acid is a very effective treatment for acne because of its antimicrobial properties that kill bacteria as well as being an effective comedolytic agent (i.e., clears blocked pores). *"Comedolytic"* is the term used to describe a product or medication that inhibits the formation of comedones, which are blemishes that form when oil and skin cells become trapped in the pore. It is also used as a treatment for rosacea.

As a treatment for hair loss, azelaic acid has been shown to be an effective 5-alpha-reductase inhibitor. This fact was determined by a study entitled *"Inhibition of 5α-Reductase Activity in Human Skin by Zinc and Azelaic acid"* conducted by Stamatiadis, Bulteau-Portois, and Mowszowicz in 1988. Dr. Stamatiadis and his research team, determined that azelaic acid could completely inhibit 5-alpha-reductase activity at a concentration of 3 millimoles per liter. Furthermore, the researchers also found that when azelaic acid, zinc, and vitamin B6 were combined at very low concentrations, it resulted in a 90% inhibition of 5-alpha-reductase. Dr. Stamatiadis concluded that zinc sulfate combined with azelaic acid could potentially be an effective treatment modality for androgenetic-related ailments.

Based on Stamatiadis et al. (1988) findings, azelaic acid has now been included in a multitude of topical hair-loss formulations for its presumed synergistic mode of action with other active ingredients, including minoxidil. Minoxidil is included to stimulate hair growth, while the azelaic acid is included to inhibit the DHT, which causes hair loss. However, despite the favorable results from Stamatiadis' study, it is important to note that his study had certain limitations in the way the researchers conducted the study. For example, the research was performed *in vitro* (i.e., outside a living organism), which means that the results obtained may not correspond to the circumstances occurring within a living organism.

Xandrox.

The Xandrox hair-loss formula was the first commercially available product to combine the benefits of the FDA-approved hair-growth stimulant minoxidil with the assumed 5-alpha-reductase DHT inhibitor azelaic acid. Xandrox is a product developed by Dr. Richard Lee, a hair-loss restoration physician. Xandrox is currently available in a 15%, 10%, and 5% minoxidil concentrations. The 15% Xandrox solution is one of the only hair-loss products that combines a high concentration of minoxidil with a formulation that the manufacturer claim acts as a DHT inhibitor that includes azelaic acid, retinol, and caffeine in a concentration of 5%, 0.025%, and 0.001%, respectively. The users of these stronger formulations should be aware that the 15% and 10% minoxidil concentration solutions can increase the chances of scalp irritation and may carry other negative side effects if misused.

The claim made by the manufacturers of the products that have been described is that they either inhibit or block the enzyme 5-alpha-reductase and thus prevent the conversion of testosterone to DHT. Dihydrotestosterone acts like a catalyst for the hair-loss process as it binds with the receptor sites in hair follicles that are genetically predisposed to hair loss. If it is allowed to continue unrestricted, this hair-loss process will result in the miniaturization of the hair follicle, which will impede the ability to grow healthy hair.

The goal of topically inhibiting, or blocking, the circulating DHT at the scalp level rather than systemically as with the use of Propecia® or Avodart® is that it is a more desirable approach because of the diminished likelihood of experiencing side effects with a topical solution. However, the success of these topical treatment modalities in reducing DHT levels in the scalp has not been clinically proven or approved by the FDA. Therefore, their efficacy in hair-loss restoration or reversal is questionable.

As previously mentioned, it is important to reemphasize that there are only two FDA-approved medications on the market that have been scientifically proven to be relatively effective in treating hair loss in some patients. They are Propecia® (finasteride) and Rogaine® (minoxidil). The reader should also be aware that hair loss is a medical condition that should be addressed medically by a physician. This means that if afflicted with hair loss, a doctor who specializes in hair-loss disorders should be consulted to evaluate and treat the condition.

A good rule to follow that will save users time and money when selecting any hair-loss product is only use FDA-approved products or ones that have been recommended by reputable consumer- protection organizations like the AHLA. However, it is totally acceptable for users to experiment with the various hair loss formulations available if they do not mind investing some money into the process. Notwithstanding any desired experimentation by users, the practice of *caveat emptor*—let the buyer beware—is applicable when searching for any hair-loss remedy.

Hair Growth Stimulants

The products and treatment modalities in this category stimulate hair growth. Because the objective of these treatment modalities is the stimulation of hair growth, they cannot stop hair loss completely since they do not address the root causes of hair loss. Stimulating hair growth is only possible by making sure that the hair is in a healthy state, which will only occur by understanding and maintaining proper dietary nutrition.

Maintaining healthy hair is all about ensuring that the body can provide the hair-growth cycle with the necessary nutrients to create the optimum nutritional environment to stimulate and enhance hair growth. Therefore, the best way to stimulate hair growth is to supply the proper amounts of vitamins, minerals, carbohydrates, and proteins necessary, so the hair follicles have the nutrients they need to lengthen the hair-growth cycle (Goldberg & Lenzy, 2010).

The following products are claimed to be stimulants for hair regrowth:

- Minoxidil (Rogaine®).
- Tricomin® follicular therapy spray (copper peptides).
- Folligen® therapy spray (copper peptides).
- Proxiphen®, Proxiphen-N, and NANO shampoo.
- Tretinoin (Retin-A®).
- Bimatoprost (Latisse®).

Minoxidil (Rogaine®).

Historically, before minoxidil was serendipitously discovered as a potential anti-baldness medication, it was a vasodilator used to treat high blood pressure. It was marketed under the FDA-approved brand name *Loniten.* Minoxidil is a potent peripheral vasodilator introduced in the early 1970s as an oral medication to treat refractory (resistant) hypertension. Refractory hypertension is defined as blood pressure that remained uncontrolled despite using 3 to 5 antihypertensive agents of different classes, including a long-acting thiazide-like diuretic and a mineralocorticoid receptor (MR) antagonist taken at maximally tolerated doses. In other words, refractory hypertension is high blood pressure that is not responsive to maximum medical therapy (Acelajado et al., 2013). A reported side effect of minoxidil, when administered to patients, resulted in *hypertrichosis,* a condition in which hair grows excessively all over the body (Zappacosta, 1980).

Minoxidil's initial developer and patent owner was Upjohn Pharmaceutical and subsequently Pfizer. However, the discoverer of minoxidil as a topical solution for treating hair loss was the late Dr. Guinter Kahn, a practicing dermatologist in North Miami, Florida. In 1971, Dr. Kahn, along with colleagues Dr. Charles Chidsey and his then-resident student Dr. Paul Grant, Kahn tested a new compound called minoxidil which initially was meant for treating refractory hypertension. As it turned out, one particular side effect of this drug was an overabundance of hair growth (hypertrichosis) on its subjects. This hypertrichosis side effect was perceived as a setback by Upjohn's chances of developing a successful hypertension drug. However, Dr. Kahn saw an opportunity for developing an effective hair loss medication. In fact, recounted by Dr. Paul Grant, his assistant at the time who stated that Kahn said, " *Boy, this would be a great stuff if we could apply it to the tops of heads.* "

This 1971 observation by Kahn led to the launch— 17 years later— of the first anti-baldness cream approved by the US Food and Drug Administration (FDA). Minoxidil is currently owned by Johnson & Johnson, under the trade name Rogaine or Regaine, depending on the country it is been sold. This serendipitous discovery by Dr. Kahn remains one of the few scientifically credible products in an industry with less than a stellar reputation.

In 1986 Dr. Kahn and his colleagues became the first team to go on record to get a patent for a hair loss medication. Kahn's serendipitous discovery eventually garnered him a fortune. However, he had to battle through the courts for more than a decade before formally recognizing him as one of its inventors. According to Dr. Grant, this was essentially the fight between "David and Goliath," when Kahn went against Upjohn's ranks of corporate lawyers (Andrew Ward, 2014).

Fortunately, with the use of minoxidil, the excessive hair growth occurred mainly close to the application areas. This was a welcome side effect when applied to the scalp. However, in some cases, the hair growth also occurred on the arms, back, chest, and other areas. Because of the resultant hypertrichosis associated with minoxidil, the drug was extensively studied in the United States, France, England, and Sweden. The conclusion from most of those investigative studies showed impressive results in hair growth, especially in androgenetic alopecia and alopecia areata.

These observations led to the development of a topical formulation of minoxidil to treat androgenetic alopecia (AGA) in men and subsequently in women. The 2% product was first marketed for hair regrowth in men in 1986 in the United States, and the 5% solution became available in 1993 (Messenger & Rundegren, 2004). Thus, in 1986, a Rogaine® topical lotion became the first FDA-approved medication for the treatment of genetic hair loss available only by prescription.

Subsequently, in 1995, the FDA decided that the minoxidil lotion was sufficiently safe for use without a prescription. Minoxidil soon became available over-the-counter in pharmacies and grocery stores following this FDA decision. Then the generic versions of minoxidil became available when the patent on Rogaine® expired. Over-the-counter Rogaine® is generally available in a 5% concentration solution for men and a 2% concentration solution for women. However, currently, Rogaine® is available as a 5% topical foam for both men and women, which, according to users, is less greasy and easier to apply.

From a historical perspective, the reason for the different minoxidil concentrations for men and women was attributed to tests that found women to be more susceptible to certain side effects of minoxidil, most notably lowered blood pressure, lightheadedness, and allergic skin reactions like contact dermatitis. Those were the reasons why the 2% concentration was initially approved for use by women. Additionally, minoxidil also caused facial hair growth, especially if the drug ran down the women's temples or forehead after it was applied. Although this condition usually resolved itself when the drug was discontinued. However, occasionally the hair needs to be removed. This observation was seen to occur more frequently when the 5% formulation was used off-label, which was another reason why women were discouraged from using the 5% solution (Bernstein, 2013).

However, in a study undertaken by Lucky et al. (2004) entitled *"A Randomized, Placebo-Controlled Trial of 5% and 2% Topical Minoxidil Solutions in the Treatment of Female Pattern Hair Loss"* the research team conducted a 48-week study of 381 women participants afflicted with androgenetic alopecia (AGA) or female pattern hair loss (FPHL). Dr. Lucky's study concluded that at week 48 of the study, the 5% topical minoxidil group demonstrated statistical superiority over the 2% group. The women in this study tolerated both concentrations of topical minoxidil without evidence of systemic adverse effects. Subsequently, as a result of research studies like this one, a 5% minoxidil foam became available for women's use in 2014.

Pharmacologic mechanism of minoxidil.

It has been known for more than thirty years that minoxidil stimulates hair growth; however, our understanding of its pharmacological mechanism of action on the hair follicle is still limited. Animal studies have shown that topical minoxidil shortens the telogen cycle, causing premature entry of resting hair follicles into the anagen stage. It is postulated that minoxidil probably has a similar action in human hair. One theory regarding the function of minoxidil is that the topical solution causes a substantial increase in DNA synthesis in hair follicle cells. When applied to the scalp and absorbed into the skin, it is converted to an active, unstable product called minoxidil sulfate.

Our bodies produce a catalyst — a substance that precipitates a change — called sulfonyl transferase, or sulfotransferase, which converts the inactive minoxidil into the active minoxidil sulfate. Minoxidil sulfate is 14 times more potent than minoxidil in stimulating cysteine incorporation in cultured follicles, which in turn activates potassium channels in the cells, and this is thought to lead to hair growth (Messenger & Rundegren, 2004). Therefore, there seems to be some evidence that the stimulatory effect of minoxidil on hair growth might be due to the opening of potassium (KATP) channels by minoxidil sulfate. Still, this idea has been difficult to prove, and to date, there has been no clear demonstration that KATP channels are expressed in the hair follicle (Messenger & Rundegren, 2004).

What is known is that minoxidil is a potent vasodilator. Some experts believe that minoxidil works by dilating the blood vessels around hair follicles, which should improve scalp circulation, thereby increasing the nutrients supplied to the papilla, and encouraging increased hair growth. However, this is still an unproven hypothesis, especially because there are other vasodilator drugs that do not seem to promote hair growth. As mentioned before, the exact science that results in hair growth from minoxidil is not known. *What is known is that it does not affect DHT levels in the blood.*

Minoxidil lotion seems to work only on active hair follicles that are still capable of producing some hair, even if they produce vellus hair. Androgenetic alopecia is characterized by a progressive miniaturization of hair follicles at the end of each hair-growth cycle, resulting in the production of finer and finer hairs. It appears that minoxidil can reduce the rate of hair follicle miniaturization and can cause hair follicles that formerly produced full-size hairs— but have recently become miniaturized— to increase in size and begin to regrow terminal-type hair again. Furthermore, the enlarged follicles seem to remain in the anagen (growth) stage for a longer period of time. A prolonged anagen period time results in the production of longer hairs and the appearance of having more hair. Thus, it appears that minoxidil acts in a supportive way to maintain the health of the hair follicles (Messenger & Rundegren, 2004).

Minoxidil can be used to stimulate hair growth in both adult men and women who possess a certain type of baldness. It has been observed that it is most effective for people younger than 40 years of age with recent hair loss. Contrary to current belief, minoxidil works in any area where there is fine or miniaturized hair, including the hairline. The source of confusion regarding this topic originates from the FDA, which limited the application of Rogaine® to the crown in accordance with the drug package insert. The FDA did this because Upjohn, the original maker of Rogaine®, specifically tested it on the crown in the clinical trials. Since this earlier study on minoxidil focused only on the crown, it gave consumers the impression that the product worked strictly on this area (Bernstein, 2014; Leyden et al., 1999).

According to Dr. Robert Bernstein (2014), he felt that it was regrettable that some physicians, and many patients, still believe that minoxidil is not efficacious on the front of the scalp. Bernstein contends that it is unfortunate that many hair-restoration surgeons have not done enough to educate the public to dispel this myth. However, it is essential to understand that the product still does not work on completely bald areas or will it lower an existing hairline. Moreover, if the drug is stopped, the new hair growth, if any, is lost within a few months. Therefore, for this medication to work effectively, the patient must use it for life. In essence, it is a lifetime commitment.

The most noticeable results from minoxidil will occur between six months and two years from the commencement of the treatment regime. Following that application regime, the user may begin to notice the drug's efficacy subsiding steadily. Patients are expected to lose hair but at a slower rate than if they were not on the medication. Patients should anticipate that hair will regress to its original pattern within three months if they stop the application of minoxidil. Starting and stopping the application regime is not advisable because any subsequent hair growth may not be as robust as the earlier phase before the medication was stopped. Therefore, as stated previously, the use of minoxidil as a hair-loss treatment is a lifelong commitment.

Experiential results from topical minoxidil.

The results that users have had with the application of topical minoxidil have been quite variable. In some individuals, minoxidil has had no effect whatsoever. For others, there has been a decrease in the hair-loss rate with no significant new hair growth. However, for some users, both men and women, the experience have been a minimal degree of new hair growth but insufficient to be an adequate cover for thinning hair areas. In some fortunate few, the new hair growth has been dense enough that the density achieved was similar to areas that had not been affected by hair loss.

Although minoxidil is an FDA-approved hair-loss medication with proven science behind its application, the reality is that minoxidil has not been efficacious for everyone. According to numerous medical studies undertaken to determine the efficacy and safety of minoxidil, it appears that the over-the-counter (OTC) minoxidil only works effectively in approximately 35%-40% of patients.

Sulfotransferase (SULT 1A1) Enzyme.

Research studies have determined that the reason for minoxidil's limited efficacy is because most users lack an active enzyme called *sulfotransferase 1A1, which is* encoded by the protein coding gene SULT 1A1. The enzyme sulfotransferase is found in the liver and the outer root sheath of the hair follicles (Dias et al., 2018*)*. For hair follicles to respond to the application of the *pro-drug minoxidil*, it needs the *sulfotransferase* enzyme to convert the topically applied minoxidil into the active metabolite *minoxidil sulfate*, which is the active drug that actually stimulates the growth of the hair follicles (Buhl, et al., 1990). A pro-drug must undergo chemical conversion by metabolic processes before becoming an active pharmacological agent. Therefore, minoxidil as a pro-drug is converted by the body through sulfotransferase into a pharmacologically active drug, minoxidil sulfate.

Clinical research studies have determined that not every minoxidil user has sufficient *sulfotransferase 1A1* enzyme to facilitate the conversion to the active metabolite minoxidil sulfate. Additionally, other biological factors may also affect the action of minoxidil, such as inflammation at or around the hair follicles on the scalp. Because of all these impediments, minoxidil is only effective in approximately 35%-40% of the users. In essence, 60%-65% of minoxidil users are considered non-respondents.

It is a well-known fact that it takes approximately 6 to 9 months of minoxidil application to determine if the user will have a favorable response to the treatment. Because of this expensive and prolonged treatment time to assess minoxidil effectiveness, a ***Minoxidil Response Test (MRT)*** was developed to determine if the potential user has the enzyme sulfotransferase 1A1. The availability of such a diagnostic test for ***ruling out non-responders*** would have a significant clinical utility and a cost-saving benefit for the patient.

As of 2020, a ***Minoxidil Response Test*** is available, which was patented and developed by Applied Biology. The Minoxidil Response Test is currently available for men and women through Daniel Alain, the world's leading hair loss and hair enhancement company. Applied Biology, headquartered in Irvine, California, is a biotechnology company specializing in hair science research. Their Minoxidil Response Test (MRT) aims to identify non-responders before initiating therapy with the topical minoxidil solution.

The expression of the sulfotransferase enzyme is variable among individuals. Therefore, Applied Biology has demonstrated in two feasibility studies that the sulfotransferase enzyme activity in plucked hair follicles correlates with minoxidil's response in the treatment of androgenetic alopecia (AGA) and thus can serve as a predictive biomarker. Their study analysis confirmed the clinical utility of a sulfotransferase enzyme test in successfully ruling out 95.9% of non-responders to topical minoxidil for the treatment of AGA. Since the availability of the ***Minoxidil Response Test,*** the potential minoxidil user does not have to invest time and money to assess if they will respond to the treatment (Applied Biology, 2020).

Now that it is understood that minoxidil will not be effective if there is a lack of the sulfotransferase enzyme. The issue then becomes how can the enzyme levels be increased so that minoxidil can be used effectively by everyone. To address this problem, ***Applied Biology*** has undertaken a study in an attempt to determine how to increase ***follicular sulfotransferase activity***. They have developed a topical formulation for that purpose. The topical formulation is classified as a *Minoxidil Adjuvant Therapy*, called AB-103. The study aims to evaluate the efficacy of AB-103 as an adjuvant therapy to 5% topical minoxidil foam in treating female pattern hair loss (FPHL). Two adjuvant therapies that can be used now while customers wait for Applied Biotechnology's development of AB-103 to come to the market are Tretinoin and microneedling (dermaroller).

In a study entitled *"Tretinoin enhances minoxidil response in androgenetic alopecia patients by upregulating follicular sulfotransferase enzymes,"* conducted by Sharma et al. (2019).

Dr. Sharma successfully demonstrated that a topical tretinoin application influences the expression of the follicular sulfotransferase enzyme. The clinical significance of the experiment was that 43% of the study participants were minoxidil nonresponders. Subsequently, the entire group participants (cohort) converted to minoxidil responders after five days of applying the tretinoin solution.

Microneedling (MN) or Dermarolling is a minimally invasive dermatological procedure that involves using a derma roller, a device that has small fine needles that cause minor skin injuries (Fig. 15.1 and 15.2). This cosmetic treatment is used to induce or produce collagen formation, neovascularization (growth of new blood vessels), and growth factor production in treated areas. Proponents of microneedling believe the skin damage created by the needling process (derma roller) can help induce stem cell stimulation in the hair follicles that may lead to hair growth. In a study by Dhurat et al., 2013 entitled *"A Randomized Evaluator Blinded Study of Effect of Microneedling in Androgenetic Alopecia: A Pilot Study,"* the researchers discovered that the dermal papilla (DP) is the site of expression of various hair growth-related genes. Moreover, other researchers have also demonstrated the importance of the Wnt proteins and the wound growth factors in stimulating the stem cells associated with the dermal papilla. Thus, microneedling works by stimulating stem cells and inducing the activation of growth factors.

Microneedling has been successfully paired with other hair growth-promoting therapies, such as minoxidil, platelet-rich plasma, and topical steroids. It is thought that microneedling facilitates penetration of such first-line medications, and this is one mechanism by which it promotes hair growth. Microneedling initially became popular as a scar treatment during the 1990s, and since then, it has been studied as an adjunctive treatment for androgenetic alopecia (AGA) and alopecia areata (AA), which is the area of most success (Ferting et al., 2018).

Fig.15.1: Derma roller instrument

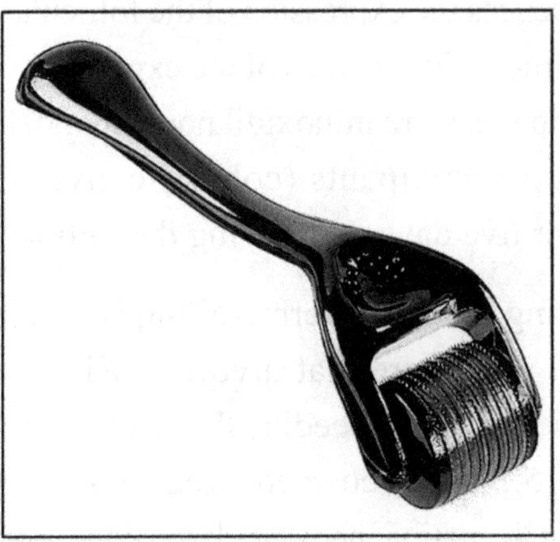

Image Source: https://zoeayla.com/products/copy-of-professional-micro-needling-derma-roller-in-black

Fig. 15.2: Scalp microneedling to treat hair loss

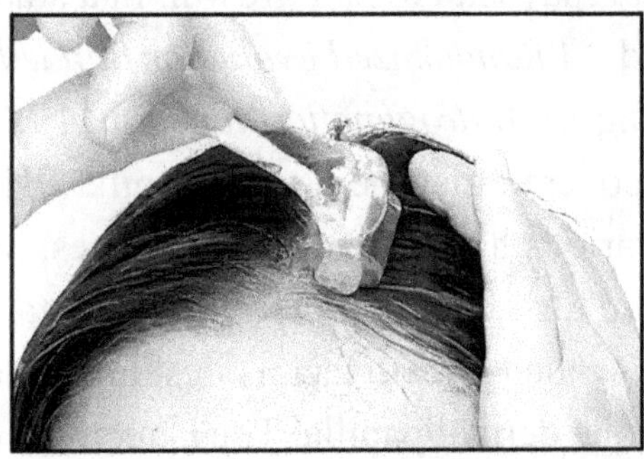

Image Source: https://www.couplesmassageorangecounty.com/derma-roller-on-scalp-for-hair-loss-massage-monday-440/

Proper use of topical minoxidil.

Minoxidil is a drug intended for external use on the scalp only, and it is accompanied by a patient instruction insert. It is important that these instructions be read carefully and followed as indicated. The hair and scalp should be completely dry before the drug is applied. The scalp and hair should be dry because a wet scalp potentiates, or enhances, the penetration of topical medications several times, typically two to five times its original strength (McAndrews, 2012). Because there can be side effects from minoxidil use, keeping the hair and scalp dry will prevent increasing the potency of the drug, thereby mitigating the potential for side effects.

However, suppose the user does not experience any side effects after the application of minoxidil. In that case, the person may try applying it to a wet scalp if a more potent effect from the drug is desired. If this is done, someone should be present in the event that the user experiences side effects. Finally, it is important to note that hair does not need to be shampooed before each application.

Minoxidil comes in a liquid or foam form, which is applied directly to the affected area of the scalp. Its recommended use is twice a day, in the morning and at bedtime. It should not be used more often than as directed. In fact, exceeding the recommended dosage will not produce greater or faster hair growth. However, it may cause increased side effects. Some physicians have recommended the use of once-a-day minoxidil because they claim it increases compliance and decreases the risk of contact allergy (Rogers & Avram, 2008).

Other physicians claim that applying once-a-day minoxidil— either the 2% or 5% solution or foam— seems to be almost as effective as using it twice a day. The rationale behind this claim is that although minoxidil has a relatively short half-life of 4.2 hours when administered orally. When topically applied, it has a half-life of 22 hours in the skin. This long half-life suggests that a once-a-day dosing is a reasonable option (Bernstein, 2014). However, it is important to understand that Johnson & Johnson, the current manufacturer of Rogaine®, has a vested interest in a higher consumption of the medication. Johnson & Johnson specifically states that Rogaine® will be less effective if the product is used only once a day. The manufacturer's recommendation as it relates to a missed application of minoxidil is to use it as soon as possible. If it is almost time for the next dose, use only that dose. Do not use double or extra doses since using more product is not better.

Adverse interactions are not expected from minoxidil use. However, do not use any other medicines on the scalp while using Rogaine® without first consulting with a doctor or healthcare professional. If the scalp becomes abraded, irritated, or sunburned, the patient should check with their doctor before applying minoxidil. This medication must be used regularly for hair to regrow. It may take two to four months of regular use before any noticeable improvement is observed. As previously mentioned, it is essential to continue using this product for life to ensure that hair regrowth is maintained. Once the treatment is stopped, the regrown hair will start to fall out within three months. If the user does not see any new hair growth after four months of continuous use, minoxidil use should be stopped, and the user should contact the doctor. It might be appropriate at this time to have a ***Minoxidil Response Test*** done.

Potential side effects of minoxidil.

As with most other drugs, there can be side effects from the use of minoxidil. The following side effects should be reported to a doctor or healthcare professional by the user as soon as they occur:

- Chest pain or palpitations.
- Dizziness or fainting.
- Skin rash, blisters, or itching.
- Sudden weight gain.
- Swelling of the hands or feet.

The following side effects usually do not require medical attention; however, if they do occur and become bothersome, they should also be reported to the doctor or healthcare professional by the user:

- Headaches.
- Redness, irritation, or itching at the site of application.
- Unusual hair growth on the face, arm, or back.

Proper storage of minoxidil.

Minoxidil should be stored at room temperature between 68°-77° Fahrenheit (20°-25° degrees Celsius). Some products may be flammable; therefore, they should be kept away from heat, fire, or flame. Any unused minoxidil should be thrown away after its expiration date. It is important to remember to keep this and all other medications out of the reach of children, to never share your medicines with others, and to use this medication only for the indication prescribed.

Tricomin® Follicular Therapy Spray.

Tricomin® is another hair growth stimulant that the manufacturer claim can be safely used by men and women. It is a topical hair spray that has undergone some scientific testing. The main ingredient in this product is *copper peptides*, which have been proven to have some beneficial effects on hair growth stimulation. Copper has been found to be particularly useful to the body when it is attached to amino acids. These are called *copper peptides*, and Tricomin® incorporates these amino acids within all its products in what it calls a triamino copper complex. The three amino acids used in Tricomin® follicular therapy spray are L-histidine, L-lysine, and

L-alanine. This combination facilitates the efficient delivery of the copper peptides to the scalp follicles (Pickart, 2002, 2003).

According to the manufacturer of this product, the presence of copper peptides has been shown to inhibit 5-alpha-reductase (5AR), which is the enzyme responsible for the formation of DHT. The claim is that as we grow older, these peptides in the body begin to decrease, thereby allowing the 5-AR enzyme to help form DHT in the hair follicle. Dr. Pickart, the discoverer of GHK-Cu, which is a particular type of copper peptide, has demonstrated that this peptide stimulates the development of the basic ingredients that comprise a healthy hair follicle.

Copper peptides occur naturally in the human body and are normally present in fluids such as blood plasma. Both proteins and peptides are chains of amino acids, except that peptide chains are much shorter— less than 70 links— and thus have a significantly lower molecular mass. During the hair growth (anagen) phase, substances at the base of the hair follicle, such as collagen and various proteins, are actively produced. However, during the telogen (resting) phase, they are virtually inactive. Tricomin® has been shown to stimulate these substances into production by delivering copper peptides to the base of the hair follicle.

Tricomin® has undergone partial FDA clinical studies. During the trials, subjects applied treatment twice per day for a period of 24 weeks. The results were generally very positive. However, despite these positive results, the makers of this product decided to bypass the FDA- approval process because it was too costly and took too long to get the product on the market. Therefore, the company released Tricomin® as an over-the-counter product without a hair-loss treatment claim. Thus, Tricomin® was introduced to the market as a cosmetic product, which does not require FDA approval.

In a study entitled *"Chemical Agents and Peptides Affect Hair Growth,"* researchers Uno and Kurata (1993) explored the possibility of some chemical agents having an effect on follicular growth. The chemical agents under study were minoxidil and diazoxide, which are known to be potent hypotensive agents that act as peripheral vasodilators known to have a hypertrichotic (i.e., hair growth excess) side effect. The topical use of both agents, minoxidil, and diazoxide, was found to induce significant hair regrowth in the bald scalps of macaque monkeys in the study.

The study also explored using a copper peptide (PC1031) that showed effects of follicular enlargement on the back skin of fuzzy rats, covering the vellus follicles. The study also concluded that copper peptide application had a similar effect on the hair like that of topical minoxidil. Hence, this study demonstrated that the use of copper peptides does have a positive hair-growth effect. In fact, copper peptides may have a synergistic effect when used concomitantly with minoxidil, as the makers of Tricomin® suggest. It appears that Tricomin® may be an effective option for those who want a treatment that has undergone scientific testing but is not drug-based.

Potential side effects of Tricomin® follicular therapy spray.

The manufacturer of Tricomin® claims that it is a natural product that may be used safely by men and women. It has also been proven that it is non-irritating, and to date, it has not manifested any known side effects. According to the manufacturer, Tricomin® is recommended for use with any type of hair loss. And as mentioned before, it has shown a synergistic effect when used in combination with minoxidil (Fig. 15.3).

Fig.15.3: The synergistic effect of using minoxidil and copper peptides

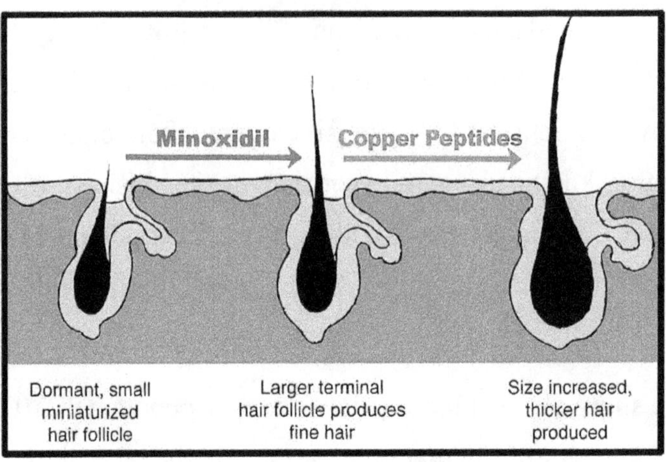

Image Source: http://folligen.com/healthy-hair-growth.html

Proper use of Tricomin® follicular therapy spray.

Tricomin® follicular therapy spray can be applied to damp or dry hair twice daily. However, if another topical treatment is utilized, such as minoxidil, the user should wait a few hours before applying Tricomin®, because minoxidil is recommended to be used on a dry scalp. Additionally, the scalp may turn a greenish color (because of the copper) when mixed with other products. However, this discoloration is not permanent and can be removed simply by washing the hair. Tricomin® is available as a follicular spray, shampoo, and conditioner. The Tricomin® shampoo and conditioner should be used in addition to the spray lotion and not as a replacement.

Tricomin®, like most other hair-loss treatments, should be used regularly to maintain its therapeutic effects. Therefore, its application is a lifelong commitment, as with most other hair-loss treatment products. Lifelong use of these products is understandable given that the underlying cause of the user's hair loss remains present.

However, a lifetime commitment to any product is very appealing to manufacturers of these hair-loss products.

Folligen® therapy spray (copper peptides).

Folligen® is another copper-peptide product similar to Tricomin®. However, Folligen® is sold at a more economical price than Tricomin®. The product is available as a cream, a lotion, or spray. It was originally designed as a skin-repair cream in the dermatology department at the University of California, San Francisco. However, because the product serendipitously regrew the hair of a 41-year-old woman who was afflicted with severe hair loss in approximately two and a half months, Skin Biology, the manufacturer of the product, has marketed Folligen® as a hair-loss treatment. This product contains blue-colored copper-peptide complexes and—according to the manufacturer— does not contain any blue dyes, scalp damaging detergents, alcohol, or any other harmful ingredients. The product's purpose is to improve the vitality of the hair and the health of the scalp and hair follicles.

Folligen products are marketed for both men and women. They feature a cream for hairline application, a spray for overall use, and a lotion for bald spots. According to the manufacturer, Folligen® is effective as a stand-alone treatment modality. However, it yields optimal results when used synergistically with other products like minoxidil.

Essentially, Folligen® products are indicated for soothing an irritated scalp. Moreover, they also relieve the occasional itching and burning associated with the application of the minoxidil topical solution. However, the Folligen® therapy spray may cause some itching or burning, and because the cream and lotion are bright blue-green, it is best to use them at night and cover the pillow to avoid staining it. In addition, while Folligen® can be washed off quite easily, it is not advisable for people with very light blonde hair to use the product; they may develop a greenish tinge to their hair.

Along with some credible scientific studies, such as the Uno and Kurata (1993) study, anecdotal evidence also seems to support the idea that copper peptides can improve the condition of the scalp, which encourages hair regrowth. Long-term users frequently swear by their success with the line of Folligen® products, citing healthier, thicker hair where the product is applied. In fact, since the benefits of copper peptides are not limited to just hair-loss prevention, the same users also frequently use the creams and lotions on their faces for firmer, more youthful skin (Pickart, Vasquez-Soltero, & Margolina, 2015).

Proxiphen®, Proxiphen-N, and NANO shampoo.

Proxiphen®

Proxiphen® is a non-FDA-approved topical cream formulation that requires a physician prescription. The reason the product is a cream is that many of the formulation components are insoluble in liquid, which can cause the precipitation of the other ingredients. The formulation essentially combines minoxidil at a higher dosage (5.5%) than the FDA-approved, commercially available medication. Additionally, it contains the prescription agent phenytoin (Dilantin®), an anticonvulsant drug that has the well-known side effect of inciting hair growth. It also contains spironolactone, a potent, topically effective antiandrogen, and tretinoin, which is the pharmaceutical form of retinoic acid. Tretinoin has been explored as a treatment for hair loss, as a way to potentially increase the ability of minoxidil to penetrate the scalp, but the evidence is weak and contradictory (Trüeb, 2015; Rogers & Avram, 2008).

Some of the other ingredients contained in Proxiphen are superoxide dismutase (SOD), a powerful antioxidant enzyme with potent anti-inflammatory properties. It also has 3-carboxylic acid pyridine-N-oxide (NANO), a natural minoxidil-like hair-growth stimulator, copper peptides as a DHT-inhibitor, and the amino acid

L-arginine as a hair-growth-promoting substance. It also contains L-arginine, which has several characteristics that may benefit hair follicles by boosting nitric oxide levels, promoting circulation, and aiding in releasing human growth hormone (HGH). The formulation also contains allantoin and NAC, among others. The user should apply the cream every day for the first eight to twelve months and, after that, every other day. Proxiphen® can only be dispensed with a physician prescription with a diagnosis of hair loss.

Proxiphen-N.

Proxiphen-N, also called Prox-N, is similar to Proxiphen® but without certain ingredients, such as tretinoin, minoxidil, phenytoin, and spironolactone. It is a topical formulation comprised of many non-prescription hair loss treatment agents, including various SODs, copper-binding peptides, and NANO hair-growth stimulators. Therefore, Proxiphen-N is the non-prescription formulation of Proxiphen®, which is a less expensive and weaker formulation. Since Prox-N does not contain minoxidil, it is recommended that patients use minoxidil with Proxiphen-N.

NANO shampoo.

NANO Shampoo is a hair regrowth shampoo that contains 3-carboxylic acids, pyridine n-oxide (NANO), and SODs, which is supposedly a very powerful hair growth stimulator with a high degree of safety, according to the developer. It is recommended that the companion conditioner be used with the NANO shampoo, which is supposedly an excellent complement. According to the product developer, these products are beneficial when used synergistically with Proxiphen® and Proxiphen-N.

The developer of these hair-loss product lines is Peter Proctor, M.D., Ph.D., a world-renowned authority on hair loss who has developed unique, patented, multi-ingredient hair formulas that address all the known factors in the balding process. According to Proctor, the patient needs to diligently use these products for at least eight to twelve months to see results.

Tretinoin (Retin-A®).

Tretinoin is a topical treatment primarily used by dermatologists to treat mild to moderate acne and other skin problems, such as sun damage and wrinkles. Therefore, it is used principally to rejuvenate the skin. Tretinoin is essentially a derivative of vitamin A that is available in liquid, cream, and gel forms, and it is typically applied daily at bedtime, or once every two or three days. This medication is also known as retinoic acid, and it is the active ingredient in the FDA-approved product Retin-A®.

Tretinoin mechanism of action.

Tretinoin is a *biologic response modifier*. It is a potent cell mitogen that promotes and regulates epithelial cell growth and differentiation. It promotes angiogenesis— the formation of new blood vessels— and increases percutaneous absorption by affecting the fluidity and lipid composition of cell membranes (androgeneticalopecia.com, n.d.). Moreover, some studies have shown that tretinoin stimulates stem cells in the hair follicle and scalp, allowing them to repair the damaged hair follicles and surrounding structures (Balañá, Charreau, & Leirós, 2015).

As a retinoid that regulates the growth and differentiation of epithelial cells, topical tretinoin can be used to help enhance the penetration and absorption of minoxidil for the treatment of hair loss. While tretinoin (Retin-A®) may have some hair growth properties by itself, its real purpose is to *triple the absorption rate of minoxidil (Lindsey, 2008)*. This increased absorption is most likely due to the increased percutaneous absorption of minoxidil through alteration of the horny outer layer of the epidermis, *the stratum corneum*. However, the manufactured formulations of tretinoin and minoxidil are incompatible and become ineffective if compounded into one formulation; therefore, tretinoin must be used separately as an off-label treatment (Androgeneticalopecia.com, n.d.).

Retin-A® should be applied in a thin layer with a gauze pad or cotton swab to the affected areas at bedtime. The user must remember to wash their hands immediately after using the product. The user should not get any Retin-A® near the eyes, mouth, or open cuts because the medication can irritate sensitive skin. It should also be mentioned that if Retin-A® is used more often than prescribed, the results will not be enhanced. Instead, side effects will increase. Side effects to the skin may include peeling, itching, scaling, redness, mild stinging, and immediate warming of the skin. However, once the skin adjusts to the medication, these effects should subside; if not, the user should stop the medication.

The use of Retin-A® may also result in increased sensitivity to sunlight, wind, and cold. For these reasons, the user should avoid prolonged exposure to the sun and sunlamps. The user should also use effective sunscreen and wear protective clothing. Research has not shown any risk of birth defects for pregnant women. Nevertheless, the use of Retin-A® should be avoided during pregnancy. If it must be used, the user should consult with a doctor before attempting to breastfeed.

Bimatoprost (Latisse®) for Eyelashes and Eyebrows.

Bimatoprost ophthalmic solution 0.03% was approved for medical use in the United States in 2001. It is sold under the brand names *Lumigan, Bitoma, Careprost and Intraprost*. It is an eyedrop medication primarily developed to treat increased intraocular pressure (IOP) or high pressure inside the eye, including glaucoma. Bimatoprost is used explicitly for open-angle glaucoma when other medications are not sufficient. Open-angle glaucoma is the most common form of the disease. The drainage angle formed by the cornea and iris remains open, but the trabecular meshwork is partially blocked.

As usually occurs during research studies, the researchers serendipitously discovered that Bimatoprost had a hypertrichosis side effect. Hypertrichosis is defined as excessive hair growth anywhere on the body in either males or females (Saleh et al., 2021). It is crucial to differentiate hypertrichosis from hirsutism, which is a term reserved for females who have excessive hair growth in areas where typically no hair usually grows. The hair growth observed in hirsutism is considered to be androgen-dependent. For a more extensive explanation of hirsutism, see chapter 6.

Bimatoprost followed a similar path or trajectory to minoxidil, a medication developed to treat refractory hypertension, but researchers subsequently discovered minoxidil also had a hypertrichosis side effect. Following that discovery, minoxidil was developed as Rogaine®, becoming the first hair loss medication to receive approval by the FDA. In the case of bimatoprost, researchers observed that the eyelashes unexpectantly began to grow when using the ophthalmic eyedrops. As a result of this discovery, in December 2008, topical bimatoprost was approved by the FDA to treat eyelash hypotrichosis under the brand name Latisse®. ***Hypotrichosis*** is a rare condition in which there is little or no hair growth on the scalp, including the eyebrows, eyelashes, or other areas of the body where hair usually grows.

Applying Latisse® along the upper eyelid lash line will gradually encourage the growth of longer, thicker, and darker eyelashes. Latisse® is not meant to be applied to the lower eyelid because it may cause excess hair growth in unwanted areas. Latisse® must be used daily for at least two months to see any results. Eyelash improvements remain as long as the patient continues to use the medication. If the drug is stopped, the eyelashes will eventually return to their original appearance; in the same way, scalp hair stops if minoxidil is not used consistently.

Besides stimulating eyelash growth, several research studies have demonstrated that Latisse® also positively affects eyebrow hair growth. The effectiveness of Latisse® is dependent on many factors, such as how often it is applied and whether there are underlying causes for eyebrow hair loss (hypotrichosis). Since Latisse® FDA approval for eyelash use, some physicians have been advocating its use *"off label"* for hair growth in other areas, such as the scalp and eyebrows. Currently, the drug is in clinical trials for FDA approval as a topical scalp hair loss treatment. If it proves efficacious during these trials, it could be available in a few years.

Bimatoprost (Latisse®) mechanism of action.

The precise mechanism of action for Latisse® is unknown. Just like scalp hair, eyelashes, and eyebrows, growth is cyclical. The normal eyelash growth cycle involves the same four phases observed in scalp hair: they are the anagen (growth), catagen (transitional), telogen (resting), and exogen (shedding) hair growth cycles. Thus, the regular eyelash and eyebrow growth cycle involves the same four hair growth phases and occurs over several months. It is postulated that bimatoprost (Latisse®) most likely works by interacting with the prostaglandin receptors in the hair follicle and stimulating the resting follicles (telogen phase) to grow follicles (anagen phase). Increasing the anagen (growth) phase cycle may increase eyelash and eyebrow growth, length, thickness, and darkness. Furthermore, in clinical trials, bimatoprost (Latisse®) has been reported to stimulate blood flow to the hair follicles, inducing hair growth. Bimatoprost (Latisse®) also increases the production of molecules in the dermal papilla, which helps to activate the transition from the telogen (shedding) to the anagen (growth) phase and to increase the duration of the anagen phase leading to hair growth.

***Disclaimer:** The product information described regarding the various hair-loss products discussed is intended as an educational aid only. It is not intended as medical advice for any individual condition(s) or treatment. Moreover, it is not a substitute for a medical exam, nor does it replace the need for services provided by healthcare professionals. The users or patients should understand that they should consult with a doctor or pharmacist before taking any prescription or over-the-counter (OTC) medication (including any herbal medicines or supplements) or following any treatment or regimen. Only a physician or pharmacist can provide the prospective patient with advice on what is safe and effective for them.

Hair Loss Thickening Fiber Concealers

Hair loss thickening fibers concealer or hair fibers concealers are products that employ keratin fibers in powder or spray form to conceal hair loss. These concealers have become a trendy alternative to camouflage hair loss or as a supplementary adjunct product to enhance and improve the appearance of hair loss or hair transplants that do not have enough hair density. These products are excellent because they create an instant and effective illusion of a full head of hair at a reasonable cost to the consumer. These hair-building fibers are a completely different approach to building thicker, more abundant hair while immediately providing the illusion of a full head of hair (Figs. 15.4 and 15.5).

Fig. 15.4: The principle behind hair fiber concealers application

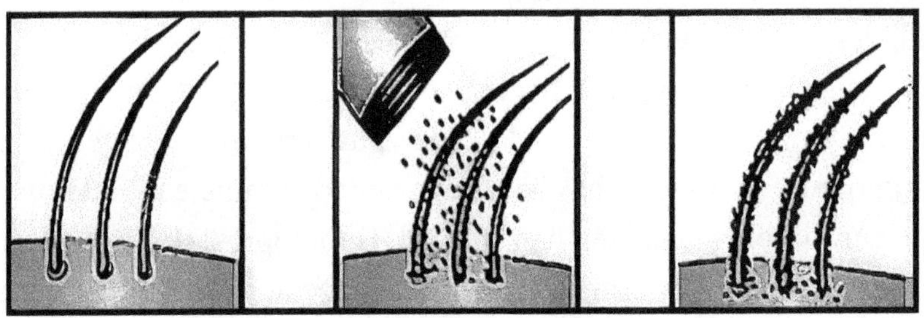

Image Source: http://hairlosscureguide.com/12-best-hair-loss-concealers-and-fibers-to-hide-baldness/

Hair thickening fibers are made from all-natural plant or keratin fibers. However, the higher-quality products are made of keratin fibers only. Once applied, these microscopic fibers bond statically to the existing hair, creating a much thicker and fuller appearance. Because this product has become very successful, the industry has become highly competitive. The competition has resulted in creating a variety of new products at very reasonable prices. The approximate cost of this product is $25.00 to $46.00 for a two-month supply.

Currently, there are approximately 12 different brands of hair fiber concealers on the market. Therefore, this increase in competition has made the hair fiber concealers market very competitive, which should further lower prices. Additionally, the quality of these hair-loss concealers has continued to improve significantly over the past few years.

Fig. 15.5: The effect hair fiber concealers can create after application

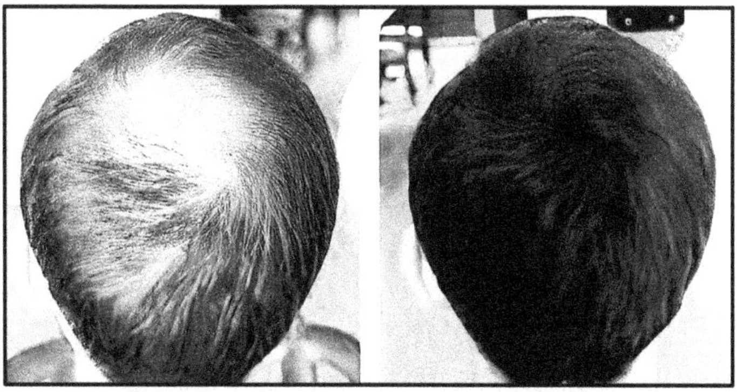

Image Source: https://www.newswire.com/news/allure-hair-building-fibers-recently-launched-their-website-offering-14626152

Scalp Micropigmentation (SMP) Procedure

Scalp micropigmentation (SMP) is a highly sophisticated and popular medical tattooing process used to improve the appearance of balding or thinning hair. SMP, also called *scalp ink*, is a scalp tattooing procedure that seems relatively simple to perform but is not. The procedure is extremely time-consuming; the SMP must be customized for each client since each patient's skin differs with regard to how the scalp reacts as it holds on to the tattoo dye. The SMP process is actually more of an art form than a science because of the many variables involved with performing the procedure. SMP is a very labor-intensive process that could require multiple tattooing sessions lasting up to 20 hours or more to create the look that will satisfy the patient (Rassman, Pak, & Kim, 2013). The SMP technique is a specialized procedure that uses conventional cosmetic tattooing instruments and pigments in a stippling pattern on the scalp. A stippling pattern is basically the creation of a pattern simulating varying degrees of solidity or shading by using small dots, which in the case of SMP, is the creation of dots to represent the appearance or illusion of hair (Fig.15.6).

Fig. 15.6: Appearance of a scalp micropigmentation (SMP) procedure

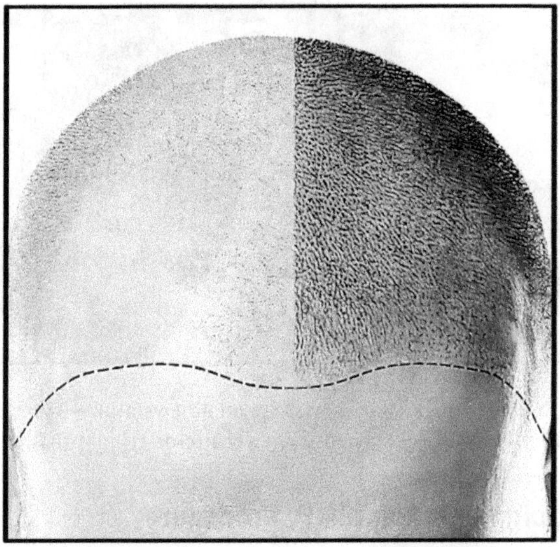

Image Source: https://www.dermaplusclinic.in/micropigmentation

Although this procedure was developed to improve the appearance of alopecia (hair loss), which was unresponsive to treatment and for the correction of hair transplants with aesthetically unacceptable outcomes, the procedure has also become quite popular with bald individuals who like the very short-hair look. Therefore, the scalp micropigmentation procedure (SMP) offers a good, non-surgical alternative treatment for hair loss and the correction of scalp deformities.

The tattoo industry is amid a cultural expansion, growing by nearly 10 percent every year for more than a decade now. Industry analysts believe that this trend will continue well into the 2020s making SMP and tattoos in general a more socially acceptable cosmetic solution for covering the appropriate scalp and hair-loss problems (Rassman et al., 2013). Conversely, according to the latest tattoo removal statistics, the tattoo removal industry is now outpacing the growth of tattoo studios. Tattoo removal services are expected to increase by 18% annually for the next few years. Moreover, a Harris Poll found that in the United States, 46% of adults have at least one tattoo in 2021. Tattoos have become an unprecedentedly extensive revolution. According to *tattoo statistics,* this 12,000 years old tradition is now a thriving $3 billion industry (TattooPro, 2021).

Psychological Effects of Hair Loss

Humanity has always admired one specific part of the human body as the symbol of beauty for centuries: the hair. Hair loss is a problem for millions of men and women, both young and old. Hair plays a vital role in determining self-image, social perceptions, and psychosocial functioning. It can decrease self-esteem and confidence and limit the ability to enjoy life to the fullest. Balding or hair loss affects people in different ways, but certain emotional reactions seem to be shared by many (Bernstein, 2014). Contrary to popular belief that bald men do not care about losing their hair as much as women, there are millions of unhappy, alopecia-afflicted men who would welcome a solution to their hair loss problems.

Body Dysmorphic Disorder (BDD)

In recent years, more attention has been paid to ***Body Dysmorphic Disorder (BDD)***, also known as Body Dysmorphia. This illness was once largely ignored by the public and was commonly lumped in with generalized anxiety, depression, and other mental issues. However, scientists have begun to recognize the specific symptoms and traits associated with BDD. Dysmorphia is a chronic (long-term) illness characterized by an obsession with a perceived bodily flaw. Body dysmorphic disorder affects people of any gender. It tends to begin during the teen years or early adulthood. That is the age when children start comparing themselves to others.

Without treatment, Body Dysmorphic Disorder can get worse as people get older. The afflicted become even more unhappy with the physical changes of aging, such as wrinkles and gray hair. This disorder can also include what's called ***Hair Dysmorphic Disorder (HDD),*** a branch of Body Dysmorphic Disorder. HDD is considered the second most common issue for patients exhibiting this disorder (Kacar et al., 2015).

Body dysmorphia is a mental condition in which you focus heavily on a perceived physical flaw that appears minor or nonexistent to everyone else. Body dysmorphia can sometimes cause someone so much anxiety about their physical appearance that they begin avoiding social interactions and outings. These BDD afflicted individuals may constantly check their appearance in the mirror or seek constant validation from others. Those individuals who experience hair loss might be more likely to suffer from body dysmorphia than other people. For example, according to a study entitled *"Body Dysmorphic Disorder Among Patients with Complaints of Hair Loss,"* dermatologists observed body dysmorphia in almost 30% of patients who experienced hair loss (Kacar et al., 2015). The study concluded that the incidence of body dysmorphic disorders (BDD) is approximately ten times higher in patients with complaints of hair loss than it is in general dermatology patients and is higher in males. Physicians agree that awareness of the condition and the referral of selected patients to mental health professionals is crucial for their well-being.

Alopecia can have serious psychosocial consequences, causing intense emotional suffering and personal, social, and work-related problems. Surveys have shown that around 40% of women with alopecia have had marital problems, and approximately 63% claim to have career-related problems (Hunt & McHale, 2004). There is also evidence that stressful life events play an essential role in triggering episodes of alopecia (Garcia-Hernandez et al., 1999).

For example, women who experience high-stress levels are eleven times more likely to experience hair loss than those who do not report high-stress levels (York et al., 1998). Compared with the general population, increased prevalence rates of psychiatric disorders are associated with alopecia, suggesting that people with hair loss may be at higher risk of developing a major depressive episode, anxiety disorder, social phobia, or paranoid disorder (Koo et al., 1994). Overall, there has been little systematic research into alopecia's psychological consequences (Hunt & McHale, 2005).

Unfortunately, there are few psychologically acceptable solutions for hair loss short of undergoing hair transplant surgery, which is the only proven method that can regrow hair on the patient's scalp to any significant degree. However, for this hair restoration method to be effective, the patient must be considered a good candidate. To be regarded as a good hair transplant candidate, the patient needs an excellent donor area to facilitate sufficient density in the bald area.

In the opinion of numerous well-known and highly respected hair restoration surgeons, hair-transplantation surgery is currently the best psychological solution for individuals afflicted with hair loss. The reason for this opinion is that the hair-transplantation solution will be relatively permanent and aesthetically acceptable if the patient is a good hair transplant candidate. At best, all other hair restoration and replacement methods can only provide a temporary psychological improvement because their results are essentially limited.

Hair restoration treatments can be frustrating, expensive, and time-consuming, but they are pursued hoping that something will work. However, the reality is that after years of trying all sorts of hair-loss remedies without any satisfactory results, most patients will give up and reluctantly accept their undesired fate. Notwithstanding this disappointment, men and women should never resign themselves to look less than what they were meant to be. Everyone's life objective should be to strive to improve both intellectually and physically in order to a achieve proper physical and psychological balance and thus live the most fulfilling and satisfying life possible. A critical component of reaching this psychological balance is keeping and preserving one's hair.

Currently, there is no conclusive evidence that explains all the causative factors that lead to male and female pattern hair loss or androgenetic alopecia (AGA). However, there are many possible solutions or options available to address the problem of hair loss. Fortunately, some interesting research reports have revealed promising and exciting results in the field of male and female alopecia that could potentially uncover the causes of androgenetic alopecia.

Significant scientific progress has been made regarding potential treatments to solve the hair-loss problem. Presently, numerous prestigious institutions are researching novel methods of hair restoration. For example, stem cell research has been undertaken in places such as Sanford-Burnham Medical Research Institute, San Francisco Veterans Affairs Medical Center, Harvard Medical School, John Hopkins University, and the University of Pennsylvania. The preliminary results are raising hope for millions of men and women that a possible cure for hair loss is forthcoming in the not-too-distant future.

16

Hygiene and Hair Care

Hygiene and regular care of the hair and scalp are extremely important aspects of the total concept of understanding hair loss, or for that matter, retaining the hair. Care of the hair and care to the scalp skin may appear separate functions. However, they are not. In fact, they are intertwined because hair grows from underneath the skin. The living parts of the hair, which are comprised of the hair follicle, hair root, root sheath, and sebaceous gland, are actually beneath the skin, or dermis. Conversely, the hair shaft that emerges through the skin, which is composed of the cuticle that covers the cortex and medulla, has no living processes.

In other words, hair is not considered living tissue with a nervous system, blood supply, or living cells, which are essential elements for regeneration. Thus, hair cannot heal itself (Rosebrook, 2016). Therefore, damage or changes made to the visible hair shaft cannot be repaired by a biological process, though much can be done to manage the hair and ensure that the cuticle remains intact. That is why hygiene and regular hair and scalp care are essential aspects in the care and prevention of hair loss.

Hair and scalp care were the physician's responsibility some 50 years ago, a role that became relegated almost entirely to trichologists, beauty parlors, barbers, and hair restoration clinics. The likely reason for this change of responsibility is that most physicians view hair care as a trivial matter unless it is associated with a disease process.

The imparting of knowledge regarding hygiene and regular scalp and hair care must commence in early childhood. The dissemination of this knowledge should be the responsibility of the family physician or nurse practitioner and the child's parents. Therefore, the involvement of the family healthcare practitioner is essential for instilling in children the proper practices of hair and scalp hygiene. Family healthcare providers should not ignore their fundamental role in hair and scalp care. Although it appears a trivial matter, it is a crucial function in developing a healthy scalp and hair. Moreover, it is essential information that needs to be provided to ensure the development of well-rounded children.

It has been well documented that the primary prerequisite for healthy, strong hair growth is a clean scalp. The first step for maintaining beautiful, shining hair is ensuring that the scalp is healthy and that no pores are clogged. A healthy scalp ensures that hair will also be healthy. It has been proven that when hair is too dry, it has the tendency to become frail, split, or break off, subsequently becoming less abundant. Conversely, when the scalp is oily, hairs have a marked tendency to fall out. Therefore, healthy, normal, long-lived hairs ideally are neither too dry nor too oily (Rosebrook, 2016).

Contrary to popular belief, frequent cleansing of the scalp is absolutely necessary for people who possess a natural tendency to have oily hair and for those individuals whose occupations subject them to dust, dirt, excessive perspiration, and air pollution. If the hair must be cleaned every day, then the mildest type of shampoo should be used. Subsequently, in another section of this chapter, there are explanations regarding the proper way of shampooing the hair and vital information regarding the different types of shampoos ideal for various hair types (e.g., dry, oily, or combination).

Adequate hygiene and regular hair and scalp care are vital during the child's formative years. Because although the scalps of young adolescents may appear to be clean and healthy, requiring only routine shampooing, many children will manifest *Pityriasis Capitis,* which is commonly known as dandruff.

It has been documented that dandruff is generally the forerunner of disease that will ultimately lead to hair loss in later years, even if it does not seem to cause immediate hair damage at an early age. The appearance of dandruff at any age, but especially in childhood, must be recognized as a warning sign for the scalp's need for medical treatment. The discussion that follows in the next section will address topics such as brushing and combing the hair, scalp massaging and shampooing the hair.

Brushing the Hair

A vital component of hygiene and hair care is the proper selection of a hairbrush. The hairbrush should not only be selected with care but should be kept scrupulously clean. Therefore, hairbrushes should never be used by anyone except the owner to avoid a possible scalp infection, especially dandruff, which can lead to hair loss if not stopped in time.

It is widely accepted that the best brushes for men and women are those with stiff or firm bristles of various lengths set widely apart or in widely spaced oval groups. In this type of arrangement, the brush can penetrate the hair and reach the scalp, a task that would be impossible if the bristles were of equal length and not widely spaced. The basic principle behind hair-brushing is the tonic influences this mild type of massage gives the hair follicles. Brushing also prevents snarling, and it polishes and increases the normal luster of the hair. The friction provided by the brushing action is considered the equivalent of shampooing since thoroughly brushing the hair with a suitable scalp brush will remove dirt and grime and stimulate scalp circulation. It is recommended that the hair be brushed at least once a day, preferably in the morning when the circulation is not up to par, and the scalp requires stimulation.

It has been hypothesized that the practice of regularly massaging the scalp improves scalp circulatory blood flow, which will result in hair growth and hair loss prevention. This postulation has been controversial for many years among physicians specializing in hair loss. However, current research studies have demonstrated that improving the scalp blood supply does, in fact, have a positive influence in preventing hair loss (Hay, Jamieson, & Omerod, 1998). Whether improving scalp circulation effectively elicits hair growth or not, most researchers concur that scalp massaging has a beneficial effect on the hair. As the analogy goes, if massage revitalizes the body's muscles, it should also help to rejuvenate and tone the hair, and it certainly cannot hurt.

When correctly performed, hair-brushing will aid in the removal of dirt and grime but will also help evenly distribute the natural oil produced by the sebaceous glands. This oily substance called sebum is actually the hair's natural conditioner. A fine head of hair enhances an individual's appearance, whether male or female. Sometimes this lesson is learned too late in life. That is why it is crucial to teach about hygiene and proper care of the hair and scalp to start in early childhood to prevent the catastrophic results one pays for ignorance.

Benjamin Franklin once said, *"An ounce of prevention is worth a pound of cure."* These words of wisdom should be a philosophy we embrace for everything we do in life, but especially for health-related issues. Another profound phrase that we should live by to ensure the prevention of health issues is: *"Genetics loads the gun, but lifestyle pulls the trigger."*

Cleaning the Hairbrushes

Like any other personal article, hairbrushes must be disinfected and cleaned frequently, a task seldom performed. They should be cleaned with soap and warm water first, placed in a disinfecting solution for 30-45 minutes, and then thoroughly rinsed with warm water once again. Performing this simple task should keep the hairbrush clean and prevent bacterial growth, leading to a possible scalp infection or dandruff. Dermatologist and hair-loss researcher Dr. M. Piliang (2016) of the Cleveland Clinic recommends that hairbrushes be cleaned every one to two weeks. Piliang recommends cleaning the brushes more frequently for people with longer hair, typically every week. It is well documented that unclean brushes are a dangerous source of potential infection. As previously mentioned, no hairbrush should be common to several people; to do this is surely asking for trouble. Hairbrushes should be treated with the same scrupulous attitude as we treat our toothbrushes and other personal articles.

Combing the Hair

Most people consider hair combing a routine activity. Correct hair-combing is essential for beautiful and healthy-looking hair. The wrong methods lead to breakage and hair damage, affecting its vitality. The comb is another instrument used for parting and unsnarling tangled hair. Combs should be made with teeth that are smooth and evenly spaced to facilitate cleaning between the teeth. It is imperative that the ends of the comb's teeth are sufficiently blunt and rounded to avoid scratching the scalp. It is possible to transmit a disease due to trauma produced by scratching the scalp. If the comb irritates the scalp, it can provide an entry port for bacteria that could lead to an infection. The comb should be cleaned before and after use to prevent hair and dirt deposits in the gap. The same practice holds for combs and hairbrushes; they should not be shared with others. Adhering to this practice should prevent any fungal or bacterial infections.

It is recommended that hair be combed twice daily—morning and evening—for about one minute so it can stay shiny, healthy, and free from tangled ends. Combing stimulates the scalp's microcirculation and helps it relax, cleans dirt accumulated from the environment during the day, and adds volume to the hair. However, one should be mindful that excessive combing is unnecessarily aggressive and may cause hair strain, stimulating the sebaceous glands and making the hair greasy faster.

Massaging the Scalp

It is a foregone conclusion for many hair-loss researchers that there is no definitive proof that poor scalp circulation results in hair loss. However, as mentioned previously, several research studies have proven that poor circulation to the scalp does lead to increased shedding of the hair, which, if left unattended, will result in permanent hair loss or baldness (Hay, Jamieson, & Omerod, 1998). The premise behind this assumption is that if the scalp is stiff, tense, and possesses little mobility, this tightness can depress the circulatory blood flow of the scalp, thus diminishing vital nutrients needed for the health of the hair follicles. This premise seems to be grounded on an old theory about the cause of male pattern baldness proposed by Dr. Lars Engstrand of Sweden in the 1960s—the tight scalp theory, or more appropriately, the tight galea theory (Seagrave, 1996). This tight galea theory is the primary reason for the popularity of scalp massage, the purpose of which is to relieve the increased tension of the scalp upon the circulatory system.

Researchers Hay et al. (1998) from the department of dermatology at the Aberdeen Royal Infirmary in Scotland, United Kingdom, conducted a randomized, seven-month research study to investigate the effectiveness of scalp massage for the treatment of people with alopecia areata (AA). This study was subsequently reported in the Archives of Dermatology in 1998. The study was composed of 86 participants who had been diagnosed with alopecia areata, an autoimmune disease process in which hair loss is apparent on some or all parts of the human body, particularly the scalp. The Hay (1998) study participants were divided into two groups. The first group, referred to as the active group, received a daily massage for hair loss for seven months. Essential oils like— lavender, cedarwood, thyme, and rosemary were blended with jojoba and grape seed oil as carrier oils. This mixture was then used to massage the participants' scalps in the first group. The second group, referred to as the control group, received a daily massage with only the carrier oils of jojoba and grape seed over the same seven months period.

Hay et al. (1998) evaluated the success of massage for hair loss by using computerized analysis of the traced areas of hair loss shown on photographs taken throughout the research study. The investigators used a six-point scale to measure the effectiveness of massage for hair loss in the two groups in the study. The results showed an improvement in 44% of the forty-three participants making up the active group. In contrast, the study showed that there was a 15% improvement in the forty-one participants that made up the study control group. These results indicate that scalp massage for hair loss combined with essential oils, like lavender, cedarwood, thyme, and rosemary, possess hair growth–promoting properties. In fact, scalp massage with restorative oils has been anecdotally used to treat alopecia for more than 100 years. The study further demonstrated that scalp massage—besides improving the circulatory blood flow of the scalp and increasing the probability of healthy hair growth—can also be soothing, can help prevent headaches, and benefit sleep patterns. Massaging the scalp can be accomplished in many different ways—with the fingertips, electric vibrators, electric combs, or ultraviolet ray lamps, just to name a few.

Notwithstanding all the positive reports by Hay et al. (1998) and Kiichiro et al. (2001) regarding scalp circulation and hair-loss prevention, it is important to bear in mind the 1951 research findings of renowned researcher Dr. Hamilton, who categorically denied that hair loss was the result of poor scalp circulation. However, common sense indicates that prudent hygiene and hair care cannot possibly hurt, and scalp massage could function as a beneficial complement to these practices.

In a fascinating study conducted by Freund and Schwartz (2010) entitled *"Treatment of Male Pattern Baldness with Botulinum Toxin: A Pilot Study,"* the investigators contended that the process of testosterone conversion to DHT occurs in low-oxygen (hypoxic) environments. Currently, it is a well-established and accepted theory that DHT is the primary contributing factor to androgenetic alopecia (AGA) or male pattern baldness. The discovery by Freund and Schwartz is significant because if the scalp muscles or anything else that constricts circulatory blood flow to the scalp will also reduce the availability of oxygen to the scalp and dermal papilla. This reduction of blood flow and lack of oxygen will increase DHT conversion because of the hypoxic (reduced oxygen) environment.

Freund and Schwartz (2010) contend that relaxing these scalp muscles through Botox® administration prevents or alleviates this low-oxygen environment. This finding would seem to confirm that improving scalp circulation by whatever means necessary, such as scalp massage, is helpful to men and women with hair loss resulting from a genetic sensitivity to DHT.

Despite this new evidence from Freund and Schwartz (2010), some investigators are against scalp massage because, according to their findings, the scalp possesses a rich supply of blood vessels and does not require any stimulating massaging action to improve it. These investigators further claim that vigorous scalp massage could damage the hair. However, it is becoming clear from some of the favorable research studies that improving scalp circulation might, in fact, be an effective hair-growth method.

Shampooing the Hair

Although shampooing the hair appears to be a relatively simple task, there is actually a method of performing it correctly. The hair should never be shampooed hurriedly, especially for women. If time is unavailable, shampooing should be postponed to a more convenient time. A properly applied shampoo promotes healthy hair, but if it is improperly applied, or if the wrong kind of shampoo is used, it can be very destructive to the hair.

The following steps should be followed to ensure a properly applied shampoo:

1. Give the hair a good, stiff brushing to activate the oil (sebaceous) glands and loosen any dead scales in the scalp.

2. Massage the scalp gently with the fingertips in a circular motion, starting at the temples and working toward the back of the scalp.

3. If an oil treatment is needed because of a dry scalp, this is the time to do it.

4. Thoroughly wet the hair using warm water. If hairsprays have been used, wet the hair with hot water to remove any spray residue.

5. Apply the shampoo. Massage the scalp with the round part of the fingertips, paying special attention to the hairline. Do not use your fingernails, thus avoiding irritating the scalp. If the hair is inordinately long, make sure that the ends are well shampooed.

6. Rinse well to avoid any soap residue remaining on the scalp. An improperly rinsed scalp could lead to disaster. Usually, this is the step most people follow incorrectly.

7. The last rinse should be with cold water. This helps to give the hair a shine and stops the sebaceous (oil) glands from producing any more oil. In an area where there is hard water, use a softener in the water system if available.

8. If you like to use a cream rinse or add color, this is the time to do it.

9. Towel-dry the hair without rubbing. Then comb it starting at the ends, working up to the roots to untangle the hair. This process is crucial for people with long hair.

10. It is extremely important to keep all brushes, combs, and any hair equipment scrupulously clean and do not lend them to anyone.

Different Types of Hair

Before selecting the appropriate type of shampoo to clean the hair and scalp, the hair type should be determined. Three types of hair will determine the kind of shampoo to select:

- Oily hair.
- Dry hair.
- Combination hair.

Oily Hair.

People that possess oily hair are individuals with overactive sebaceous glands. The oil or sebum produced by these sebaceous glands is a built-in conditioning and lubricating system for the hair. Oily or greasy hair is more evident in individuals with fine hair since the hair is so thin that it cannot absorb excess oil as coarse hair can.

If an individual possesses this type of hair, there is very little that can be done to reverse the process other than keeping it clean and free from excess oil. Oily hair requires frequent shampooing. Provided that the mildest kinds of shampoos are used, no hair damage will occur. The most crucial treatment for oily hair is washing the hair as frequently as necessary. Just do not leave the oil on the scalp. Since oily hair must be cleaned often or even daily—this also applies to individuals whose occupation exposes them to excessive amounts of dust and perspiration—the mildest kind of shampoos must be used. An important point to remember is that most shampoos recommended for oily hair are too strong and harsh, especially if used daily.

It would probably be surprising to most people that the mildest kinds of shampoos are shampoos for dry hair; therefore, this kind is recommended over the shampoos made for oily hair if daily cleaning is necessary. Furthermore, if the hair must be shampooed daily, it is strongly recommended to lather just one time; it is better for the hair to be shampooed frequently with one lather than less frequently with two.

Dry Hair.

Dry hair is generally the direct result of mistreating the hair or not protecting it appropriately. If this is the case, then the dryness results from an inadequate amount of sebum (oil) excreted from the sebaceous glands. It can be safely stated that possessing naturally dry hair is an extremely rare condition since most dry hair is self-inflicted through one or all of the following mechanisms:

- Perming the hair.
- Tinting the hair.
- Frosting the hair.
- Blow-drying (done improperly).
- Electric rollers.
- Curling irons.
- Hot combs.
- Flat irons.

The last five situations on the list will only result in dry hair if applied too frequently or without proper knowledge and care. Moreover, other situations that can result in dry hair are exposure to salty seawater, chlorinated water in swimming pools, and too-frequent shampooing resulting from today's environment, which is characterized by high levels of air pollution. This dirt can accumulate on the scalp and clog the hair follicle, preventing sebum excretion from the sebaceous glands and making the hair even drier. Once again, it is essential to remember that the mildest form of shampoos should be used. Furthermore, just one lathering is recommended unless the hair is extremely dirty. Dry hair requires a conditioner or a cream rinse following the shampoo, and a regular, deep, penetrating conditioning treatment (i.e., once every two to three weeks should be sufficient).

Combination Hair.

Combination hair should be treated exactly as dry hair, meaning that a mild shampoo should be used. When shampooing this type of hair, the primary emphasis is to concentrate on the roots and less on the ends since combination hair usually implies that the roots are greasy while the ends remain dry. The shampoo should be applied primarily to the roots, and just before rinsing the hair, massage and shampoo the entire scalp.

The emphasis when shampooing is to do it as often as necessary; because it is more hygienic and healthier for the hair to have a clean scalp environment. The individual should always be mindful that the mildest types of shampoo be used, especially if the hair is washed frequently.

Blow-Drying the Hair

A very popular method of drying the hair today is the handheld blow-dryer. These dryers are a versatile instrument essential for creating today's numerous hairstyles. Since this instrument utilizes hot air to dry the hair, it has the potential to damage the hair by simply overdrying it, thus making the hair weak and brittle, which can lead to hair loss.

When using the hand-dryer, care must be taken not to utilize too much heat or apply it directly to the scalp. A warm setting is recommended to prevent overdrying. It has been said that the utilization of handheld dryers leads to hair loss, but this is simply not the case since not all individuals who use the instrument lose their hair.

When these instruments are used, the situation that leads to hair loss is when they are misused and when extremely hot temperatures are applied directly onto the scalp and hair. It is recommended that when using the handheld dryer, the user should cool the scalp and hair down by applying cool air to the entire head after the hair has been dried. This simple technique can reduce the degree of hair damage resulting from too much heat exposure and reduce the static electricity that is sometimes created by brushing the hair with hot air.

17

Nutritional Aspects of the Hair

The term nutrition is defined as a biological process in humans, animals, and plants involving the intake of food and its subsequent assimilation into the tissues. During the twentieth century, scientists identified the various nutrients that constitute food and defined nutritional standards and recommendations to prevent deficiencies and promote human health. Now, entering the twenty-first century, for industrialized countries, the emphasis for nutritional science is on increasing life expectancy by offering new strategies to improve the quality of human life. Nutritional supplements are defined as concentrated and essential sources of nutrients or other substances with a nutritional or physiological effect that supplements the standard diet (Piccardi & Manissier, 2009).

Hair, like any other part of the body, requires certain nutrients to ensure its proper health. These nutrients are provided to the hair bulb for cellular replication through the scalp circulatory system after being processed into their proper chemical composition by the liver. That is why hair problems can be manifested in the presence of liver disease even if an individual is well nourished. Therefore, in general, healthy-looking hair is a sign of good health and good hair-care practices (Goldberg & Lenzy, 2010). Although vitamin and mineral imbalances have been postulated causes of hair loss, the nutritional parameters that might regulate hair production have not been evaluated comprehensively. Much of the focus has been on zinc, vitamin D, and protein (Rushton, 2002).

However, in the past decade, many scientific reports have supported nutraceuticals as an effective and safe treatment option for general hair loss. A nutraceutical is a food or naturally occurring food supplement thought to prevent disease or have other beneficial effects on human health. Nutraceuticals have also been called *functional foods.* Today, there seems to be a growing trend toward the use of nutritional supplementation compared to the use of prescription or over-the-counter (OTC) medications. A famous quote attributed to Hippocrates, the father of western medicine, who in 400 B.C. stated, "Let food be thy medicine, and medicine thy food." This quote by Hippocrates exemplifies that society might be realizing that the body has the ability to rejuvenate or restore itself if given the proper nutrition. Some isolated research reports have evaluated the influence of varying dietary supplements (e.g., millet extracts, biotin, pantothenic acid, and other B-complex vitamins, minerals like zinc and iron, omega-3, omega-7, and omega-6 fatty acids, and antioxidants like lycopene) on hair loss of various origins, with different results. Unfortunately, these studies have infrequently focused on evaluating the efficacy or effectiveness of these nutraceuticals in preventing or resolving androgenetic alopecia (Sonthaliam, Daulatabad, & Tosti, 2015).

Since hair is primarily composed of keratin protein, it requires protein as a nutrient for proper health. Hair keratin is formed from 16 amino acids that become keratinized (i.e., they create keratin) in the scalp before hair emerges from the scalp's surface. A diet deficient in protein can lead to a temporary change of color (depigmentation) and texture, resulting in thin, dry, easily shed hair. It has been observed that protein deficiency can result in a higher proportion of hairs being in the telogen (resting) or exogen (shedding) stage of the hair-growth cycle.

If this protein deficiency is corrected in time, the hair will return to its normal condition. If not, it could lead to permanent hair loss. Carbohydrates are needed to provide energy for protein utilization and improve the mitotic activity (cell replication) in the hair follicles. Fats are also essential nutrients, especially for the proper function of the sebaceous glands, which produce the hair's natural conditioner, sebum. In fact, the normal function of the sebaceous glands is that of fat formation or adipogenesis, with the manufactured fat having a special composition of its own.

It has been observed that keratin contains a greater proportion of the amino acid cysteine than most other proteins and a higher sulfur content as well. Cysteine is a sulfur-containing amino acid found in foods like poultry, eggs, dairy, red peppers, garlic, and onions. It works as an antioxidant in collagen production— a component of hair, skin, and nails— and is also used in the body to create glutathione, another important antioxidant.

It is essential to understand the difference between the amino acids ***cysteine*** and ***cystine***, which are frequently mistaken as being the same amino acid. Although they are invaluable to hair growth, they are two different things. ***Cysteine*** is the single most crucial amino acid for hair growth. It helps prevent damage to existing hair from external factors in addition to promoting new hair growth. Conversely, ***cystine,*** which is formed from two cysteine molecules joined together, is a more stable amino acid than *cysteine* but may not be as absorbable. The amino acid cystine is also a component of hair, skin, and nails. However, there is no conclusive evidence that supplementing with ***cystine*** improves hair, skin, or nail health; thus, it is rarely used as a dietary supplement.

It is believed that where there is some degree of scaling from the scalp and body (exfoliative dermatitis), increased ingestion of the sulfur-containing amino acids (i.e., cysteine or methionine) could be beneficial. Tyrosine is another essential amino acid that makes hair grow faster. A significant factor that affects hair loss is stress, and L-tyrosine helps reduce stress. L-tyrosine lowers stress hormones such as adrenaline, cortisol, and norepinephrine, reducing the risk of hair loss from stress (Young, 2007; Sood, 2013).

The L in front of the amino acid means that the amino acid is in its free form. Being in its free form means that the amino acid is not attached to other amino acids, with peptide bonds forming a protein chain. For some reason, the amino acids that make up the proteins in our bodies are all L-amino acids. Thus, only L-amino acids are building blocks of proteins. Additionally, the L designation tells us that the amino acid is on its own and in the form absorbable by the cells to synthesize proteins.

While the two amino acids mentioned above are important to maintaining healthy hair, all amino acids are crucial for the entire body. Amino acids are organic compounds that combine to form proteins. Thus, they are called the building blocks of proteins, which play many critical roles in the body. Amino acids are organic compounds composed mainly of nitrogen, carbon, hydrogen, and oxygen. Essentially amino acids are the source of life; they are crucial. They are needed for vital processes such as building proteins, hormones, and neurotransmitters. In other words, our muscles, hair, nails, and skin, as well as our blood, hormones, and our immune system, are all made up of proteins, namely amino acids. Our bodies could not exist without them.

Only twenty amino acids are necessary for human health. Therefore, the body needs 20 different amino acids to maintain good health and normal functioning. Of these twenty, only eleven can be produced by the body. These eleven are classified as *nonessential amino acids*. The remaining nine amino acids are classified as ***essential amino acids***, which must be obtained from the food we eat. These essential amino acids must come from a person's diet, as the human body lacks the metabolic pathways required to synthesize these amino acids. Essential amino acids are also known as ***indispensable amino acids.*** A lack of even one of these essential amino acids can, over time, affect both the physical body and mental health of the individual. The nine essential amino acids that our bodies cannot make are the following:

- Histidine.
- Isoleucine.

- Leucine.
- Lysine.
- Methionine.
- Phenylalanine.
- Threonine.
- Tryptophan.
- Valine.

In the human body, amino acids are the foundation or underpinning for all the body's vital functions. Amino acids build muscles, cause chemical reactions in the body, transport nutrients, prevent illness, and carry out other functions. Amino acid deficiency can decrease immunity, digestive problems, depression, fertility issues, lower mental alertness, slowed growth in children, and many other health issues. Amino acids can produce over 100,000 different proteins. In other words, those 100,000 proteins are all made up of various combinations of the twenty different amino acids. The blueprint that determines the exact number and arrangement of amino acids in each protein is encoded in the DNA (Morishima, N.D.). Understanding how vital amino acids are to every bodily function, it is a wise practice to supplement with a predigested essential amino acid formulation. These amino acid products have an absorbability rate of 99% and effectively ensure that none of the essential nine amino acids are deficient in the diet.

Vitamins are also crucial for proper scalp and hair health. For example, a vitamin-A deficiency can result in dull, dry, and lusterless hair. It could even lead to hair loss if the deficiency becomes more pronounced. Vitamin A and its derivatives (retinoids) are critically important for developing and maintaining multiple epithelial tissues, including skin, hair, and sebaceous glands, as shown by the detrimental effects of either vitamin-A deficiency or toxicity

(Everts, 2012). Not only does vitamin-A deficiency lead to hair problems, but excessive ingestion of vitamin A (hypervitaminosis A) can also lead to scalp problems. In fact, hair loss is a consistent finding observed during vitamin-A toxicity (Ries & Hess, 1999). The problems with excessive ingestion of vitamin A are similar to those seen with vitamin-A deficiency.

Vitamin A also called retinol, regulates retinoic acid synthesis in the hair follicle. It is believed that changes in the hair attributed to a vitamin-A deficiency are caused by the atrophy of some hair bulbs and by the cystic degeneration of others. Under the microscope, it has been observed that changes in the skin and scalp due to a vitamin-A deficiency consist of superficial hyperkeratosis (i.e., overgrowth of the horny layer of the outer layer of the skin). This hyperkeratosis typically extends into the mouth of the pilosebaceous follicles.

This condition could lead to obstruction of the follicular orifices due to the progressive keratinization process that is taking place. The follicular orifices can become widely distended, which could impair hair growth and obstruct the outflow of sebum. If it persists, this keratinization process could lead to the formation of keratin plugs (keratosis pilaris, or KP), which can encapsulate the hair and impede it from coming out, and the sebaceous glands will atrophy (Fig. 17.1).

Fig. 17.1: Formation of a keratin plug (keratosis pilaris)

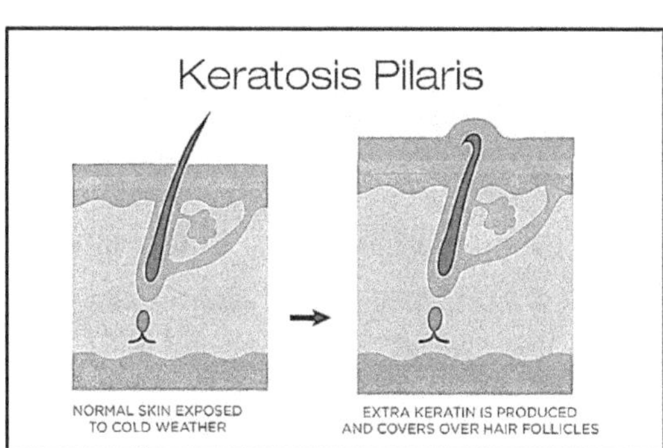

Image Source: http://treatingkeratosispilaris.blogspot.com/p/contact.html

Keratosis pilaris (KP) is a genetic keratinization disorder of the hair follicles of the skin. It is a commonly occurring, benign condition that manifests as small, rough, folliculocentric, keratotic papules. A papule is a raised area of skin tissue that is less than one centimeter around. These papules are often described as chicken bumps, chicken skin, or goose-bumps in specific areas of the body, particularly the outer-upper arms, thighs, cheeks, back, and buttocks. Keratosis pilaris creates havoc with the skin's surface as a raised, rough, bumpy texture and uneven, nutmeg-grater appearances. It is often quite noticeable. Inflammation within each hair follicle can cause the formation of embarrassing, pinpoint, red, or brown polka dots beneath each miniature mound of keratin.

This condition has been described as a genetic condition likely to worsen with age as more keratin builds up in the follicle. Because of the possible genetic etiology of KP, no cure or universally effective treatment modality is available to arrest the condition effectively. However, treatment is all about smoothing away the bumps. Therapy can eliminate the bumps, improve the texture, eliminate acne-causing plugs, and improve the skin's overall appearance. Prescription medications that contain exfoliants like lactic acid, salicylic acid, and urea can be helpful, along with moisturizing creams. Worldwide, over 50% of the population will suffer from KP at some point in their life. Typically, KP affects 50%-80% of adolescents and 40% of adults at some point in any given year. In general, keratosis pilaris (KP) is frequently cosmetically displeasing but medically harmless (Alai & Elston, 2016).

Other vitamin deficiencies such as B-complex and vitamin C can also lead to hair and scalp problems. Iodine and iron deficiencies can also be causative factors in producing hair loss. It has been observed that iron-deficiency anemia—a common problem seen in middle-aged women—is a contributing factor associated with poor hair growth in this group of patients.

Nutrients That May Be Beneficial in Treating Hair Loss

It is safe to say that emphasis should be placed on building a sound nutritional foundation consisting of the following nutrients that may be beneficial in the treatment of hair loss:

- Carbohydrates.
- Proteins.
- Fat.
- Vitamins A, B-complex, C, D, E, biotin.
- Minerals such as zinc, iodine, and iron.
- Amino acids such as cysteine.

These nutrients become even more critical when dieting; therefore, supplementation is strongly recommended when the amount of food intake is reduced. One health factor that can lead to an increased bodily demand for these vital nutrients is stress, including distressing factors of modern-day living such as environmental pollutants and processed foods. A well-balanced diet is considered necessary in maintaining a healthy, full head of hair. Although hereditary hair loss cannot be entirely prevented by nutritional means only, it can at least slow down the process. The slowing down of the process can be further improved when accompanied by a synergistic approach. This synergistic approach can be attained when all the FDA-approved hair-loss medications, like minoxidil, finasteride, and low-level laser therapy (LLLT), are combined with hair transplantation and proper hygiene and care of the hair and scalp.

In the last decade, many companies and hair-restoration clinics have popularized the nutrient biotin, a compound in the vitamin B-complex family also known as vitamin H, vitamin B7, and coenzyme R. Although biotin is a member of the B-complex family, it is not actually a vitamin. It is a coenzyme that works with vitamins. The discovery of biotin has a similar history to other vitamins insofar as no one single person can be credited with its identification. However, in 1916 W.G. Bateman became one of the first notable contributors to the discovery of biotin after finding toxic levels of biotin within an organism following the addition of excess raw egg white to a nutritionally adequate diet. It was not until 1935 that scientists Fritz Kogl and Paul Gyorgy suggested the name *"Biotin"* for the pure vitamin concentrations that they extracted (Chinwe et al., 2010).

The nutrient biotin performs various roles, both individually and in combination with other B vitamins. The functions of biotin include the metabolism of carbohydrates, fats, and amino acids, and hence, protein production. It is also believed that biotin helps maintain control of blood sugar (glucose) levels in people suffering from diabetes types 1 and 2. However, no concrete evidence has been demonstrated to prove this theory. Furthermore, biotin supports hair and nail health and normal embryonic growth during pregnancy. In fact, biotin is also known as vitamin H, which stems from the German words *Haar and Haut,* which mean "hair" and "skin," respectively (Axe, 2016).

According to Chinwe et al. (2010), biotin can be found naturally in the body, where it is produced or synthesized by a bacterium found in the human intestine. The intestine is exposed to two sources of biotin: a dietary source that is mainly processed in the small intestine and a bacterial source wherein it is synthesized by the normal microflora of the large intestine (Said, 2009). Theoretically, as it relates to hair loss, biotin is thought to accelerate the metabolic breakdown of the hormone DHT, which is the androgenic substance believed to be responsible for hair loss in androgenetic alopecia (AGA). Some studies have documented the effectiveness of biotin creams and solutions in preventing excessive hair loss (Ablon, 2012). However, there is no strong evidence favoring the role of oral and topical biotin in arresting hair loss or stimulating regrowth. In fact, considering that biotin cannot be readily absorbed through the hair or skin, any company that promises hair and skin improvement through the topical application of biotin is promoting an ineffective product (Chinwe et al., 2010).

Notwithstanding the lack of research, biotin remains one of the most prescribed nutritional supplements for any hair-loss affliction. In fact, biotin is frequently an integral component in any hair mesotherapy treatment solution. Mesotherapy treatment is a non-surgical cosmetic solution aimed at diminishing problem areas on the body (Sonthaliam, Daulatabad, & Tosti, 2015). However, whether or not these Biotin creams, topical solutions, and capsules are effective is open to debate. While biotin is a vital micronutrient in maintaining healthy hair, it has been overpromoted to the point that it is included in everything from shampoos, hairsprays, and hair conditioners to topical hair solutions. Although there is no recommended dietary allowance for biotin, proponents of Biotin usage often recommend taking 2-5 milligrams (2000-5000 micrograms) in supplement form daily in an attempt to strengthen hair shafts and hopefully achieve results (Rajput, 2010; Daniels & Hardy, 2010; Wong, 2015).

Regarding zinc, the relation between zinc deficiency and hair growth has been the subject of debate for the past 30 years. Zinc is a mineral essential for a healthy immune system, producing certain hormones, wound healing, bone formation, and clear skin. In fact, the normal growth and development of the body cannot occur without zinc. It is required in minimal amounts and is thus known as a trace mineral. Despite the low requirement, zinc is found in nearly every cell of the body, and it is key to the proper function of more than 300 enzymes, including the crucial superoxide dismutase (SOD). The SOD enzyme is one of the body's most potent, natural antioxidant enzymes present both inside and outside cell membranes. SOD is one of the body's primary internal antioxidants that effectively treat inflammatory and degenerative disease processes (Kiefer, 2006).

In numerous research studies, researchers repeatedly discovered that SODs have a stimulatory effect on hair growth and decreased hair loss. Because of these findings, several hair-loss products on the market now contain copper peptides, which are SOD mimetics. While not a panacea, researchers have noted that these SOD-containing products stimulate hair growth and block hair loss in mice (Sampayo, Gill, & Lithgow, 2003). Recent study data on the hair loss product Tricomin®, a copper peptide SOD, demonstrate increased hair growth in androgenetic alopecia (AGA). Among other beneficial effects, SODs appear to help spare growth-stimulating nitric oxide, reduce damaging inflammation, and help reverse scarring hair loss.

In the hair-loss field, zinc is known as a potent inhibitor of hair follicle regression and an accelerator of hair follicle recovery. Although the relationship between zinc and hair loss is contentious among hair-loss experts, it has been observed that a zinc deficiency has been present in almost all forms of non-scarring alopecia. Zinc is also known to have some 5-alpha-reductase *(5AR)* inhibitory activity. Therefore, it is not surprising that zinc-containing supplements, like biotin, have become a regular and routine prescription by trichologists for androgenetic alopecia (male pattern baldness) patients (Sonthaliam, Daulatabad, & Tosti, 2015).

It might be worth the effort for hair-loss afflicted individuals to try these substances, especially if their nutrition has been subpar. However, they are usually a waste of time and money. The author came to this conclusion based on experimentation with the majority of these types of nutritional supplements for several years without any significant hair-loss improvement. Notwithstanding the author's experience with most of these treatment modalities, anyone desiring to have their own personal experiences should not feel deterred.

It is a well-known principle that what does not work for one person could potentially work for another. Therefore, a well-informed approach with careful, personal experimentation is an appropriate practice when searching for what works. Moreover, one should be mindful when perusing the statistical reports provided by hair-restoration clinics and hair-product manufacturers. The data provided are frequently their own data, not a double-blinded peered-reviewed study.

Currently, there are several drugs under investigation that promise some degree of effectiveness in preventing AGA. Most of these drugs focus on either inhibiting or blocking the conversion of testosterone to dihydrotestosterone (DHT). It is important to note that of the many factors affecting hair loss, it is currently believed that the only factor considered amenable or responsive to medical treatment is the testosterone-DHT conversion process.

Topical Nutrition

Topical nutrition relates to the substances or products consumers apply to their hair for the purpose of improving its health. A myriad of topical remedies promising to restore hair to the balding scalp has been around since antiquity. Currently, the tradition continues unabated. The consumer is still offered a multitude of topical hair solutions that promise to restore their hair. The unfortunate reality is that most of these products are ineffective in reversing hair loss. A few of the topical solution products marketed to improve hair health are:

- Specially formulated shampoos.
- Hair conditioners.
- Protein treatment packs.
- Hot oil treatment.
- Hair growth serums.
- Fermented rice water serum.

Today, consumers' philosophy is that if the product is natural or organic, it must be good, which gives rise to an enormous market potential for the sale of such products. It is doubtful that most of these products can improve the nutritional status of the hair through topical application since none of their unique ingredients can effectively alter the chemical composition of the hair. However, while these products may not improve the nutritional status of the hair, they can improve its appearance and prevent damage to the existing hair. Therefore, selecting quality products for scalp and hair care is a good idea. Moreover, it is essential to remember that nutrition starts from within, which is why a proper diet is crucial in maintaining hair and scalp health. Let us remember the quote by the father of western medicine, Hippocrates: "Let food be thy medicine and medicine be thy food."

Hair Analysis

Historically, the importance of examining hair or fiber was recognized in the early stages of forensic science. In France in 1857, one of the first forensic science reports was published involving the scientific study of hair. This study introduced the idea of hair and fiber analysis. The field expanded rapidly after microscopic hair examination became known in the early twentieth century. In 1931, Professor John Glaister published a book entitled "*Hairs of Mammalia from the Medico-Legal Aspect,*" which became a renowned and widely used resource for hair analysis information. Forensic hair analysis has played a significant role in the court system since the beginning of the 1900s. In the United States, Paul L. Kirk established the fundamentals of microscopic hair analysis used by scientists today. His textbook "*Crime Investigation*" is still an important text and resource in the criminal investigation.

Hair analysis is the most recently introduced procedure for evaluating the nutritional status of hair. It has become a thriving, multi-million-dollar industry. The claim regarding hair analysis is that it can— for a fee— tell whether an individual is suffering from a deficiency or excess of vitamins or minerals. Some claim that it can also tell whether a patient is suffering from metal toxicity, such as lead poisoning, and that it provides helpful information for suggesting dietary changes. The technique for testing hair involves washing the hair sample and heating it at a very high temperature so that the metals contained in the hair will give off light at different wavelengths. By recording the emitted spectrum of light, technicians can determine the mineral content of the hair, which— according to the claims— reflects the mineral content of the body.

Some critics of hair analysis consider this test to be the equivalent of modern-day fortune-telling, and it is viewed as a scam by some since the mineral composition of the hair can be affected by several factors, including:

- age.
- hair color.
- rate of hair growth.
- use of hair dyes.
- use of bleach.
- use of shampoo.

For example, some shampoos and hair dyes contain minerals such as zinc, selenium, and lead, which could possibly give a false diagnosis when the hair is analyzed. This test, although useful, cannot be viewed as a panacea.

In 2001, the Agency for Toxic Substances and Disease Registry (ATSDR) convened a seven-member panel in Atlanta, Georgia, to review and discuss the current state of the science related to hair analysis. The panel's objective was to determine if their use of hair analysis in assessing environmental exposure was effective in supporting the agency's public health assessment activities. In other words, the panel's goal was to determine the overall utility of hair analysis as a tool for evaluating exposure at hazardous waste sites.

The main lesson learned from the meeting was that, for most substances, data are insufficient to predict health effects from the concentration of substances in the hair. The presence of a substance in the hair may indicate exposure— both internal and external— but this observation does not necessarily indicate the source of exposure. Therefore, before hair analysis can be considered a valid tool for assessing a particular substance's exposure and health impact, more research is needed to establish standardized reference ranges. Moreover, we also need to better understand the biologic variation of hair growth with age, gender, race, ethnicity, and pharmacokinetics; and further explore possible dose-response relationships (Harkins & Susten, 2003).

In another study to determine the reliability and effectiveness of hair analysis, some hair samples from two healthy teenagers were submitted— under assumed names— to 13 commercial laboratories that perform multimineral hair analysis. The reported levels of most minerals varied considerably between the identical samples sent to the same laboratory and from laboratory to laboratory. The laboratories also disagreed about what was normal or usual for many of the minerals. The conclusion was that commercial use of hair analysis in this manner is unscientific, economically wasteful, unethical, and probably illegal (Barrett, 1985).

Currently, hair follicle analysis or testing is used to determine substance abuse (drugs and alcohol use). Some corporate, legal, medical, and educational institutions have embraced hair follicle drug testing as a complementary approach to traditional urine-based testing. The growing interest in hair follicle testing is because drug metabolites can remain present in hair from a person's scalp for up to three months. Conversely, urine tests have a detection window of up to ten hours to about one week for most drugs except marijuana, which can remain present in a person's urine for up to 30 days. However, the hair follicle test involves a two-step testing process to minimize the risk of false-positive results. Hair follicle testing has been embraced by many institutions because the test can help identify individuals who participate in regular, long-term drug use (Hadland & Levy, 2016; Gryczynski et al., 2014).

It is crucial to know that hair follicle tests can detect the presence of some prescription medications, which can result in false-positive results. Therefore, individuals undergoing a hair follicle test who are taking prescription medications should share this information with their employer or test administrator to mitigate any misinterpretation.

18

The Graying Hair Process

According to Tobin and Paus (2001), researchers of graying hair, the visual appearance of humans is derived predominantly from their skin and hair color, which is attributed to melanin levels. The pigment melanin is produced in melanosomes by melanocytes in a complex biochemical pathway termed *melanogenesis*. Thus, melanogenesis is the production of melanin by specialized cells called melanocytes. These melanin cells are located in the skin, hair, and eyes. Therefore, melanin is the primary determinant of skin, hair, and eye color.

Besides defining an important human phenotypic trait, melanin also plays a critical role in photoprotection due to its ability to absorb ultraviolet (UV) radiation. While melanin pigmentation from epidermal melanocytes clearly protects the skin by screening harmful UV radiation, the biological value of hair pigmentation is not as clear (Costin & Hearing, 2007; Tobin et al., 2001). In addition to important roles in social-sexual communication, one potential benefit of pigmented scalp hair in humans may be the rapid excretion of heavy metals, chemicals, and toxins from the body by their selective binding to melanin.

The hair follicle pigmentary unit is perhaps one of the most visible and accurate predictor of aging in the human body because it reflects a significant dilution of pigment intensity (graying) that occurs long before we see any aging changes in the skin (epidermis). While the hair follicle and skin (epidermal) melanogenic systems may share a common origin, their biology is regulated to some degree differently. For example, the follicular melanocytes engage in intermittent or periodic activity driven by changes in the hair-growth (anagen) cycle. In contrast, epidermal (skin) melanocyte activity remains, for the most part, continuous (Van Neste & Tobin, 2004). In fact, the primary distinguishing characteristic of the follicular melanogenesis system is its dependency or tight coupling of the hair follicle melanogenesis process to the hair-growth cycle.

According to Professor Tobin et al. (2001), the hair-growth cycle appears to involve periods of melanocyte proliferation during early anagen, maturation of melanocytes during mid to late anagen, and melanocyte apoptosis (cellular death) during early catagen. Therefore, each hair-growth cycle is associated with the reconstruction of an intact hair follicle pigmentary unit at least for the first ten hair-growth cycles. In other words, this cyclic reconstruction of an intact hair follicle pigmentary unit works optimally in scalp follicles during the first ten hair-growth cycles, which means approximately 40 years of age (Van Neste et al., 2004). After these ten hair-growth cycles, there appears to be a genetically regulated exhaustion (depletion) of the pigmentary potential of each individual follicle, leading to hair graying (Figs.18.1 and 18.2).

Fig.18.1: Complete premature graying of the hair

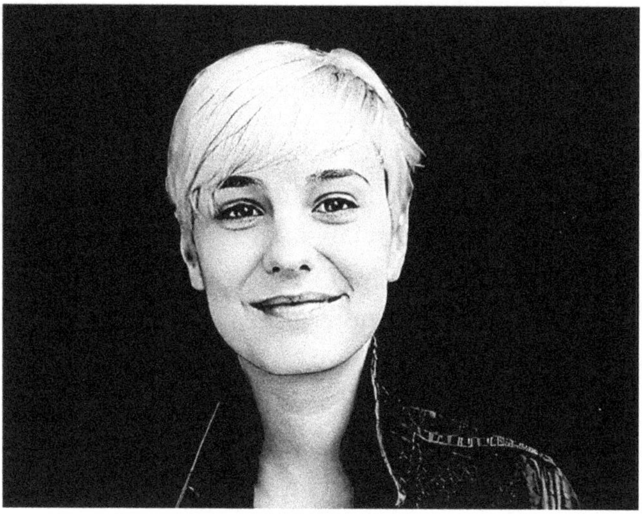

Image Source: http://www.istockphoto.com/photo/cute-girl-gm477445845-35685840

Fig. 18.2: Diagram of graying hair

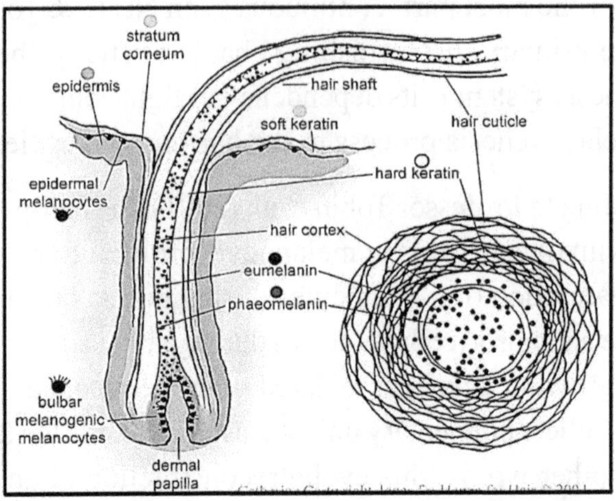

Image Source: By Catherine Cartwright-Jones for Henna for Hair © 2004. Contributions to http://skindisorders3.wikispaces.com/ are licensed under a Creative Commons Attribution Share-Alike 3.0 License. http://www.hennaforhair.com/gray/

There are three types of melanin: eumelanin, pheomelanin, and neuromelanin. The most common is eumelanin, of which there are two types: brown and black (or dark) insoluble polymers. Thus, eumelanin is the major type of melanin in individuals with dark skin and dark hair and is more efficient in photoprotection. Photoprotection is the biochemical process that helps organisms cope with molecular damage caused by sunlight.

Pheomelanin is a red-yellow, soluble polymer formed by the conjugation of cysteine or glutathione. This type of melanin is predominantly found in individuals with red hair and a Fitzpatrick skin phototype scale of I and II (Table18.1). Individuals with these skin phototypes are usually more susceptible to tumors. Blond hair can have almost any proportion of pheomelanin and eumelanin, but only in small amounts of both. More pheomelanin creates a more golden or strawberry blond color, and more eumelanin creates an ash or sandy blond color (Tsatmi, Ancans, & Thody, 2002; Rouzaud, Kadekaro, Abdel-Malek, & Hearing, 2005; Fitzpatrick, 1975). Pheomelanin imparts a pink to red hue depending on its concentration. This type of melanin is typically concentrated in the lips, nipples, glans of the penis, and vagina (Hearing & Tsakamoto, 1991). Pheomelanin is also present in the skin, and redheaded individuals—or those carrying the red-hair gene— often have a more pinkish hue to their skin.

Neuromelanin is a dark, insoluble polymer pigment found in the brain and is structurally related to melanin. It is expressed in large quantities in the catecholaminergic cells of the *substantia nigra pars compacta* and *locus coeruleus,* giving the structures their dark color (Fedorow et al., 2005). Humans have the largest amount of neuromelanin, which is present in lesser amounts in other primates and is totally absent in many other species (Lillie, 1957). However, the biological function of neuromelanin remains unknown, although human neuromelanin has been shown to efficiently bind transition metals, such as iron and other potentially toxic molecules. Therefore, it may play a crucial role in apoptosis (cell death) and the related Parkinson's disease (Double, 2006).

Table 18.1: Skin phototypes depend on the amount of melanin pigment in the skin

Skin Phototypes	Typical Features	Tanning ability
I	Pale white skin, blue/hazel eyes, blond/red hair	Always burns, does not tan
II	Fair skin, blue eyes	Burns easily, tans poorly
III	Darker white skin	Tans after initial burn
IV	Light brown skin	Burns minimally, tans easily
V	Brown skin	Rarely burns, tans darkly easily
VI	Dark brown or black skin	Never burns, always tans darkly

Source: Fitzpatrick, T. B. The Validity and Practicality of Sun-Reactive Skin Types I Through VI.

While the perception of gray hair largely derives from the admixture of pigmented and white hair, it is important to note that individual hair follicles can exhibit pigment dilution or true hair grayness (Tobin et al., 2001). Tobin contends that this pigment dilution is essentially attributed to:

- A reduction in tyrosine activity of hair bulbar melanocytes.
- Sub-optimal melanocyte-cortical keratinocyte interactions.
- Defective migration of melanocytes from a reservoir in the upper-outer root sheath to the pigment-permitting microenvironment close to the dermal papilla of the hair bulb.

According to Tobin (2009), the pigmentary unit of the hair follicle is highly susceptible to age-related change, and this is especially visible in people of European ancestry. Hair color is at its lightest in early childhood and becomes progressively darker before puberty and darkens further during adolescence and young adulthood until the onset of hair graying, or *canities senilis* (Allende, 1972; Costin & Hearing, 2007).

It has been observed that the epidermal (skin) melanin pigmentary unit succumbs to a 10%-20% reduction in pigment-producing epidermal melanocytes— whether in sun-exposed or unexposed skin— every decade after 30 years of age (Whiteman, Parsons, & Green, 1999). Therefore, according to the American Academy of Dermatology, the chance of getting gray hair increases by 10%-20% every ten years after the individual reaches the age of 30. This fact suggests that possibly 30 years of age might be a helpful time point to operationally assess the effects of chronologic skin aging in humans (Tobin, 2009).

Reasons for Gray Hair

According to the world's leading expert on graying hair, Dr. Desmond Tobin (2010), from the University of Bradford in England, the most common reason for the graying of human hair is because of our biological clock and preset genetic factors within the body. Tobin contends that melanocyte stem cells eventually fail after a predetermined period, resulting in decreased melanin production. Nishimura et al. (2005) have also observed this melanocyte stem-cell failure. Their study proposed that the failure of melanocyte stem cells (MSC) to maintain the production of melanocytes could be the cause of graying hair. This failure of MSC maintenance may result in the breakdown of signals that produce hair color. In other words, these researchers suggest that the hair follicle has a "melanogenic time clock" that slows down or stops melanocyte activity, resulting in a decrease in the amount of pigment our hair receives. This process has been observed to occur just before the hair is preparing to fall out or shed, so the roots always look pale.

Another interesting and important study entitled *"Senile Hair Graying: H2O2-Mediated Oxidative Stress Affect Human Hair Color by Blunting Methionine Sulfoxide Repair"* was published by the peer-reviewed Journal of the Federation of American Societies for Experimental Biology (FASEB). The research team of Wood et al. (2009) demonstrated how hair follicles produce small amounts of hydrogen peroxide. This chemical— H2O2— builds on the hair shafts, which can lead to a gradual loss of hair color. In other words, people who become gray develop massive oxidative stress via the accumulation of hydrogen peroxide (H2O2) in the hair follicle, which essentially causes hair to bleach itself from the inside out.

In a subsequent study also published by the Journal of the FASEB, researchers demonstrated that the accumulation of hydrogen peroxide could be cured with a proprietary treatment they had developed. The treatment is described as a topical, ultraviolet B-activated— or sunlight activated—compound that the researchers claim can correct loss of skin or hair color (vitiligo). The formulated compound is a modified pseudocatalase (PC-KUS) that is supposed to reverse the oxidative process that leads to the accumulation of hydrogen peroxide in the hair follicle. This process of hydrogen peroxide accumulation affects most people as they move into middle age and beyond. The hydrogen peroxide essentially acts as a bleaching agent on the new hair growing from the follicles (Schallreuter, Mohammed, Salem, Holtz, & Panske, 2013).

Other Factors That Can Change the Pigmentation of the Hair

Sometimes, gray hair in men and women can be produced by environmental factors instead of genetic sources. For example, factors such as climate, pollutants, toxins, and chemical exposure can cause gray hair by altering the melanin cells (melanocytes) in the hair that produce the coloring pigment (Borreli, 2015). Moreover, many researchers have been concerned about the possible association of graying hair with systemic disease. They believe that certain diseases could be responsible for the premature graying of the hair. Some responsible diseases include thyroid dysfunction, multiple sclerosis, and conditions that produce physical abnormalities. Starvation and diets low in vitamins and minerals can also cause the hair to lose its pigmentation. However, according to Hyoseung et al. (2014), the common factors associated with hair graying and systemic disease have not been well established or elucidated.

Reversal Solutions for Graying Hair

Contrary to popular belief, graying hair is not always an age-related condition. Hair graying can occur as young as in our teens and range into our late fifties or older. For some individuals, the graying process can start to manifest in their early twenties or thirties, a condition called *premature canities or graying.* As previously mentioned, people with graying hair have little or no melanin, which is the hair pigment that produces hair color. Gray or white hair is not actually a true gray or white pigment; the hair is clear or transparent due to a lack of pigmentation and melanin. The transparent hairs appear gray or white because of how light reflects from them.

The most promising graying-hair reversal research has been conducted by Woods et al., 2009 and Schallreuter et al., 2013. These researchers discovered that gray hair results when naturally occurring hydrogen peroxide— H2O2— builds up in hair follicles, causing oxidative stress, which ultimately bleaches out the color of the hair.

It is well known that younger people possess an enzyme called *catalase*, whose function is the breakdown of the accumulation of hydrogen peroxide into water and oxygen. This enzyme often stops performing its function as we age. Schallreuter et al. (2013) formulated a PC-KUS, which is a pseudocatalase compound that, once activated by exposure to the sun, adds new catalase enzymes and converts hydrogen peroxide in the hair follicle to the harmless solution of water and oxygen, thereby blocking it from accumulating in the follicle and skin. This discovery, if successful, will result not only in the reversal of graying hair but also in a cure for vitiligo, a disease that causes the loss of skin color in blotches (Fig. 18.3).

In fact, the original research from Schallreuter et al. (2013) focused on vitiligo intervention. However, serendipitously, as can usually occur with any research study, the researchers discovered that the catalase replacement treatment was effective in restoring color to the vitiliginous (loss of pigmentation) skin. Following this finding, the researchers realized that the catalase cream might also prove efficacious on graying hair. In the most recent study, the investigators applied the PC-KUS (catalase) cream to both the skin and eyelashes of 2400 people afflicted with vitiligo. They found that both the discolored skin and graying eyelashes responded favorably to the treatment. However, even though a formulation of the PC-KUS catalase cream has now become commercially available to treat graying hair, the reviews from users have not been favorable.

Fig. 18.3: Vitiligo of the skin and hair

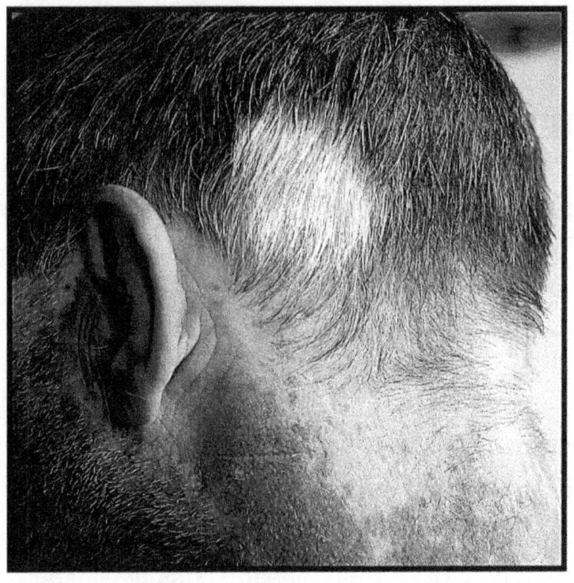

Image Source: By Klaus D. Peter, Gummersbach, Germany (Own work) [CC BY 3.0 de (http://creativecommons.org/licenses/by/3.0/de/deed.en)], via Wikimedia Commonshttps://commons.wikimedia.org/wiki/File%3AVitiligo_and_Poliosis.jpg

Graying hair in aging men and women is a perfectly natural process, although not always desirable. Currently, Tobin et al. (2001), Woods et al. (2009), and Schallreuter et al. (2013) have conducted impressive research on graying hair reversal. While people wait for a research discovery to become a viable commercial reality, currently, there are some natural products and remedies that claim to reverse graying hair or change or improve the appearance of the graying hair.

However, this is yet another marketing area where *caveat emptor*— let the buyer beware— is applicable. In fact, in 2015, the Federal Trade Commission (FTC) filed suit against multiple defendants who allegedly used misleading claims to convince consumers that their products, which contained the enzyme catalase, could help cure and reverse graying hair. The defendants claimed that the catalase in their products attacked hydrogen peroxide, the chemical that causes hair to turn gray. Thus, the defendants used research information from Woods et al. (2009) and Schallreuter et al. (2013) graying hair studies to claim the effectiveness of their product.

It is apparent that the Federal Trade Commission (FTC), in conjunction with the Department of Justice (DOJ), Department of Defense (DOD), Food and Drug Administration (FDA), and other agencies are making a concerted effort to make the dietary supplement manufacturers and advertisers a focal point for enforcement to prevent consumer fraud.

19

Future Trends in Hair Restoration Solutions

The hair transplantation and restoration industry has evolved significantly over the past quarter- century. The improvements achieved in instrumentation and developments of new surgical procedures have resulted in more natural and aesthetically pleasing hair transplant outcomes for patients. However, to achieve an aesthetically acceptable hair transplant, the patient must have a donor area with enough hair to create the necessary density. In fact, the current standard in hair transplantation surgery is the use and redistribution of already existing hair follicles.

Therefore, for patients with severe baldness that do not have a sufficient supply of hair in their donor area, the option for attaining a dense and copious hair transplant is quite limited. Because of this hair supply limitation in patients who have extensive baldness, an increasing number of hair-transplant surgeons now believe that the future of hair restoration will not be in surgery but rather in the biosciences. Therefore, stem cell therapy and gene therapy, such as hair cloning and hair multiplication, maybe the future of hair-restoration therapy (Chan & Ducic, 2015).

Hair Cloning Theory

It is well known that most of hair-loss treatments currently available possess serious limitations. It is highly disappointing that most hair-loss products are essentially ineffective at addressing the problem of balding. In contrast, hair-transplant surgery can be quite effective in resolving hair loss if the prospective patient has an adequately dense donor area and a skilled and competent hair-restoration surgeon performs the procedure. However, most people would prefer not to undergo surgery to restore their hair. This dilemma gives rise to the demand for alternative methods of hair restoration. Two promising methods that people anxiously await are hair cloning (HC) and hair multiplication (HM).

Hair cloning is a promising, hypothetical treatment modality that involves extracting healthy hair follicle cells (dermal papillae cells) and growing or multiplying them outside the body. Hair cloning, also known as *hair regeneration, hair multiplication, or follicular neogenesis,* is a technique that attempts to elicit new hair growth using a person's own hair-forming cells, which are then implanted into the bald area of the scalp (Fig.19.1). The expectation or objective of this process is that once the cells are implanted, they will become or grow into hair follicles, resulting in new and permanent hair growth. The research being undertaken in this field is very exciting because hair-cloning methods have the potential to create a treatment that could effectively cure or resolve common pattern hair loss. Actually, this is precisely the goal that scientists and hair-restoration physicians have been seeking for decades.

Fig. 19.1: The critical property steps in hair cloning

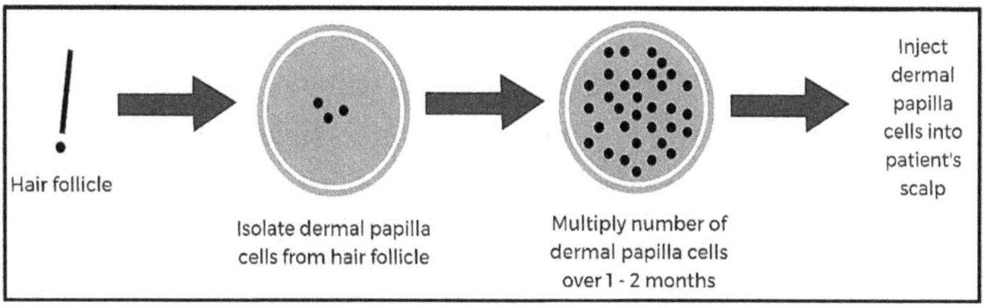

Image Source: By https://tophairlosstreatments.com/when-will-hair-cloning-be-available/ (Use with Permission)

To date, the most difficult challenge facing researchers investigating hair cloning or hair regeneration therapies is achieving consistent results. According to the research team of Higgins et al. (2010), there are two central problems in developing an effective cloning hair-loss therapy. The first problem is the difficulty in getting human dermal papillae cells to self-aggregate (clump together), which is an essential process to elicit human follicle neogenesis. The dilemma discovered by these researchers is that when human dermal papillae cells are removed from their hair-follicle microenvironment and grown in culture, they immediately lose their contextual and positional signals or cues (inductive properties) from the surrounding epithelial cells. Therefore, inhibiting follicle neogenesis or growth of new hair.

In other words, scientists have had a hard time cloning dermal papilla cells because the cells simply revert back to basic skin cells when they are put into a culture. Conversely, rodent papillae cells do not have that problem because they can clump together (self-aggregate), making it easier for the cells to communicate with each other and grow hair. However, Higgins et al. (2013), in a new research study entitled *"Microenvironmental Reprogramming by Three-Dimensional (3D) Culture Enables Dermal Papilla Cells to Induce de Novo Human Hair-Follicle Growth,"* demonstrated that by manipulating cell culture conditions to establish 3D papilla spheroids, the research team was able to restore dermal papilla inductivity. Inductivity is the ability of one cell to direct the development of neighboring cells.

The second challenging problem with hair cloning is the inability of scientists to generate normal hairs and follicles. In other words, it is a matter of hair quality. When it comes to dermal papillae cell implantation, there is no guarantee that the hair will possess the correct color, proper texture, or grow in the appropriate direction or angulation. These findings imply that cloned hair will more likely be used as filler-type hair to be used after a hair transplantation surgery. Furthermore, it is believed that these hair follicles may only grow first-generation hair, which would eventually be shed over time. Moreover, as previously mentioned, there is the concern that the newly injected or implanted dermal papilla cells will dedifferentiate and lose any characteristics of hair altogether.

Current State of Hair Cloning Research

Despite the challenges that hair-cloning research faces, the process continues in search of an efficacious solution. The quest to uncover the key to an effective hair cloning method has not been easy for several companies that enthusiastically have embraced the challenge. One of the first companies to recognize the potential of developing a hair-cloning therapy was the British regenerative medicine company *Intercytex.* Their hair multiplication and cloning research initially showed promise. Reaching FDA phase II trials, but unfortunately, after a long uphill battle attempting to develop a hair-cloning and hair-multiplication solution, the company announced in 2008 that the therapy was not efficacious enough to continue with the research. Japanese company Aderans Research Institute (ARI), a subdivision of the Aderans Organization, also had a similar story. Despite showing initial promise, the company announced in 2013 that it would stop funding its hair-cloning research due to a lack of success.

Another company in the field of regenerative medicine that is pursuing research for a treatment to correct androgenetic alopecia is RepliCel™ Life Sciences, Inc., based in Vancouver, British Columbia. RepliCel™ is showing far greater promise than the two companies mentioned above. The product that RepriCel™ is using to treat AGA is RCH-01, which is a similar methodology to the ones described by the other companies. The product *RCH-01-hair-regeneration* is an autologous cell therapy utilizing dermal sheath cup cells (DSC) that are isolated from a small punch biopsy taken from the back of the subject's scalp. These cells are replicated and then reintroduced through injection into the balding areas on the subject's scalp (Fig.19.2).

Fig. 19.2: The critical steps in hair cloning

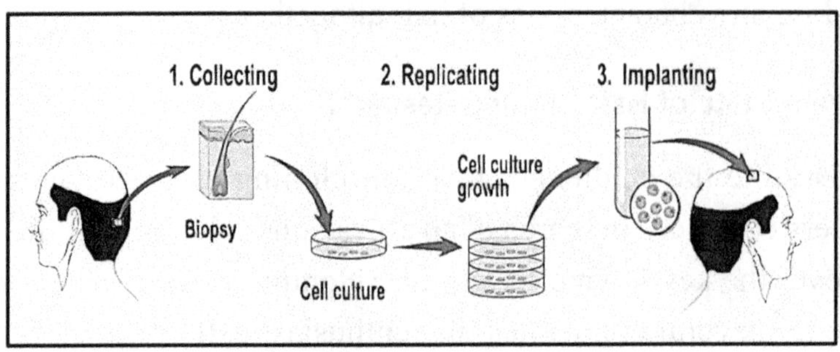

Image Source: By Bishan Mahadevia, M.D. Use with Permission. http://goodbyehairloss.blogspot.com/2010/03/hair-cloning-hair-multiplication-hm.html/Modified image.

The goal of RepliCel™ is to use the injected, cultured DSC cells therapy in an attempt to immunize hair follicles prone to DHT sensitivity, which is the enzymatic system believed to be the cause of androgenetic alopecia (AGA). Currently, RepliCel™ is conducting a phase III trial. RCH-01 is being co-developed by Shiseido Company and RepliCel™. RepliCel™ continues to own the rights exclusively for the rest of the world. Currently, the product is anticipated to launch first in Japan, with Shiseido, while it continues to be developed elsewhere. The clinical study is being conducted at Tokyo Medical University Hospital and Toho University Ohasi Medical Center by Drs. Tsuboi and Niiyama (Replicel.com, n.d.).

Clinical endpoints will include measures of safety and efficacy based on hair fiber thickness and density. The study is being financed by Shiseido, which is the fourth largest cosmetic company in the world. Consequently, each product injected will be manufactured by Shiseido at their SPEC (Cell-Processing and Expansion Center) facility in Kobe, Japan. RepliCel™ helped the Shiseido corporation design, validate, and prepare the SPEC facility for certification by Japan's PMDA (Pharmaceuticals and Medical Device Agency), which is Japan's FDA equivalency.

Given the failures of companies like Aderans and Intercytex, there is reason to be cautious regarding any claims that hair cloning or hair multiplication will be available by 2022 or 2023. Organ cloning and stem cell research are currently in their infancy. While hair cloning may sound simple in theory, there are often unexpected complications and unintended consequences with any new medical technology (Matthews, 2008). Nevertheless, research is ongoing. Lessons are being learned, and each day that passes, the solution is getting closer to a potential cure that will hopefully resolve the hair loss puzzle.

Hair Multiplication Theory

Hair Multiplication (HM) is another related potential hair-loss cure, essentially a cell-based hair-restoration treatment. The HM method also involves removing a hair follicle from the scalp and manipulating it to create more than one hair follicle. However, unlike hair cloning, the number of new follicles created from each individual follicle is not unlimited. With this method, hair follicles are cut in half, with each half going on to produce hair. The theory is that by removing some, but not all, of the dermal papillae cells should be sufficient to grow a new hair follicle without destroying the original one.

This HM process is the hair-multiplication method used in the HST transplantation method, also known as *Partial Longitudinal Follicular Unit Transplantation (PL-FUT),* as proposed by Dr. Coen Gho of the Netherlands. The HST method does not remove the entire hair follicle; instead, several hair stem cells are left in the donor area to stimulate hair regrowth and hopefully preserve the donor area.

As previously mentioned, there is another interesting hair-multiplication technique under investigation that uses plucked hair fragments rather than whole or transected follicles. In a study conducted by Chen et al. (2015) entitled *"Organ-Level Quorum Sensing Directs Regeneration in Hair Stem Cell Populations,"* the research team found that if the hair is forcibly removed or plucked out, it sends a distress signal to the surrounding cells. According to Dr. Chen, hair-plucking produces a micro-injury, which results in a sense and response reaction known as ***quorum sensing***. The quorum sensing reaction, in turn, promotes hair growth and compensates for the loss of hair by producing new growth within the area that has been plucked or injured.

This regrowth was due to the chemical distress signal produced by the initial shock of having each hair plucked out. This signal forced hairs in the telogen (resting) phase of the hair-growth cycle back into the anagen (growth) stage. Chen's study determined that the chemical signal had to reach a precise level of strength for the regrowth effect to occur. Furthermore, it was observed that if the hairs were taken or plucked from large areas, there was no regrowth, as the signal was too weak. Similarly, if the plucked area was very small, the removed hairs grew back; however, there was no further growth outside the area.

Although the potential for stem cell therapies to provide an answer for those individuals afflicted with hair loss is promising, science does not yet have a viable solution for curing baldness. In fact, even if scientists can find an efficacious solution to resolve the hair-loss problem, the industry would still have to address the obstacles of dealing with the requirements imposed by the FDA-approval process, which can take many years but is essential to guarantee the safety and effectiveness of products for the consumers.

The FDA is aware that stem cell therapies offer the potential to treat diseases or conditions for which few treatments exist, and that include hair-loss conditions. However, the FDA is concerned that the hope that patients have for cures not yet available may leave them vulnerable to unscrupulous providers of stem cell treatments that are illegal and potentially harmful. For example, according to Dr. Simek, deputy director of FDA's Office of Cellular, Tissue and Gene Therapies, there is a potential safety risk when stem cells are placed in an area where they are not performing the same biological function as they were when in their original location. Therefore, stem cells, when introduced to a different environment, may multiply, form tumors, or may leave the site they were relocated to and migrate somewhere else. As a consequence of these potential risks, the FDA warns and cautions consumers to make sure that any stem cell treatment they are considering has been approved by the FDA or is being studied under a clinical investigation that has been submitted to and allowed to proceed by FDA (FDA.org, 2015).

Therefore, until a safe and efficacious hair-cloning or hair-multiplication method is developed, patients with androgenetic alopecia will have to continue to be treated with currently available options. Meanwhile, the most effective standard in hair restoration to date is the use and redistribution of already existing hair follicles, which is hair transplant surgery. However, for patients who do not possess an adequate hair supply in the donor area, their options for an aesthetically pleasing hair restoration are quite limited.

Fortunately, stem cell research is still being undertaken by the best and brightest around the world to unlock the potential for new hair growth. Presently, some researchers are investigating novel methods to reactivate follicles that have lost their ability to grow hair due to AGA. These follicles retain their stem cells within the bulge region but lack the ability to form new hair. Hopefully, gene therapy may provide the key to reactivating these dormant follicles. Besides the future potential HC and HM research might bring to the hair restoration industry, there are currently some other novel hair-restoration therapies that are showing promising results. These are platelet-rich plasma (PRP) and ACell™ + PRP Therapy.

Platelet-Rich Plasma Therapy

Platelet-rich plasma (PRP) therapy is essentially an old therapy that has been used extensively in medical specialties like dermatology, cosmetic surgery, orthopedic surgery, cardiovascular surgery, dentistry, sports medicine, and pain management. PRP was initially developed in the 1970s and first used in Italy in 1987 in an open-heart surgery procedure. Currently, PRP therapy is being used as a hair stimulant and growth therapy that utilizes the body's own rich plasma growth factor concentrated from platelets to promote hair growth.

Consequently, PRP has become a newer method for treating various types of alopecia. PRP is blood plasma that has been enriched with platelets. As a concentrated source of autologous platelets, PRP contains several different growth factors and other cytokines that may stimulate soft tissue healing. According to researchers Eppley, Pietzak, and Blanton (2006), the activation of alpha granules of platelets releases numerous proteins, including various growth factors such as platelet-derived growth factor (PDGF), transforming growth factor (TGF), vascular endothelial growth factor (VEGF), insulin-like growth factor (IGF), epidermal growth factor (EGF), and interleukin-1 (IL-1).

It is hypothesized that the release of these growth factors from platelets may act on stem cells in the bulge area of the follicles by stimulating the development of new hair follicles and promoting ***neovascularization.*** The prefix *neo means new, and vascular refers to vessels.* Thus, the concept of neovascularization is described as the formation of functional microvascular networks with red blood cell perfusion. In other words, neovascularization is the natural formation of blood vessels, usually in the form of functional microvascular networks, capable of perfusion by red blood cells. These new blood vessels serve as collateral circulation in response to poor local perfusion or ischemia. Therefore, neovascularization differs from angiogenesis in that angiogenesis is principally characterized by the protrusion and outgrowth of capillary buds and sprouts from preexisting blood vessels (Uebel, Silva, Cantarelli, & Martins, 2006).

As a consequence of this hypothesis, platelet-rich plasma (PRP) therapy has attracted the attention of several medical fields, such as dermatology, plastic surgery, orthopedics, and cardiovascular surgery. The reason for the attraction is due to PRP's potential use in skin rejuvenation, rapid healing, reduced infection, and decreased chance of developing hypertrophic keloids and scars (Gardner et al., 2007). Plasma-rich growth factors are also known to activate the proliferative phase and transdifferentiation of hair and stem cells that can produce new follicular units (FUs) and hence, new hair growth. Thus, the beneficial effects of PRP in androgenetic alopecia (AGA) can be attributed to the various platelet-derived growth factors causing improvement in the function of the hair follicle and promotion of hair growth.

Moreover, in another study by Rinaldi, Sorbellini, and Coscera (2011) entitled *"The Role of Platelet-Rich Plasma to Control Anagen Phase: Evaluation In Vitro and in Vivo in Hair Transplant and Hair Treatments,"* the researchers performed in-vivo evaluations in 100 subjects— 50 men and 50 women— suffering from AGA in a double-blind, randomized clinical trial to evaluate the clinical effect of growth factors from PRP during an 18-month period. The research data confirmed the study's hypothesis that growth factors from PRP therapy had a significant impact on hair bulbs in vitro and in vivo without side effects during the treatment period and 12 months after the procedure.

Furthermore, PRP therapy has been demonstrated to be a safe, cost-effective, and non-allergic treatment modality that can be regarded as a useful adjuvant in managing androgenetic alopecia (Chaudhari et al., 2012; Khatu et al., 2007). However, although PRP has a sufficient theoretical and scientific basis to support its use in hair restoration, this modality is still in its infancy and requires further research. Thus, PRP hair therapy is a promising treatment option for patients afflicted with thinning hair and hair loss. The PRP process essentially follows the following steps (Fig.19.3):

- A patient's blood is collected from the arm, similar to getting a blood test. Normally, Less than two ounces (between 15 to 50 milliliters) are required for the procedure.

- The patient's blood is centrifuged to separate the blood into the platelet fraction and the nutrients in the platelets— the growth factors (GFs).
- The patient's scalp is anesthetized with some form of local freezing medications as an anesthetic to induce insensitivity to pain.
- The platelet-rich plasma (PRP) components, along with vitamins are injected or infused directly into the scalp, specifically on the area manifesting hair thinning (Figs. 19.4 and 19.5).
- Treatments are typically performed monthly for the first three to four months and then every three to six months thereafter. This schedule is optimal for stimulating hair growth factors and stem cells associated with reducing hair loss. PRP has proven to combat hair loss in more than 70% of cases.

Fig. 19.3: The steps of the PRP therapy process

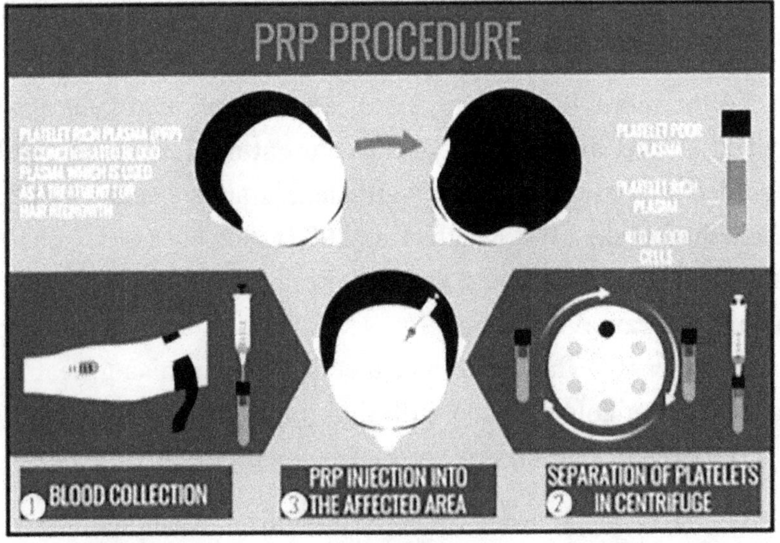

Image Source: http://www.istockphoto.com/vector/platelet-rich-plasma-procedure-gm516289090-88924135

Fig.19.4: Injecting PRP growth factors

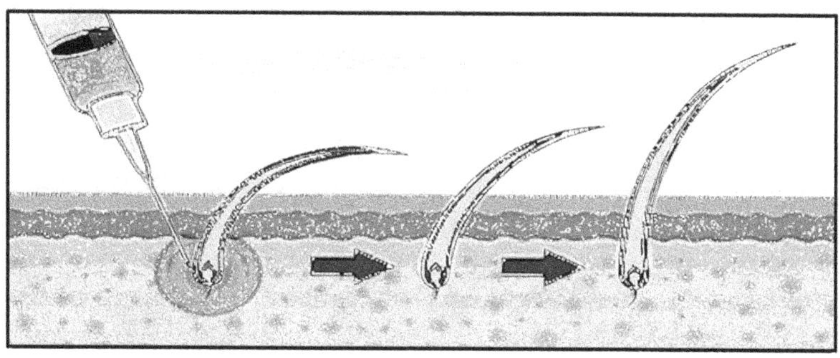

Image Source: http://www.istockphoto.com/vector/hair-follicle-treatment-with-medical-method-gm665510946-121363049? clarity=false

Fig. 19.5: PRP therapy results

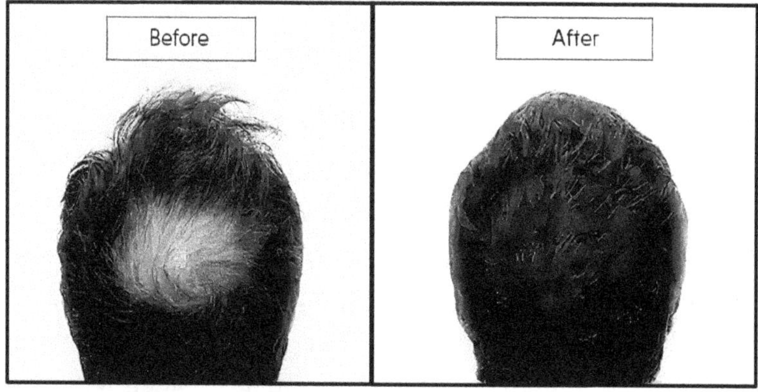

Image Source: https://www.wembleyclinic.co.za/hair-loss/can-prp-cure-hairloss/

ACell™ Regenerative Medicine Tissue Graft

ACell™ is a product that has been developed to help wound healing by encouraging adult stem cells to create their own new, healthy tissue. This regenerative medicine product is what doctors and researchers call an extra-cellular matrix (ECM) tissue graft. The ECM is derived from the naturally occurring porcine (pig's) urinary bladder, which acts as a scaffold— a supporting framework— for epithelial and progenitor cell attachment and proliferation. These cells have the potential to differentiate into numerous types of site-specific tissues where they elicit a healing function. During the healing process, the scaffold is degraded and completely dissolved and assimilated (resorbed), leaving new tissue where scar tissue would normally be expected.

Thus, the ACell™ healing matrix is an FDA-approved cellular regeneration product used for healing wounds and helping regenerate skin, muscle, tendons, and other living tissue. In fact, the ACell™-ECM products, available from various manufacturers, have been successfully used on humans to heal surgical wounds, diabetic ulcers, and damaged muscles and ligaments. These regenerative medicine products have even been used to facilitate the reconstruction of urinary tracts, rotator cuffs, and other anatomical surfaces.

ACell™ + PRP Therapy

Currently, in the hair-restoration field, ACell™ is being combined with PRP and injected into the scalp. Proponents of this hair-loss procedure claim that the application of ACell™ in combination with PRP causes miniaturized hair follicles to become healthier and larger, producing more robust hair growth. The premise of this new hair-loss therapy is that ACell™ activates follicular progenitor cells (adult stem cells), and the PRP, which is loaded with plasma growth factors, seems to promote rapid neovascularization and localized cellular growth. This type of combination therapy has been shown to be effective for both male and female pattern hair loss. ACell™ + PRP has also been efficacious in stimulating hair regrowth in alopecia areata, loss of eyebrow hair (hypotrichosis), and other non-hereditary hair loss.

Even though ACell™ + PRP therapy can and is being used as stand-alone hair-loss restoration therapy, incorporating it concomitantly with hair-transplantation surgery has produced favorable results. According to renowned hair-transplant surgeon Dr. Sam Lam (2013) of Plano, Texas, it is an excellent practice to incorporate PRP and

ACell™ with hair-transplant surgery as a synergistic complement to the procedure.

Dr. Lam claims that PRP therapy has shown a profound capability to improve the growth of the transplanted hair follicles, stating that PRP appears to act as a sort of fertilizer for the hair follicles. Moreover, adding ACell™ product to the process serves as a scaffold for the PRP to work better. The ACell™ product may also contribute unique and powerful ways to help grafts grow more finely and limit scarring in the donor and recipient areas. Dr. Lam further claims that the two processes may work synergistically.

An additional strategic consideration for the use of ACell™ + PRP therapy is hair preservation for very young individuals. For example, it is a fact that young individuals who are losing their hair are normally not considered good hair-transplant candidates. Because their baldness patterns have not yet been defined, and they might not be safe candidates for the procedure. Conversely, providing ACell™ + PRP therapy is an excellent option for these potential hair-transplant candidates to preserve and regrow some hair until the person is older with a more defined baldness pattern.

Platelet-Rich Fibrin Matrix Therapy

An enhanced platelet-rich plasma (PRP) version is currently being used to treat hair loss and wound healing. This enhanced version of PRP is called ***Platelet-Rich Fibrin Matrix*** **(PRFM). PRFM** is considered a more effective treatment modality than the original PRP. In fact, the platelet-rich fibrin matrix therapy is regarded as the next generation of PRP for cosmetic purposes. PRFM involves extracting the same blood cells and growth factors from the spun centrifuge blood but at a much slower speed than PRP.

Because the centrifuge to collect the PRFM sample is spun at a slower speed before the various cells and growth factors are extracted for cosmetic use, the end result is that more blood cells and growth factors are gathered for PRFM than are collected from a

PRP sample. Additionally, the slower spin speed causes less trauma to the individual blood cells, allowing more collection of these beneficial stem cells to remain in the final PRFM product. Because of its higher cells concentration, PRFM can be more effective and powerful compared to traditional PRP. There is also some research that shows the growth activity stimulated by platelet-rich fibrin matrix lasts longer, which may provide better results and progress with the same amount of PRP treatments.

Because both PRP and PRFM are derived from the patient's own blood cells, there is minimal risk of an allergic reaction to the treatment. If the patient is anemic or has any blood conditions, they might not be a good candidate for PRP or PRFM therapy. Both PRP and PRFM can be used to treat the following conditions:

- Hair loss and volume loss.
- Aging, sagging skin.
- Loss of elasticity or collagen.
- Scarring, acne scars, keloids.
- Stretchmarks and fine lines.
- Wrinkles.

It is appropriate to conclude this book by stating that currently, there is no definitive evidence that explains all the causative factors leading to male and female pattern hair loss or androgenetic alopecia (AGA). However, List 19.1 below enumerates some of the likely contributors to hair loss that have been described throughout the book:

List 19.1: Likely causes that may contribute to androgenetic alopecia

- Increased testosterone/DHT conversion.
- Hereditary (genetic) predisposition.

- The normal senescence (aging) process.
- Diminished scalp circulation.
- Increased prostaglandin D2 (PGD_2).
- Janus kinase (JAK) enzymes.
- Activation the Wnt/β-catenin pathway to prompt hair growth of dormant hair follicles.
- Decreased oxygen (hypoxemia) content in the blood circulating at the scalp level, leading to increased levels of DHT.
- Increased stress exposure.
- Interaction of the adrenal glands, ovaries, and liver.
- Scalp conditions resulting in hair loss.
- DHT-mediated skull bones remodeling (expansion).
- Improper scalp hygiene and hair care.
- Inadequate nutrition.
- Decrease scalp brown fat.

Notwithstanding the lack of a specific, definitive cause for hair loss, there are currently many more viable options available than ever before to address the problem of hair loss. Some interesting research reports have revealed promising and exciting results in the field of male and female alopecia that could potentially uncover some of the definitive causes of androgenetic alopecia.

Science is making noteworthy progress toward discovering potential treatment modalities to resolve the hair-loss problem. Presently, numerous prestigious institutions are researching novel methods of hair restoration. For example, stem-cell hair research is being conducted in institutions like Sanford-Burnham Medical

Research Institute, Harvard Medical School, John Hopkins University, and the University of Pennsylvania. The preliminary research results arising from these institutions are raising the hope for millions of men and women that a possible cure for hair loss is on the horizon— moreover, the research being conducted by Drs. Harel and Christiano at Columbia University on the Janus kinase (JAK) enzyme is also very exciting and is showing promise. Additionally, prostaglandin D2 (PGD_2) research has been conducted by Garza, Nieves, and Cotsarelis at the University of Pennsylvania and Johns Hopkins University, which is also creating some excitement.

Moreover, Italian biotech company Cassiopea is currently developing a topical drug called ***clascoterone*** (*Breezula*), and it promises to do something very *similar to finasteride* but in a topical solution. Clascoterone is classified as a steroidal androgen receptor antagonist which combats hair loss by blocking the androgen receptor (AR). Cassiopea claims there will be hardly any side effects with this drug. According to Cassiopea, their treatment directly blocks the negative effect of DHT on the scalp based on a mechanism of action discovered through studying the hormone's role in acne development. Appendix B demonstrates a table that shows the pipeline of all the hair growth clinical trials currently underway.

However, a caveat is appropriate at this juncture, despite some excellent news, the reality is far different from the disseminated stories. In fact, it is essential to understand that not all new medical discoveries are commercially viable as practical treatments. For example, gene therapy (GT), hair cloning (HC), hair multiplication (HM), and other "wonder" treatments have been tested successfully in laboratories. However, in reality, these discoveries are costly, and it would be nearly impossible to make them available on a mass scale. Notwithstanding these warnings and limitations, we live in an exciting and promising time for hair-loss research. The goal for all hair-loss sufferers should be to preserve and maintain their existing hair with the various treatment modalities available today.

We need to take care of our remaining hair to prepare for the day when a cure is discovered, which could be sooner than expected.

Despite the disappointment of being afflicted with hair-loss problems, men and women should never resign themselves to looking less than what they were meant to be. Everyone's life objective should be to improve intellectually, physically, and spiritually to achieve a proper physical and psychological balance and, therefore, live the most fulfilling and satisfying life possible. A critical component of reaching this balance is maintaining and preserving one's hair. This goal can be achieved with perseverance and all the hair loss treatment modalities available today.

Author's Note

Dear Reader,

Thank you for taking the time to read my book and helping me present the information behind the research that went into the creation of ***HAIR LOSS: Options for Restoration & Reversal.*** I hope learning about the crucial and extensive topic of hair loss was as exciting and valuable to you as it was for me. It is an essential topic for everyone to embrace sooner rather than later. Eventually, we all will have to address the issue of hair loss. Maintaining and preserving your hair in a healthy state is essential as we wait for more effective treatment modalities.

I hope you enjoyed reading the book and found it a worthwhile investment of time and money. If you did, I would appreciate it very much if you could leave a short review on the site where you purchased the book. Your help in spreading the word is much appreciated.

Thank you!
Gustavo J. Gomez

Official author's website: www.gustavojgomez.com
Amazon author's page: amazon.com/author/gustavojgomez

Appendices

Appendix A

Hair Loss Statistical Data by Age Group

Hair Loss

Percent of men manifesting hair loss by age

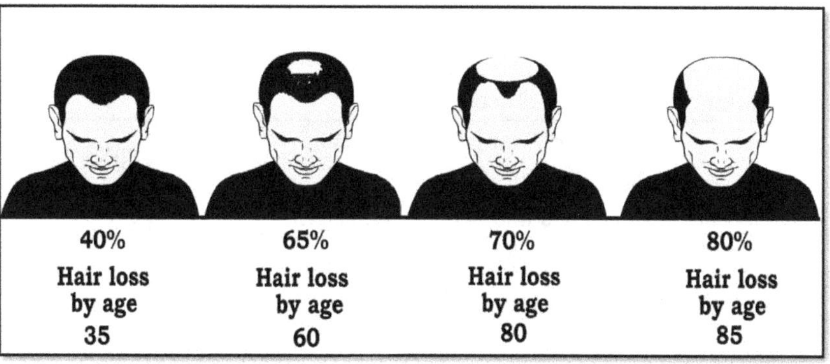

Hair Loss Statistics	Data
Number of U.S. women experiencing hair loss	21 Million
Number of hair loss sufferers worldwide seeking professional treatment	811,363
Number of U.S. men experiencing hair loss	35 Million
Percent of men who will have noticeable hair loss by age 35	40%
Percent of men who will have noticeable hair loss by age 60	65%
Percent of men who will have noticeable hair loss by age 80	70%

Percent of women who will have noticeable hair loss by age 60	80%
Average number of hair follicles on the scalp	110,000
Average number of hairs lost daily by hair-loss sufferers	100
Of the two medical treatments, minoxidil and finasteride:	
Percent of male patients that use a minoxidil (such as Rogaine®)	85%
Percent of male patients that use a finasteride (such as Propecia®)	15%
Percent of all patients that had a negative reaction to any hair-loss treatment	7%
Percent of hair-loss sufferers who would spend their life savings to regain a full head of hair	47%
Percent of hair-loss sufferers who said they would rather have more hair than money or friends	60%
Percent of hair-loss sufferers who said they would give up sex if it meant they would get their hair back	30%
Surgical Hair Restoration:	
Number of surgical hair-restoration procedures in the U.S. (2010)	101,252
Number of surgical hair-restoration procedures worldwide (2010)	279,381
Surgical hair restoration worldwide revenue	$1.87 Billion
Under 20 Years Old	1.4%
Ages 20 – 29	19.3%
Ages 30 – 39	30.4%
Ages 40 – 49	26.3%
Ages 50 – 59	15.4%

60 +	7.1%
Patients who needed 1 procedure to achieve desired results	57%
Patients who needed 2 procedures to achieve desired results	37%
Patients who needed 3 or more procedures to achieve desired results	6%
Percent who needed 1- 999 grafts to achieve desired results	4%
Percent who needed 1,000 – 1,999 grafts to achieve desired results	50%
Percent who needed 2,000 – 2,999 grafts to achieve desired results	41%
Percent who needed 3,000+ grafts to achieve desired results	5%
Non-Surgical Patient Prescription Usage:	
Propecia®	27.5%
Rogaine® Foam	14.8%
Minoxidil	13.4%
Proscar® or generic finasteride	4.3%
Nizoral shampoo	6.1%
Other herbs / vitamins	3.2%
Home low-level laser therapy (LLLT)	3.7%
Other special shampoo	5.5%
Head and Shoulders	2.7%
Biotin	4.9%

Compounded minoxidil with additives	3.8%
Clinical low-level laser therapy	1.4%
Avodart	1%
Nioxin Shampoo	1%

Data Source: http://www.statisticbrain.com/hair-loss-statistics/
Relevant Research, Inc.
International Society of Hair Restoration Surgery

Appendix B

Ongoing Hair Growth Research Pipeline

Hair Growth Clinical Therapies Pipeline -- 2022

Company	Product	Description	Preclinical	Phase 1	Phase 2a	Phase3/ Pivotal	Esti- mated Market Launch
Shiseido/ RepliCel	RCH-01	Multiplied Dermal Sheath Cup Cell Injection				X	2024- 2025 (Japan)
Follica	FOL-004	Micro- Wounding +Topical Compound					2023- 2025 (USA)
Cassiopea	Breezula	Androgen Receptor Antagonist Topical					2024- 2025 (EU)
Kintor Phar- maceutical	KX-826	Androgen Receptor Antagonist Topical			X		2023- 2025 (USA)

TechnoDerma Medicines	TDM-105795	Novel Small Molecule		X			2027-2029 (USA)
Kintor Pharmaceutical	GT20029	Androgen Receptor Degraded PROTAC		X			2027-2029 (China)
Hope Medicine	HMI-115	PRL Receptor Antibody					2027-2029 (USA/ China)
HairClone	TBD	Multiplied DP Cell Therapy Injection					2022-2033 (UK Specials*)
Stemson Therapeutics	TBD	IPSCs > De Novo Hair Follicles With Scaffold					2029-2033 (TBA)
Epibiotech	EPI-001	Multiplied DP Cell Injections					2025-2027 (Korea)
						* = Non-Market, available by doctor's discretion	
						X = In Progress	

Source: FollicleThought.com

Glossary

A

Abnormal: Outside the expected norm, or uncharacteristic of a particular patient.

Adipogenesis: A term relating to the formation of fat. In this book, it relates to the normal function of the sebaceous glands those of fat formation (sebum).

Aging: The process of becoming older, a process that is genetically determined and environmentally modulated.

Alopecia: This was a term used by Aristotle in 384 BCE to describe the condition of hair loss or baldness. Alopecia is derived from the Greek word meaning "fox." The reason for using this term was that foxes had bare spots on their skin due to a parasitic skin condition (i. e. mange) with which they were afflicted. The term as it is used today means baldness or hair loss. Alopecia may result from serious illness, drugs, endocrine disorders, dermatitis, hereditary factors, radiation, or physiological changes during aging (senescence).

When this term is used concomitantly with another term (e. g. alopecia prematura or alopecia seborrheica), it means that the hair loss is the result of a specific condition: hair loss due to a seborrheic condition or premature baldness.

Alopecia Androgenetica: Hair loss resulting from a genetic predisposition of the hair follicles to be affected by the conversion of testosterone to dihydrotestosterone (DHT) facilitated by the enzyme 5-alpha-reductase. Androgenetic alopecia is a common form of hair loss in both men and women. It is characterized by the replacement of thick, terminal hairs with fine, miniaturized hairs that are eventually lost. Androgenetic alopecia is also termed female pattern baldness, male pattern baldness, hereditary alopecia, or simply, common baldness.

Alopecia Areata: An autoimmune condition where the body produces antibodies against its own hair follicles. It is characterized by the sudden appearance of smooth circular patches of bald spots on the scalp, beard, eyelashes, or other parts of the body. Hair transplantation is generally not indicated for this condition, and treatment consists of injections with cortisone or other medical therapies. Generally, for this condition the earlier the onset and the more extensive the hair loss, the worse the prognosis. Some characteristic features of this condition include the following:

- Exclamation point hairs—hairs tapered at the bottom due to the inflammation that causes injury to the hair shaft
- Hair pigment changes
- Grid like nail pitting
- Positive hair-pull test—showing telogen hairs and hairs with tapered, broken ends (dystrophic anagen hairs).

Alopecia Capitis Totalis: Complete or near complete loss of hair on the scalp.

Alopecia Congenitalis: Baldness due to absence of hair bulbs at birth.

Alopecia Follicularis: Baldness due to inflammation of the hair follicles of the scalp.

Alopecia Liminaris: Loss of hair along the hairline, in both the front and back of the scalp.

Alopecia Marginalis: Hair loss primarily at the hairline and temples, which is usually caused by continued traction from braids or hair extensions. If condition persists over a length of time, hair loss may become permanent, even when braiding is discontinued. Other causes of hair loss in men occurring in this distribution include a hereditary thinning in the area (unrelated to trauma) and follicular degeneration syndrome.

Alopecia Symptomatica: Loss of hair after prolonged fevers or during the course of a disease. This baldness may be due to systemic or psychogenic factors.

Alopecia Totalis: Complete or near complete loss of hair on the scalp.

Alopecia Universalis: A type of alopecia areata that involves all the hair on the body, including the eyelashes, eyebrows, nose, and hair on the trunk and extremities.

Ameliorate: To make or become better, more bearable, or satisfactory.

Amino Acids: Amino acids are molecules that combine to form proteins; they are considered the building blocks of life. When proteins are digested or broken down, amino acids is what is left.

Anagen Effluvium: Extensive hair shedding that results from damage to the hair follicles. It appears soon after exposure to the offending agent. One can see broken hair shafts and tapered, irregular hair roots. Anagen effluvium is seen with chemotherapy and radiation therapy.

Anagen Stage: The growing stage of hair development.

Androgen: Substance producing or stimulating male characteristics as the male sex hormone, testosterone.

Androgenetic or Androgenic Alopecia: Hair loss resulting from a genetic predisposition of the hair follicles to be affected by dihydrotestosterone (DHT). Androgenetic alopecia is a common form of hair loss in both men and women.

It is characterized by the replacement of thick terminal hairs with fine, miniaturized hairs that are eventually lost. Androgenic alopecia is also termed female pattern baldness, male pattern baldness, hereditary alopecia or simply, common baldness.

Anesthetic: An agent that produces insensitivity to pain or touch.

Angiogenesis: is the physiological process through which new blood vessels form from pre-existing vessels

Anti-Neoplastic Agents: Refers to drugs utilized for the treatment of cancer.

Apoptosis: A normal, genetically regulated process leading to the death of cells and triggered by the presence or absence of certain stimuli, such as DNA damage.

B

Bacitracin Ointment: An antibiotic for topical application.

Biopsy: The removal of a sample of tissue for examination under a microscope to check for cancer cells or other abnormalities.

Body dysmorphic disorder (BDD): occasionally still called **dysmorphophobia**, is a mental disorder characterized by the obsessive idea that some aspect of one's own body part or appearance is severely flawed and therefore warrants exceptional measures to hide or fix it.

Brocq Pseudopelade: In 1888, Brocq used the term pseudopelade to describe a unique form of cicatricial alopecia resembling alopecia areata. *Pelade* is the French term for alopecia areata. Over the last century, this condition has been a source of controversy. While some believe that pseudopelade is a unique entity, most now believe that it is an end-stage or clinical variant of various forms of cicatricial alopecia.

C

Catagen Stage: Intermediate or transitional phase of the hair-growth cycle, which falls after the anagen (growth) stage. Catagen is the shortest phase of the growth cycle, lasting only about two to three weeks.

Cicatricial: Scarring.

Cysteine: This a sulfur-containing amino acid found in foods like poultry, eggs, dairy, red peppers, garlic, and onions. It works as an antioxidant, in the production of collagen (a component of hair, skin and nails), and is also used in the body to create glutathione, another important antioxidant.

Cystine: Is formed from two cysteine molecules joined together, and it is more stable than cysteine but may not be absorbed as well. This amino acid is also a component of hair, skin, and nails. However, there is no evidence that supplementing with cystine improves hair, skin, or nail health, and it is rarely used as a dietary supplement.

Cytokine: Any of a group of small, short-lived proteins that are released by one cell to regulate the function of another cell, thereby serving as intercellular chemical messengers. Cytokines are any of a number of substances, such as interferon, interleukin, and growth factors that are secreted by certain cells of the immune system and have an effect on other cells. They are probably best known for the roles they play in the immune system's defense against disease-causing organisms.

Cytotoxic: Chemicals or drugs, which destroy cells or prevent their multiplication. They are a group of compounds developed for use in cancer chemotherapy.

D

Densitometry: Densitometry is a technique to help evaluate a patient's candidacy for hair transplantation and predict future hair loss. It analyzes the scalp under high-power magnification to give information on hair density, follicular unit composition, and degree of miniaturization.

Density: The number of hairs in a specific area. An accurate, quantitative evaluation of hair density can be difficult and certainly time consuming. The average hair density on an adult scalp that does not have baldness is approximately 200-300 hairs per square centimeter (cm2). Generally, the classifications of hair density are thin, medium, and thick, and they are unrelated to the texture of the hair. While there is not a true ethnic or racial determiner of hair density, it has been found that blondes tend to have the greatest hair density while redheads have the lowest. The average head has approximately 2,200 strands of hair per square inch and a total of approximately 100,000 hairs (Rushton et al., 1993).

Dermis: The skin. It is also known as the cutis vera, or true skin.

Diffuse Patterned Alopecia (DPA): A type of androgenetic hair loss characterized by diffuse thinning in the front, top, and vertex of the scalp. It is usually associated with a stable permanent zone.

Diffuse Unpatterned Alopecia (DUPA): A type of androgenetic hair loss that occurs over the entire scalp so that there is no permanent zone of hair normally present in the back and sides of the scalp. The progression of hair loss is often rapid and can result in an almost transparent look due to the low density. Diagnosing DUPA is imperative, as most patients with diffuse unpatterned alopecia should not have a surgical hair restoration, since the transplanted hair will not be permanent. DUPA is a pattern more commonly seen in women. The use of densitometry is very helpful in diagnosing this condition.

Dihydrotestosterone (DHT): A derivative of testosterone after it has been converted by the enzyme 5-alpha-reductase. It is a stronger form of testosterone, believed to be responsible for hair loss.

Donor Area: Refers to the site from which the hair plugs or strips will be taken when performing a hair transplant operation.

Donor Dominant: A term used by Orentreich, meaning that the transposed or transplanted punch graft (hair plug) of skin maintains its integrity and characteristics independent of the recipient site.

E

Embryonic State: A state pertaining to, or in the condition of, an embryo. This term is used in this book to refer to hair that regresses to a primitive state (e.g., from a terminal hair to a vellus hair).

Epidermis: The cuticle or outer layer of the skin.

Epithelial Cells: The layer of cells forming the epidermis of the skin and the surface layer of the mucous and serous membranes.

Eunuch: A castrated male, or one who has had his testicles removed.

Exogen Hair Cycle: The shedding phase of the hair-growth cycle. The hair shedding function has been assumed to be part of the telogen phase; however, it has been found that shedding actually occurs as a distinct phase.

F

Febrile Illness: An ailment associated with a feverish condition.

Female Pattern Hair Loss (FPHL): A condition associated with loss of hair in women. This condition is not uncommon.

Five-Alpha-Reductase (5AR): The enzyme responsible for the conversion of testosterone into dihydrotestosterone (DHT).

Follicular Degeneration Syndrome: A form of scarring alopecia caused by the premature shedding of the inner root sheath of the hair follicle. It eventually results in complete follicular destruction. Because it occurs in a band around the frontal part of the scalp, it had been felt that the condition was due to traction. It is now felt that the condition is idiopathic and unrelated to mechanical trauma or that it can be caused by a hot comb.

Folliculitis Decalvans: A form of alopecia characterized by scarring, redness, swelling and pustules around the hair follicle, which leads to the destruction of the follicle and consequent permanent hair loss. Folliculitis decalvans affects both men and women and may start first during adolescence or at any time in adult life. The exact cause is unknown. In most cases, staphylococcus aureus can be isolated from the pustules, but the role of the bacteria is not clear. Treatment modalities includes the following:

- Oral antibiotics (e.g., cephalosporin),
- Minocycline,
- Rifampin
- Intralesional corticosteroids

Frontal Fibrosing Alopecia (FFA): A primary lymphocytic cicatricial alopecia with a distinctive clinical pattern of hair loss characterized by progressive recession of the fronto-temporal hairline, with or without progressive loss of eyebrows.

More common in post-menopausal women, the front part of the scalp appears shiny, smooth, and devoid of hair follicles. This pattern can mimic androgenetic alopecia, but on close inspection, one notes scarring and the absence of hair follicle openings. There may be signs of inflammation, including redness and scaling. The condition may be a variant of lichen planopilaris.

G

Genetics: The science that accounts for natural differences and resemblances among organisms related by descent.

Gestation: Period of intrauterine fetal development from conception to birth.

Gonads: The embryonic sex gland before differentiation into definitive testes or ovaries. It is also a generic term referring to both, female and male sex glands.

H

Hair Bulb: Lower expanded portion of a hair root. Growth of a hair results from the proliferation of cells of the hair bulb.

Hair Follicle: An invagination of the epidermis, which forms a cylindrical depression penetrating the corium into the connective tissue, which holds the hair root.

Hair Papilla: A projection of the corium which extends into the hair bulb at the bottom of a hair follicle.

Hair Root: The part of the hair that is embedded in the dermis (skin).

Hair Shaft: The visible portion of the hair.

Hair Transplant: An operation or surgical procedure that entails the transferring of hair bearing tissue from a donor site to a recipient site on a patient's scalp.

Heredity: Innate capacity of an individual to develop traits and characteristics possessed by his/her ancestors.

Hippocratic Baldness: The most advanced type of baldness (hair loss), named after the Greek philosopher Hippocrates.

Hormones: Any member of a class of signaling molecules produced by glands in multicellular organisms that are transported by the circulatory system to target distant organs to regulate physiology and behavior. Hormones have diverse chemical structures, mainly of three classes:

- Eicosanoids
- Steroids
- Amino acid derivatives (amines, peptides, and proteins).

Therefore, hormones are regulatory substances produced in an organism and transported in tissue fluids such as blood or sap to stimulate specific cells or tissues into action. The glands that secrete hormones comprise the endocrine signaling system. The term hormone is sometimes extended to include chemicals produced by cells that affect the same cell (autocrine or intracrine signaling) or nearby cells (paracrine signalling).

Hygiene: The study of health and observance of health rules. It can also be the study of the methods and means of preserving health.

Hyperkeratosis: The overgrowth of the horny layer of the epidermis.

Hypervitaminosis A: An excessive ingestion of vitamin A.

Hypopituitarism: Diminished hormone secretion by the pituitary gland, causing dwarfism in children and premature aging in adults.

Hypotrichosis Simplex of the Scalp: Hypotrichosis simplex of the scalp (HSS) is a genetic disorder, characterized by sparse or absent scalp hair without structural defects, in the absence of other ectodermal or systemic abnormalities.

Hypovitaminosis A: Deficient ingestion of vitamin A.

Hypoxia: Lack of an adequate amount of oxygen in circulating arterial blood. It can also be called hypoxemia.

Hypoxic State: A condition referring to an inadequate amount of available oxygen.

I

Inciting Agents: Factors that stimulate or urge to action.

J

Janus Kinase (JAK) Enzyme: A family of intracellular, nonreceptor tyrosine kinases that transduce cytokine-mediated signals via the JAK-STAT pathway.

K

Kenogen Hair Cycle: The term kenogen was coined to describe the interval of the hair cycle in which the hair follicle remains empty after the telogen hair has been ejected or shed and before a new anagen hair reappears. It is normal to observe kenogen in healthy skin, but in men and women with androgenetic alopecia the frequency and duration of kenogen have been reported to be greater (Rebora & Guarrera, 2002).

Keratin: An extremely tough protein substance in hair, nails, and horny tissue.

Keratosis Pilaris: Develops when keratin forms a scaly plug that blocks the opening of the hair follicle. Usually plugs form in many hair follicles, causing patches of rough, bumpy skin.

L

Lanugo Hair: Fine downy hairs that cover the body of the fetus, especially when premature.

Latisse (bimatoprost): is a topical prostaglandin eye solution. It's not known exactly how Latisse (bimatoprost) works to grow eyelashes, but it might increase the number of eyelash hairs that are actively growing, making them longer, thicker, and darker.

Lichen Planopilaris (LPP): An uncommon inflammatory scalp disorder that is clinically characterized by perifollicular erythema, follicular hyperkeratosis, and permanent hair loss. A condition affecting the hair follicles in localized, scaly, red patches that result in scarring and hair loss in the affected areas. The disease is characterized by a band-like layer of inflammatory cells at the upper most layer of the dermis that damage the hair follicles. Treatment modalities includes the following:

- Potent topical corticosteroids
- Intralesional corticosteroids
- Systemic corticosteroids
- Oral retinoids
- Anti-malarials
- Oral cyclosporine

Loose Anagen Hair Syndrome: This is a very rare condition but seen more often in females than males, presenting early in childhood, usually between the ages of two and nine as diffuse patches of hair loss. This syndrome is characterized by a defective inner root sheath (abnormal keratinization) that prevents it from grasping the hair shaft cuticle. As a result, the newly growing hair shaft falls out. The hair is usually blonde, feels matted or sticky, is lusterless, and does not require cutting. A hair-pull test is positive for anagen hairs. No systemic abnormality is associated with it. With adolescence, the hair grows longer, denser, and darker, but the hair pull remains positive.

Ludwig Classification: Classification of female pattern hair loss. It encompasses three stages: mild (type 1), moderate (type II) and extensive (type III). In all three stages, there is loss on the front and top of the scalp, with preservation of the frontal hairline in the majority of cases. If the person's donor hair is stable at the back and sides of the scalp, women of all three types of Ludwig classification may be candidates for hair transplantation.

M

Male Pattern Hair Loss (MPHL): Premature loss of hair, sometimes called common baldness. It is believed to be dependent on hereditary factors and the influence of androgen stimulation as well as the normal aging process.

Medulla: The inner or central portion of an organ in contrast to the outer portion or cortex.

Melanin: A dark brown to black pigment occurring in the hair, skin, and iris of the eye in people and animals. Melanin is responsible for tanning of skin exposed to sunlight.

Melanocytes: Melanin forming or producing cells.

Mitotic Process: A method of action involving indirect cellular division.

Myxedema: Is swelling of the skin and underlying tissues giving a waxy consistency, typical of patients with underactive thyroid glands.

N

Neovascularization: Has been described as the formation of functional, microvascular networks with red blood cell perfusion. Neovascularization differs from angiogenesis in that angiogenesis is principally characterized by the protrusion and outgrowth of capillary buds and sprouts from preexisting blood vessels.

Norwood Classification: Published by Dr. O'tar Norwood in 1975, this is the most common classification for describing genetic hair loss in men. The regular Norwood classification pattern has seven stages that begin with recession at the temples and thinning in the crown. The Norwood Class A patterns or variants has five stages and is characterized by a predominantly front to back progression of hair loss.

Nutrients: Foods that supply the body with its necessary elements.

Nutrition: The sum total of the processes involved in the ingestion and utilization of food substances by which growth, repair, and maintenance of activities within the body as a whole or in any of its parts is accomplished. Nutrition includes the following three processes:

- Ingestion
- Absorption
- Assimilation (metabolism)

O

P

Palliate: To alleviate or lessen the pain or severity without curing.

Parturition: Act of giving birth.

Pigmented: Having pigmentation or possessing color.

Pilosebaceous: Concerning the hair and sebaceous glands.

Pityriasis: A skin disease characterized by the shedding of fine, flaky scales.

Pityriasis Capitis: Dandruff.

Pityriasis Seborrheica: Oily dandruff.

Pityriasis Sicca: Dry dandruff.

Postnatal: After birth.

Postpartum: Following childbirth or the birth of young.

Pseudo Palade of Braque: A non-specific scarring alopecia of unknown cause. It also may represent the end stage of other inflammatory scalp conditions. It presents with white or flesh-colored atrophic plaques, without active inflammation.

Punch Graft: Another term for hair plug.

Q

Quorum Sensing: Is a system of stimuli and response correlated to population density. Many species of bacteria use quorum sensing to coordinate gene expression according to the density of their local population.

R

Receptor: A group of cells functioning in reception of stimuli. An end organ or a group of end organs of sensory or afferent neurons specialized to be sensitive to stimulating agents, such as touch or heat.

Recipient Area: The site that will receive the hair plugs or follicular units removed from the donor area during hair transplant surgery.

Recipient Dominant: A term used by Orentreich, meaning that the transposed or transplanted punch graft of skin takes on the characteristics of the recipient site.

S

Scarlet Fever: An acute (sudden) contagious disease characterized by sore throat, strawberry tongue, fever, punctiform scarlet rash, and rapid pulse.

Sebaceous Glands: The oil-secreting glands of the skin.

Seborrhea: Functional disease of the sebaceous glands.

Sebum: A fatty secretion of the sebaceous glands of the skin.

Secondary Stage Syphilis: The second stage of syphilis that appears from 2 to 6 months after primary infection, which is marked by lesions especially in the skin but also in organs and tissues, and that lasts from 3 to 12 weeks.

Side Effect: The action or effect, usually of a drug, other than that desired.

Systemic Lupus Erythematosus (SLE): An auto-immune disease where the immune system attacks the body's own cells, resulting in inflammation and tissue destruction. SLE can affect any part of the body, but most commonly affects the skin, joints, kidneys, heart, and blood vessels. The course of the disease is unpredictable, with periods of flares and remissions. Lupus can occur at any age and is more common in women. The skin manifestations are quite varied and can present with localized lesions (DLE), diffuse hair loss and sensitivity to the sun. The name comes from the fact that the photo-sensitive rash that occurs on the face resembles that of a wolf.

T

Telogen Effluvium: Hair loss that follows any kind of stress, such as fever, surgical operation, parturition, or emotional disturbance. This condition is usually of a temporary nature.

Telogen Stage: Resting stage of the growth cycle.

Testosterone: An androgen isolated from the testes of a number of animals, including man; male sex hormone.

Toxic: Acting as or having the effect, of a poison; poisonous.

Traction Alopecia: Is a form of alopecia, or gradual hair loss, caused primarily by pulling; force being applied to the hair. This commonly results from the sufferer frequently wearing their hair in a particularly tight ponytail, pigtails, or braids.

Trichologist: A specialist who studies the hair and its care and treatment.

Trichology: The branch of medical and cosmetic study and practice concerned with the hair and scalp.

Trichotillomania: The unnatural impulse to pull out one's own hair.

V

Vellus Hair: This type of hair replaces lanugo hair in the postnatal period. It will cover the entire body surface. It is soft, fine, and unmedullated, sometimes pigmented.

Vertex: The corona capitis or crown; top of the head.

X

Z

References

Abimelec, P. (2016). Hair transplant; hair restoration. Abimelec Dermatologist. Retrieved October 27, 2016 from, http://www.abimelec.com/dermatologist/hair-transplant.html

Ablon, G. (2012). A Double-blind, placebo-controlled study evaluating the efficacy of an oral supplement in women with self-perceived Thinning Hair. J Clin Aesthet Dermatol v.5 (11); Nov PMC3509882, Retrieved August 3, 2016, from, http://www.ncbi.nlm.nih.gov/pmc/articles/PMC3509882/

Acelajado, M. C., Pisoni, R., Dudenbostel, T., Dell'Italia, L., Cartmill, F., Zhang, B., Cofield, S. S., Oparil, S. and Calhoun, D. A. (2013). Refractory hypertension: Definition, Prevalence And Patient Characteristics. J Clin Hypertens (Greenwich). 2012 Jan; 14(1): 7–12. Published online 2011 Nov 15. Doi: 10.1111/j.1751-7176.2011.00556. x. Retrieved May 23, 2014, from, http://www.ncbi.nlm.nih.gov/pmc/articles/PMC3400427/

Acvi, P., Gupta, G. K., Clark, J., Wikonkal, N. and Hamblin, M.R. (2013). Low-level laser (light) therapy (LLLT) for treatment of Hair Loss. Lasers Surg Med. 2014 Feb; 46(2): 144–151. Retrieved July 24, 2014, from, http://www.ncbi.nlm.nih.gov/pmc/articles/PMC3944668/

Agarwal, S., Godse, k., Mahajan, A., Patil, S. and Nadkarni, N. (2013). Application of the basic and specific classification on patterned hair loss in Indians. Int J of Trichol 2013; 5:126-31. Retrieved January 29, 2017, from, http://www.ijtrichology.com/text.asp?2013/5/3/126/125606

Agrawal, M. (2008). Modern artificial hair implantation: a pilot study of 10 patients. J Cosmet Dermatol. 2008;7: 315–23. Retrieved July 23, 2015, from, http://www.ncbi.nlm.nih.gov/pubmed/19146611

AHLA.org (n. d.). Hair shafts defects. Retrieved April 30, 2016, from, http://www.americanhairloss.org/types_of_hair_loss/hair_shaft_defects.asp

Ahmed, A., Almohanna, H., Griggs, J., and Tosti, A. (2019). Genetic Hair Disorders: A Review. Dermatology and Therapy volume 9. Retrieved April 30, 2022, from, https://link.springer.com/article/10.1007/s13555-019-0313-2

Alai, N. A., and Elston, M. D. (2016). Keratosis pilaris. Retrieved September 20, 2015, from, http://emedicine.medscape.com/article/1070651-overvi

American Hair Loss Association (n.d.). Hair Loss Treatment. Retrieved April 15, 2016, from, https://www.americanhairloss.org/hair_loss_treatment/default.html

Androgeneticalopecia.com (n. d.). Savin scale for diagnosis of androgenetic alopecia in women. Retrieved September 1, 2013, from, http://www.androgeneticalopecia.com/hair-loss-men- women/hair-loss-baldness-savin-scale.shtml

Androgeneticalopecia.com (n.d.). Topical tretinoin for the treatment of pattern hair loss. Retrieved September 1, 2013, from, http://www.androgeneticalopecia.com/hair-loss-treatments/tretinoin-pattern-baldness.shtml

Applied Biology, Inc. (2016). Minoxidil response testing in males with androgenetic alopecia. Retrieved August 19, 2016, from, https://clinicaltrials.gov/ct2/show/NCT02198261

Araújo, R., Fernandes, Margarida Cavaco-Paulo, A. and Gomes, A. (2010). Biology of human hair: Know Your Hair to Control It. Adv Biochem Engin/Biotechnol. Retrieved September 21, 2015, from, https://repositorium.sdum.uminho.pt/bitstream/1822/15299/1/2010%20Biology%20of%20Human%20Hair%20Know%20Your%20Hair.pdf

Axe, J. (2016). Biotin benefits: Thicken Hair, Nails and Beautify Skin. Retrieved November 2, 2016 from, https://draxe.com/biotin-benefits/

Balañá, M. E., Charreau, H. E. and Leirós, G. J. (2015). Epidermal stem cells and skin tissue engineering in hair follicle regeneration. World J Stem Cells. 2015 May 26; 7(4): 711–727. Retrieved August 25, 2016, from, https://www.ncbi.nlm.nih.gov/pmc/articles/PMC4444612/

Barrett, S. (1985). Commercial hair analysis: Science or scam? JAMA, 254(8):1041-5. Retrieved August 2, 2016, from, http://www.ncbi.nlm.nih.gov/pubmed/4021042

Battmann, T., Bonfils, A., Branche, C., Humbert, J., Goubet, F., Teutsch, G. and Philibert, D. (1994). RU 58841, a new specific topical antiandrogen: a candidate of choice for the treatment of acne, androgenetic alopecia, and hirsutism. J Steroid Biochem Mol Biol. 1994 Jan;48(1):55-60. Retrieved August 23, 2014, from, https://www.ncbi.nlm.nih.gov/pubmed/8136306

Bernstein, R. (2013). Miniaturization. Retrieved January 26, 2016, from, http://www.bernsteinmedical.com/hair loss/miniaturization/

Bernstein, R. (2014). Psychological aspects of balding. Bernstein Medical Center for Hair Restoration. Retrieved January 6, 2014, from, http://www.bernsteinmedical.com/hair-loss/fqamyths more/psychological-aspects-of-balding/

Bland, K. I., Sarr, M. G., Csendes, A. (2008). General Surgery: Principles and International Practice, Volume 1. Springer. pp. 1,534. ISBN: 9781846288326.

Blatchley, C. (2017). Do topical finasteride and dutasteride help prevent male pattern hair loss, and if so what is the minimum concentration to prevent systemic effects? Retrieved May 2, 2017, from, https://www.researchgate.net/post/Do_topical_finasteride_and_dutasteride_help_prevent_male_pattern_hair_loss_and_if_so_what_is_the_minimum_concentration_to_prevent_systemic_effect

Blattner, C., Polley, D. C., Ferritto, F. and Dirk M. Elston, D. M. (2013). Central centrifugal cicatricial alopecia. Indian Dermatol Online J. 2013 Jan-Mar; 4(1): 50–51. doi:10.4103/2229-5178.105484. Retrieved January 12, 2016, from, https://www.ncbi.nlm.nih.gov/pmc/articles/PMC3573455/

Blume-Peytavi, U., Whiting, D. A. and Trüeb, R. M. (2008). Hair Growth and Disorders. Springer Science & Business Media. pp. 182, 369. ISBN 978-3-540-46911-7. Retrieved August 12, 2014, from, https://books.google.com/books?id=pHrX2-huQCoC&pg=PA369#v=onepage&q&f=false

Boersma, I. H., Oranje, A. P., Grimalt, R., Iorizzo, M., Piraccini, B. M. and Verdonschot, E.H. (2014). The effectiveness of finasteride and dutasteride used for 3 years in women with androgenetic alopecia. Indian J Dermatol Venereol Leprol., 80(6):521-5. doi: 10.4103/0378-6323.144162. Retrieved September 24, 2015, from, https://www.ncbi.nlm.nih.gov/pubmed/25382509

Borreli, L. (2015). What causes gray hair? The Influence of Genetics and other factors on hair color. Retrieved November 20, 2016, from, http://www.medicaldaily.com/pulse/what-causes-gray-hair-influence-genetics-and-other-factors-hair-color-324622

Botchkareva, N. V., Ahluwalia, G. and Shander, D. (2006). Apoptosis in the hair follicle. J Invest Dermatol.126(2):258-64. Retrieved September 3, 2014, from, http://www.ncbi.nlm.nih.gov/pubmed/16418734

Bou-Abboud, C. F., Nemec, F, & Toffel, F. (1990). Reversal of androgenetic alopecia in a male. A Spironolactone Effect. Acta erm Venerol; 70 (4):342-3. Retrieved December 1, 2015, from, http://www.ncbi.nlm.nih.gov/pubmed/1977262

Bruchovsky, N., and Wilson, J. D. (1968). The inter-nuclear binding of testosterone and 5-alpha-androstan-17-beta-ol-3-one by rat prostate. *J Biol. Chem.* 243(22):5953–5960. Retrieved December 15, 2015, from, http://www.ncbi.nlm.nih.gov/pubmed/?term=Bruchovsky+N%2C+Wilson+JD.+The+intranuclear+binding+of+testosterone+and+5-alpha-androstan-17-beta-ol-3-one+by+rat+prostate.

Buffoli, B., Rinaldi, F., Labanca, M., Sorbellini, E., Trink, A., Guanziroli, E., Rezzani, R., and Rodella, L. F. (2013). The human hair: from anatomy to physiology. International Society of Dermatology. Retrieved February 9, 2016, from, http://onlinelibrary.wiley.com/doi/10.1111/ijd.12362/abstract? User Is Authenticated=false & denied Access Customized Message =

Buhl, A. E., Waldon, D. J., Baker, C. A. and Johnson, G. A. (1990). Minoxidil sulfate is the active metabolite that stimulates hair follicles. J Invest Dermatol, 95(5):553-7. Retrieved May 23, 2015, from, http://www.ncbi.nlm.nih.gov/pubmed/2230218

BusinessWire. (2011). ARTAS system receives FDA clearance approval for ground-breaking technology for treating hair loss. BusinessWire. Retrieved October 28, 2016, from, http://www.businesswire.com/news/home/20110414005869/en/ARTAS-System-Receives-FDA-Clearance-Ground-Breaking-Technology.

Camacho, F. and Montagna, W. (1998). Trichology: Diseases of the pilosebaceous follicle. S. Karger Publishers Inc. Farmington, USA. ISBN: 3-8055-6672-7

Carf.org (2016). Cicatricial alopecia. Retrieved November 21, 2015, from, http://www.carfintl.org/faq.php

Carmichael, S. W. (2014). The tangled web of Langer's lines. Clin Anat, 27(2):162-8. doi: 10.1002/ca.22278. Retrieved November 1, 2015, from, https://www.ncbi.nlm.nih.gov/pubmed/24038134

Cash, T. F., Price, V. H., and Savin, R. C. (1993). Psychological effects of androgenetic alopecia on women: Comparisons with balding men and with female control subjects. J Am Acad Dermatol, 29:568–75. Retrieved January 22, 2015, from, http://www.ncbi.nlm.nih.gov/pubmed/8408792

Cather, J.C., Lane, D., Heaphy, M.R., Jr., Nelson, B.R. (1999). Finasteride – an update and review. Cutis. 1999;64:167–172. Retrieved November 12, 2017, from, https://pubmed.ncbi.nlm.nih.gov/10500917/https://pascal-francis.inist.fr/vibad/index.php?action=getRecordDetail&idt=1930104

Chan, D. and Ducic, Y. (2015). An update on hair restoration. Journal of Aesthetic and Reconstructive Surgery. Retrieved January 15, 2016, from, http://aesthetic-reconstructive-surgery.imedpub.com/an-update-on-hair-restoration.php?aid=7956

Chase, B. H. (1954). Growth of the hair. Physiological reviews, 34 (1): 113-126. Retrieved December 2, 2014, from, http://physrev.physiology.org/content/34/1/11

Chaudhari, N. D., Sharma, Y. K., Dash, K. and Deshmukh, P. (2012). Role of platelet-rich plasma in the management of androgenetic alopecia. Int J Trichology, 4(4): 291–292. doi:10.4103/0974-7753.111222. Retrieved October 23, 2014, from, https://www.ncbi.nlm.nih.gov/pmc/articles/PMC3681120/

Chen, C. C., Wang, L., Plikus, M. V., Jiang, T. X., Murray, P. J., Ramos, R., Guerrero-Suarez, C.F., Hughes, M. W., Lee, O. K., Shi, S., Widelitz, R.B., Lander, A. D. and Chuong, C. M. (2015). Organ-level quorum sensing directs regeneration in hair stem cell populations. Cell 161 (2): p 277–290. Retrieved December 5, 2016, from, http://www.cell.com/cell/fulltext/S0092-8674(15)00182-8

Cheng, A.S. and Bayliss, S.J. (2008). The genetics of hair shaft disorders. J Am Acad Dermatol 2008; 59(1):1-22. Retrieved October 15, 2015, from, http://www.ncbi.nlm.nih.gov/pubmed/18571596

Chinwe, C., Bowers, E., Cox, T., Jewell, R., Johnson, B., Overman, D., Thakkar, J., Alcaraz, C., and Davis, K. (2010). Biotin. Retrieved August 23, 2014, from, http://www4.ncsu.edu/~knopp/BCH451/Biotin.htm

Choi, G. S., Kim, J.H., Oh, S. Y., Park, J. M., Hong, J. S., Lee, Y. S. and Won-Soo Lee, W. S. (2016). Safety and Tolerability of the Dual 5-Alpha Reductase Inhibitor Dutasteride in the Treatment of Androgenetic Alopecia. Ann Dermatol., 28(4): 444–450. Retrieved October 20, 2016, from, https://www.ncbi.nlm.nih.gov/pmc/articles/PMC4969473/

Choi, Y. S., Zhang, Y., Xu, M., Yang, Y., Ito, M., Peng, T., Cui, Z., Nagy, A., Hadjantonakis, A. K., Lang, R. A., Cotsarelis, G. Andl, T., Morrisey, E. E. and Millar, S. E. (2013). Distinct functions for Wnt/β-catenin in hair follicle stem cell proliferation and survival and interfollicular epidermal homeostasis. Cell Stem Cell. 13(6):720-33. doi: 10.1016/j.stem.2013.10.003. Retrieved November 12, 2016, from, https://www.ncbi.nlm.nih.gov/pubmed/24315444

Clark, R.V., Hermann, D.J., Cunningham, G.R., Wilson, T. H., H., B. Morrill, B.B., and Hobbs, S. (2004). Marked suppression of dihydrotestosterone in men with benign prostatic hyperplasia by dutasteride a dual 5α-reductase inhibitor. Journal of Clinical Endocrinology and Metabolism, vol. 89, no. 5, pp. 2179–2184. Retrieved December 17, 2015, from, http://www.ncbi.nlm.nih.gov/pubmed/15126539. Retrieved December 9, 2014, from, http://press.endocrine.org/doi/abs/10.1210/jc.2003-030330. DOI: http://dx.doi.org/10.1210/jc.2003-030330

Cleary, M. L., Smith, S. D. and Sklar, J. (1986). Cloning and structural analysis of cDNAs for bcl-2 and a hybrid bcl-2/immunoglobulin transcript resulting from the t (14;18) translocation". Cell, 47 (1): 19–28. doi:10.1016/0092-8674(86)90362-4. Retrieved September 3, 2014, from, http://www.cell.com/cell/abstract/0092-8674(86)90362 4? returnURL=http%3A%2F%2Flinkinghub.elsevier.com%2Fretrieve%2Fpii%2F0092867486903624%3Fshowall%3Dtrue

Coiffman F. (1979). Use of square scalp graft for male pattern baldness. In: Unger WP, eds. Hair Transplantation, 1st ed. New York: Dekker, 1979:159-63. In: Plastic & Reconstructive Surgery: August 1977, 60(2): pp 228-232. Retrieved August 12, 2011, from, http://journals.lww.com/plasreconsurg/Citation/1977/08000/Use_of_Square_Scalp_Grafts_for_Male_Pattern.9.aspx

Cole hair Transplant Group (n. d.). Strip hair transplant. Retrieved December 6, 2015, from, http://www.forhair.com/strip-hair transplant/

Compton, S. (2016). What is gene expression? -regulation, analysis, and definition. Retrieved February 13, 2015, from, http://study.com/academy/lesson/what-is-gene-expression-regulation-analysis-definition.html

Costin, G. E. and Hearing, V. J. (2007). Human skin pigmentation: melanocytes modulate skin color in response to stress. FASEB J, 21:976-94. Retrieved July 22, 2016, from, http://www.ncbi.nlm.nih.gov/pubmed/17242160 http://www.scielo.br/scielo.php?script=sci_nlinks&pid=S0365 05962013000100076000003&lng=en

Cotsarelis, G., Millar, S. E. (2001). Towards a molecular understanding of hair loss and its treatment. Trends Mol Med, 7(7):293–301. Doi: 10.1016/S1471-4914(01)02027-5. Retrieved August 12, 2014, from, http://www.ncbi.nlm.nih.gov/pubmed/11425637

Curtis, N. J. (2004). Comparison of clinical trials with finasteride and dutasteride. Reviews in Urology 6(Suppl 9): S31–S39. Retrieved November 3, 2015, from, http://www.ncbi.nlm.nih.gov/pmc/articles/PMC1472914/ http://onlinelibrary.wiley.com/doi/10.1111/j.13497006.2007.0 0656.x/full.

Daniells, S. and Hardy, G. (2010). Hair loss in long-term or home parenteral nutrition: are micronutrient deficiencies to blame? Curr Opin Clin Nutr Metab Care, 13(6):690-7. Retrieved July 25, 2016, from, http://www.ncbi.nlm.nih.gov/pubmed/20823774

Dauer, M. (2014). Scalp reductions: A Procedure from the Past. Retrieved November 30, 2016, from, http://mdnewhair.com/scalp-reductions-procedure-past/

Davis, S. A., Narahari, S., Feldman, S. R., Huang, W., Pichardo-Geisinger, R. O. and McMichael, A. J. (2012). Top dermatologic conditions in patients of color: an analysis of nationally representative data. J Drugs Dermatol, 11(4):466-73. Retrieved October 12, 2016, from, https://www.ncbi.nlm.nih.gov/pubmed/22453583

DuBois, J., Bruce, S., Stewart, D., Kempers, S., Harutunian, C., Boodhoo, T., Weitzenfeld, A., Chang-Lin, J. E. (2021). Setipiprant for Androgenetic

Alopecia in Males: Results from a Randomized, Double-Blind, Placebo-Controlled Phase 2a Trial. Clinical, Cosmetic and Investigational Dermatology. Retrieved November 20, 2021, from, https://www.ncbi.nlm.nih.gov/pmc/articles/PMC8526366/

De Brouwer, B., Tételin, C., Leroy, T., Bonfils, A. and Van Neste, D. (1997). A controlled study of the effects of RU58841, a non-steroidal antiandrogen, on human hair production by balding scalp grafts maintained on testosterone-conditioned nude mice. Br J Dermatol., 137(5):699-702. Retrieved December 12, 2014, from, https://www.ncbi.nlm.nih.gov/pubmed/9415227

Dhurat, R., Sukesh, M. S., Avhad, G., Dandale, A., Pal, A., and Pund, P. (2013). A Randomized Evaluator Blinded Study of Effect of Microneedling in Androgenetic Alopecia: A Pilot Study. Int J Trichology; doi: 10.4103/0974-7753.114700. Retrieved, May 5, 2021, from, https://www.ncbi.nlm.nih.gov/pmc/articles/PMC3746236/

Dias P.C.R., Miot, H.R., Trüeb, R.M., and Ramos, P.M. (2018). Use of Minoxidil Sulfate versus Minoxidil Base in Androgenetic Alopecia Treatment: Friend or Foe? Skin Appendage Disorders. Retrieved October 3, 2021, from, https://www.karger.com/Article/Fulltext/488011

Dihn, Q. Q., and Sinclair, R. (2007). Female pattern hair loss: Current treatment concepts. Clin Interv Aging. Retrieved January 1, 2013, from, http://pubmedcentralcanada.ca/pmcc/articles/PMC2684510/

Dondi, D., Piccolella, M., Bisemi, A., Della Torre, S., Ramachandran, B., Locatelli, A., Rusmini, P., Sau, D., Maggi, A., Ciana, P., and Poletti, A. (2010). Estrogen receptor beta and the progression of prostate cancer: role of 5alpha-androstane-3beta,17beta-diol. Endocr Relat Cancer., 17(3): 731-42. Retrieved September 12, 2015, from, https://www.ncbi.nlm.nih.gov/pubmed/20562232

Double, K. L. (2006). Functional effects of neuromelanin and synthetic melanin in model systems. J Neural Transm. 113 (6): 751–756. doi:10.1007/s00702-006-0450-5. Retrieved December 20, 2016, from, https://www.ncbi.nlm.nih.gov/pubmed/16755379

Dry, F. W. (1926). The coat of the mouse (Mus Musculus). J. Genet. 16, 287-340. Retrieved October 20, 2015, from, https://www.hairlosstalk.com/news/education/anagen-effluvium-causes-symptoms/

Duarte, L. (2016). Wen hair products under fire after reports of hair loss. Retrieved August 20, 2016 from, http://wgntv.com/2016/01/14/wen-hair-products-under-fire-after-reports-of-hair-loss/Elitehairinstitute.com (n. d.). Female pattern hair loss. Retrieved July 12, 2014, from, http://elitehairinstitute.com/pages/female_pattern_hair_loss.php

Eppley, B. L., Pietzak, W.S. and Blanton, M. (2006). Platelet-rich plasma: A review of biology and applications in plastic surgery. Plast Reconstr Surg.118:147–59e. Retrieved November 12, 2015, from, https://www.ncbi.nlm.nih.gov/pubmed/17051095

Evans, A. (2021). Another Door Opens? New JAK Inhibitor Options on the Horizon, Including for Psoriasis. Dermatology World. Retrieved December 1, 2021, from, https://www.medpagetoday.com/reading-room/aad/psoriasis/92610

FDA.org. (2015). FDA warns about stem cell claims. Retrieved January 10, 2016, from, http://www.fda.gov/ForConsumers/ConsumerUpdates/ucm286155.htm

Ferriman, G. D. (1971). Human hair growth in health and disease. Published Springfield, Ill. Ferting, R. M., Gamret, A. C., Cervantes, J., and Tosti, A.(2017). Microneedling for the treatment of hair loss? J Eur Acad Dermatol Venereol. 2018 Apr;32(4):564-569. doi: 10.1111/jdv.14722. Retrieved March 17, 2022, from, https://pubmed.ncbi.nlm.nih.gov/29194786

Fitzpatrick, T.B. (1988). The validity and practicality of sun-reactive skin types I through VII. Archives of Dermatology, 124 (6): 869–871, doi:10.1001/archderm.1988.01670060015008. Retrieved December 26, 2016, from, http://jamanetwork.com/journals/jamadermatology/article-abstract/549509

Flesch, P. (1954). Physiology and biochemistry of the skin. Edit. by Rothman, S., 601 University of Chicago Press. Retrieved December 2, 2014, from, http://www.nature.com/nature/journal/v193/n4822/abs/193134b0.html

French, F. S., Van Wyk, J., Bagett, B., Easterling, W. E., Talbert, L. M., Johnston, F. R., Forchielli, E., and Dey, A. C. (1966). Further evidence of a target organ defect in the syndrome of testicular feminization. J. Clin.Endocr. 26, 493—503. Retrieved February 20, 2014, from, http://www.ncbi.nlm.nih.gov/pubmed/5949337

Freund, B. J. and Schwartz, M. (2010). Treatment of Male Pattern Baldness with Botulinum Toxin: A Pilot Study. Plastic Reconstructive Surgery. 126(5):246e-248e. doi:10.1097/PRS.0b013e3181ef816d. Retrieved October 10, 2015, from, http://www.ncbi.nlm.nih.gov/pubmed/21042071; http://journals.lww.com/plasreconsurg/Fulltext/2010/11000/Teatment_of_Male_Pattern_Baldness_with_Botulinum.79.aspx

Gan, D. C., and Sinclair, R.D. (2005). Prevalence of male and female pattern hair loss in Mary borough. J Investig Dermatol Symp Proc, 10:184–9. Retrieved February 23,2014 from, http://www.ncbi.nlm.nih.gov/pubmed/16382660

Gang, A.K., and Gang, S. (2018). Donor Harvesting: Follicular Unit Excision. J Cutan Aesthet Surg. 2018 Oct-Dec; 11(4): 195–201. doi: 10.4103/JCAS.JCAS_123_18. Retrieved March 8, 2022, from, https://www.ncbi.nlm.nih.gov/pmc/articles/PMC6371717/

Gardner, M.J., Demetrakopolous, D., Klepchick, P.R. and Mooar, P.A. (2007). The efficacy of autologous platelet gel in pain control and blood loss in total knee arthroplasty. An analysis of the hemoglobin, narcotic requirement, and range of motion. Int Orthop, 31:309–13. Retrieved November 3, 2013, from, https://www.ncbi.nlm.nih.gov/pubmed/16816947

Garza, L. A., Liu, Y., Yang, Z., Alagesan, B., Lawson, J. A., Norberg, S. M., Loy, D. E., Zhao, T., Blatt, H. B., Stanton, D. C., Carrasco, L., Ahluwalia, G., Fischer, S. M., FitzGerald, G. A., and Cotsarelis, G. (2012). Prostaglandin D2 inhibits hair growth and is elevated in bald scalp of men with androgenetic alopecia. Sci. Transl. Med, 4(126):126ra34. PMID: 22440736. Doi: 10.1126/scitranslmed.3003122. Retrieved January 4, 2015, from, http://www.ncbi.nlm.nih.gov/pubmed/22440736

Garza, L. A., Yang, C. C., Zhao, T., Blatt, H.B., Lee, M., He, H., Stanton, D. C., Carrasco, L., Spiegel, J. H., Tobias, J. W., and Cotsarelis, G. (2011). Bald scalp in men with androgenetic alopecia retains hair follicle stem cells but lacks CD200-rich and CD34-positive hair follicle progenitor cells. J Clin Invst, 121(2): 613-622. doi: 10.1172/JCI44478. Retrieved January 20, 2014, from, http://www.ncbi.nlm.nih.gov/pmc/articles/PMC3026732/

Genome.gov. (May 5, 2022). National Human Genome Research Institute. Retrieved May 5, 2022, from, https://www.genome.gov/genetics-glossary/Allele#

Gho, C. (2016). Hair stem cell transplantation: The HASCI Method. Retrieved October 18, 2016 from, http://www.hasci.com/hair-stem-cell-transplantation

Giacometti, L. (1982). Hair biological facts clashes with romantic fancies. American Health, vol. 1 November 4, 1982. Giacometti, L. (1969). A perspective on baldness. J Am. Med Wo Assoc, 24: 869-72. Retrieved October 23, 2015, from, http://www.ncbi.nlm.nih.gov/pubmed/?term=Giacometti%20L%5BAuthor%5D&cauthor=true&cauthor_uid=4242863

Giron, A. (2015). Seborrheic dermatitis treatment. Retrieved October 12, 2016, from, http://www.steadyhealth.com/medical-answers/seborrheic-dermatitis-treatment

Gnedeva, K., Vorotelyak, E., Cimadamore, F., Cattarossi, G., Giusto, E., and Terskikh, V. V. (2015) Derivation of Hair-Inducing Cell from Human Pluripotent Stem Cells. PLoS ONE 1 0(1): e0116892. doi: 10.1371/journal.pone.0116892. Retrieved January 8, 2016, from, http://journals.plos.org/plosone/article?id=10.1371/journal.pone.0 116892#ack

Godoy, A., Kawinski, E., Li, Y., Oka, D., Alexiev, B., Azzouni, F., Titus, M.A. and Mohler, J.L. (July 2011). 5α-reductase type 3 expression in human benign and malignant tissues: a comparative analysis during prostate cancer progression. Prostate, 71 (10): 1033–46. doi:10.1002/pros.21318. PMed 21557268. Retrieved October 4, 2015, from, http://www.ncbi.nlm.nih.gov/pubmed/21557268

Goldberg, L. J. and Lenzy, Y. (2010). Nutrition and hair. Clin Dermatol. 2010 Jul-Aug;28(4):412-9. doi: 10.1016/j.clindermatol.2010.03.038.Retrieved July 24, 2016, from, http://www.ncbi.nlm.nih.gov/pubmed/20620758

Gormley, G. http://www.ncbi.nlm.nih.gov/pubmed/20620758 J., Stoner, E., Bruskewitz, R. C., Imperato-McGinley, J. Walsh, P. C., McConnell, J. D., Andriole, G. L., Geller, J., Bracken, B.R., Tenover, J. S., et al. (1992). The effect of finasteride in men with benign prostatic hyperplasia. The Finasteride Study Group. N Engl J Med, 327(17):1185-91. Retrieved September 1, 2015, from, http://www.nejm.org/doi/full/10.1056/NEJM19921022327171

Grandinetti, L. M and Tomecki, K. J. (2010). Dermatologic signs of systemic disease. Retrieved October 15, 2016, from, http://www.clevelandclinicmeded.com/medicalpubs/diseasemanagement/dermatology/dermatologic-signs-of-systemic-disease/

Gryczynski, J., Schwartz, R. P., Mitchell, S. G., O'Grady, K. E., and Ondersma, S. J. (2014). Hair Drug Testing Results and Self-reported Drug Use among Primary Care Patients with Moderate-risk Illicit Drug Use. Drug Alcohol Depend. 2014 Aug 1; 141: 44–50. Retrieved March 29, 2022, from,https://www.ncbi.nlm.nih.gov/pmc/articles/PMC4080811/

Gupta, M. and Mysore, V. (2016). Classifications of patterned hair loss: A review. J Cutan Aesthet Surg. 2016 Jan-Mar; 9(1):3-12. doi: 10.4103/0974-2077.178536. Retrieved October 13, 2016, from, https://www.ncbi.nlm.nih.gov/pubmed/27081243

Gwinup, G., Wieland, R. G., Besch, P. K. A. and Hamwi, G. J. (1966). Studies on the mechanism of the production of the testicular feminization syndrome. Am J Med, 41(3):448-52. Retrieved February 13, 2014, from, http://www.ncbi.nlm.nih.gov/pubmed/5914115

Habif, T. P. (2010). Hair diseases. In Clinical dermatology, 5th ed. Mosby, Maryland Heights, MO

Hadland, S. E., AND Levy, S. (2016). OBJECTIVE TESTING – URINE AND OTHER DRUG TESTS. Child Adolesc Psychiatr Clin N Am. 2016 Jul; 25(3): 549–565. Retrieved March 29, 2022, from, https://www.ncbi.nlm.nih.gov/pmc/articles/PMC4920965/

Hailmann, S., Brockschmidt, F. F., Hilmer, A.M., Hanneken, S., Eigelshoven, S., Ludwig, K. U., Herold, C., Mangold, E.M., Becker, T., Krusse, R., Knapp, M., and Nöthen, M. M. (2013). Evidence for a polygenic contribution to androgenetic alopecia. Br J Dermatol. 2013 Oct; 169(4):927-30. Doi: 10 Retrieved August 2, 2016, from, http://www.ncbi.nlm.nih.gov/pubmed/23701444.1111/bjd.12443.

Hair Loss Learning Center.org. (2006). Copper peptides: The Overlooked Hair Loss Treatment. Retrieved August 3, 2015from, http://www.regrowhair.com/non-surgical-hair-loss-treatments/copper-peptides-the-overlooked-hair-loss-treatment/

Hair loss Library (n.d.). Hair loss information and treatments. Retrieved January 16th, 2014, from, http://www.hairlosslibrary.com/hair_growth_cycle.htm

Hair Transplant Forum International (Nov-Dec 2009). A visit: a note from Richard C. Shield, MBBS Melbourne, Australia. Retrieved April 30, 2016, from, file:///C:/Users/MyPC/Downloads/visittothehouseofokuda_ishrs-ht-forum_f6-2009% 20(5).pdf

Hair Transplant Network.com. (2016). The concept of hair transplantation is born. Retrieved December 5, 2015, from, http://www.hairtransplantnetwork.com/Hair-Loss Treatments/hair transplant-history.asp

Hall-Flavin, D. K. (2016). Can stress cause hair loss. Retrieved September 15, 2016, from, http://www.mayoclinic.org/healthy-lifestyle/stress-management/expert-answers/stress-and-hair-loss/faq-20057820

Hamblin, M. R. (2008.). Mechanisms of low level light therapy. Dept. of Dermatology, Harvard Medical School, BAR 414 Wellman Center for Photomedicine, Massachusetts General Hospital 40 Blossom Street, Boston MA. Retrieved August 18, 2015, from, http://photobiology.info/Hamblin.html

Hamilton, J. B. (1942). Male hormone stimulation is a prerequisite and an incitant in common baldness. Am J Anat. 1942; 71:451–480. Retrieved December 15, 2015, from, http://onlinelibrary.wiley.com/doi/10.1002/aja.1000710306/abstr act

Hamilton, J. B. (1946). The Relationship between common baldness and male sex hormones. Transactions of the New York Academy of Sciences. Vol. 8, Issue 3 Series II pages 101-102, Retrieved August 12, 2014, from, http://onlinelibrary.wiley.com/doi/10.1111/j.2164-0947.1946.tb00220.x/abstract

Hamilton, J. B. (1951). Male pattern hair loss in man: types and incidence. Ana N Y Acad Dermatol: 53; 708-28. Retrieved August 12, 2015, from, http://www.ncbi.nlm.nih.gov/pubmed/14819896; http://onlinelibrary.wiley.com/doi/10.1111/j.1749 6632. 1951.tb31971.x/abstract; jsessionid=FD9558A93AC24B10AB3433F0B921F96.f04t03

Hammond, G. L. and Bocchinfuso, W. P. (1996). Sex hormone-binding globulin: gene organization and structure/function analyses. Hormone Research. 45 (3–5): 197–201. doi:10.1159/000184787. PMID 8964583. Retrieved August 23, 2014, from, https://www.ncbi.nlm.nih.gov/pubmed/8964583

Handa, R. J., Pak, T. R., Kudwa, A. E., Lund, T. D., and Hinds, L. (2008). An alternate pathway for androgen regulation of brain function: Activation of estrogen receptor beta by the metabolite of dihydrotestosterone, 5α-androstane 3β, 17β diol. Horm Behav. 2008 May; 53(5): 741–752. Retrieved August 12, 2016, from, https://www.ncbi.nlm.nih.gov/pmc/articles/PMC2430080/

Hanke, C. W. and Berfeld, W. F. (1981). Fiber implantation for pattern baldness. Review of complications in forty-one patients. J Am Acad Dermatol, 4:278–83. Retrieved August 2, 2016, from, http://www.ncbi.nlm.nih.gov/pubmed/7012203

Hardy, M. H. (1949). The development of mouse hair in vitro with some observations on pigmentation. *J. Anat,* 83(4), 364.Retrieved October 12, 2014, from, http://www.ncbi.nlm.nih.gov/pubmed/15394398

Hardy, M. H. (1951). The development of pelage hairs and vibrissae from skin in tissue culture. *Ann. N.Y. Acad. Sci.* 1951 Mar 53(3), 546-61. Retrieved October 12, 2014, from, http://www.ncbi.nlm.nih.gov/pubmed/14819881

Harel, S., Higgins, C. A., Cerise, J. E., Dai, Z., Chen, J. C., Clynes, R. and Christiano, A. M. (2015). Pharmacologic inhibition of JAK-STAT signaling promotes hair growth. Science Advances: 1(9) e1500973 doi: 10.1126/sciadv.1500973. Retrieved March 2, 2016, from, http://advances.sciencemag.org/content/1/9/e1500973

Harkins, D. K. and Susten, A. S. (2003). Hair analysis: exploring the state of the science. Environ Health Perspect, 111(4): 576–578.Retrieved August 3, 2016, from, http://www.ncbi.nlm.nih.gov/pmc/articles/PMC1241447/

Harris, M. O. (2015). Hair and culture. Center for Aesthetic Modernism. Retrieved September 3, 2016, from, http://www.harrisface.com/hair-and-culture.html

Hay, I.C., Jamieson, M., and Ormerod, A.D. (1998). Randomized trial of aromatherapy. Successful Treatment for Alopecia Areata. Arch Dermatol, 134 (11):1349-52. Retrieved December 20, 2016, from, http://www.ncbi.nlm.nih.gov/pubmed/10328210; http://www.worldhairresearch.com/?p=95

Hearing, V. J. and Tsakamoto, K. (1991). Enzymatic control of pigmentation in mammals. The FASEB Journal, 5 (14): 2902–2909. Retrieved December 20, 2016, from, https://www.ncbi.nlm.nih.gov/pubmed/1752358

Hecht, A. (1985). Hair grower and hair-loss prevention drugs. FDA Consumer, 1985 April 19:1-3. Retrieved December 12, 2015, from, http://www.ncbi.nlm.nih.gov/pmc/articles/PMC1113949 /#B28

Higgins, C. A., Westgate, G. E., Jahoda, C. A. B. (2009). From Telogen to Exogen: Mechanism Underlying Formation and Subsequent Loss of the Hair Club Fiber. Journal of Investigative Dermatology; volume 129(9):2100-8. April 2009 with 114 Reads DOI: 10.1038/jid.2009.66. https://www.ncbi.nlm.nih.gov/pubmed/19340011

Higgins, C. A., Richardson, G. D., Ferdinando, D., Westgate, G. E. and Jahoda, C. A. (2010). Modelling the hair follicle dermal papilla using spheroid cell cultures. Exp Dermatol. 2010 Jun;19(6):546-8. doi: 10.1111/j.1600-0625.2009.01007.x. Epub 2010 Apr 20. Retrieved December,4, 2016 from, https://www.ncbi.nlm.nih.gov/pubmed/20456497

Higgins, C. A., Chen, J. C., Cerise, J. E., Jahoda, C. A. and Christiano, A. M. (2013). Microenvironmental reprogramming by three-dimensional culture enables dermal papilla cells to induce de novo human hair-follicle growth. Proc Natl Acad Sci U S A. 110(49): 19679–19688. doi: 10.1073/pnas.1309970110. Retrieved November 23, 2016, from, http://www.pnas.org/content/110/49/19679.full https://www.ncbi.nlm.nih.gov/pmc/articles/PMC3856847/

Hitner, H. and Nagle, B. (2016). Pharmacology: An Introduction. Published by McGraw-Hill education., 2 Penn Plaza, New York, N.Y. 10121: ISBN: 978-0-07-351381-2

Hong, H., Ji, J. H., Lee, Y., Kang, H., Choi, G. S. and Lee, W. S. (2013). Reliability of the pattern hair loss classifications: A comparison of the basic and specific and Norwood-Hamilton classifications. J Dermatol 2013; 40:102-6. Back to cited text no. 11. doi: 10.1111/1346-8138.12024. Retrieved December 23, 2016, from, https://www.ncbi.nlm.nih.gov/pubmed/23110308

Hunt, H. L. (1926). Plastic surgery of the head, face, and neck. New Philadelphia: Lea and Febiger New Philadelphia:

Hunt, N. and McHale, S. (2005). Clinical review: The psychological impact of alopecia. British Medical Journal, 331, 951–953. Doi:10.1136/bmj.331.7522.951. Retrieved May 20, 2014, from, http://www.ncbi.nlm.nih.gov/pmc/articles/PMC1261195/

Hyoseung, S., Hyeong, H. R., Junghee, Y., Seongmoon, J., Sihyeok, J., Mira, C., Ohsang, K., and Seong, J. J. (2014). Association of premature hair graying with family history, smoking, and obesity: A cross-sectional study. JAAD. DOI: http://dx.doi.org/10.1016/j.jaad, 11.008. Retrieved November 12, 2015, from, http://www.jaad.org/article/S0190-9622 (14)02140-9/fulltext.

International Society of Hair Restoration Surgery. (2015). ISHRS 2015 Practice census results. Retrieved July 26, 2016, from, http://www.ishrs.org/statistics-research.htm

i-Brain Robotics (2016). World's fastest 2 hours-robotic hair transplant technical specifications. Retrieved January 16, 2016, from, http://ibrainrobotics.com/robotic-hair-transplant-system.php

International Society of Hair Restoration Surgery. (2015). ISHRS 2015 practice census results. Retrieved July 26, 2016, from, http://www.ishrs.org/statistics-research.htm

ISO 9000 (2016). Quality management. Retrieved November 11, 2016, from, http://www.iso.org/iso/home/standards/management-standards/iso_9000.htm

Jackson, T. G. and McMurty, C, W. (1912). A treatise on diseases of the hair. Publisher: Lea & Febiger. Retrieved January 2, 2015, from, https://books.google.com/books?id=2hG0AAAAIAAJ&printsec=frontcover&dq=inauthor:%22Charles+Wood+McMurtry%22&hl=en&sa=X&ved=0ahUKEwjrqK_RmcTKAhVOzGMKHWPgCP4Q6AEIHTAA#v=onepage&q&f=false

Jimenez, J. J., Wikramanayake, T. C., Bergfeld, W., Hordinsky, M., Hickman, J. G., Hamblin, M. R. and Schachner, L. A. (2014). Efficacy and Safety of a Low-level Laser Device in the Treatment of Male and Female Pattern Hair Loss: A Multicenter, Randomized, Sham Device-controlled, Double-blind Study. Am J Clin Dermatol. 2014; 15(2): 115–127. doi: 10.1007/s40257-013-0060-6. Retrieved August 4, 2016, from,http://www.ncbi.nlm.nih.gov/pmc/articles/PMC3986893/

Jockers, D. (2011). Reversing female hair loss. Bioidentical Hormone Health. Retrieved December 29, 2016 from, http://www.bio-hormone-health.com/2011/12/12/reversing-female-hair-loss/

Johnson, G. (2013), Penn dermatologist makes breakthrough in battle against hair loss. Penn Current. Retrieved June 12, 2014, from, http://www.upenn.edu/pennnews/current/2014-03-13/research/penn-dermatologist-makes-breakthrough-battle-against-hair-loss

Jones, R. (2015). Pros and cons of ARTAS robotic hair transplants. Dr. Robert Jones Hair Transplant Center. Retrieved November 2, 2016, from, https://www.drrobertjones.com/artas-hair-transplant-pros-cons/

Juri, J. (1975). Use of parieto-occipital flaps in the surgical treatment of baldness. Plast Reconstr Surg. 1975; 55:456–460.Retrieved October 12, 2015, from, https://www.ncbi.nlm.nih.gov/pubmed/1090958

Kacar, S.D., Ozuguz, P., Bagcioglu, E., Coskun, K. S., Polat, S., Karaca, s., and Ozbulut, O. (2015).Body Dysmorphic Disorder Among Patients With Complaints of Hair Loss. International Journal of Dermatology. Retrieved March 26, 2022, fromhttps://www.practiceupdate.com/content/body-dysmorphic-disorder-among-patients-with-complaints-of-hair loss/26645#:~:text=BDD%20was%20diagnosed%20in%2029.6,in%20female%20patients%20(25.6%25).

Kaminer, M. S., Dover, J. S. and Arndt, K. A. (2002). Atlas of cosmetic surgery. W.B. Saunders Company., Philadelphia, PA, 2002, pg 248.

Keifer, D. (2006). Superoxide dismutase boosting the body's primary antioxidant defense. Retrieved November 3, 2015, from, http://www.lifeextension.com/magazine/2006/6/report_sod/page-01

Keratin.com (2015). The history of hair transplants. Retrieved Nov.29, 2015 from, http://www.keratin.com/aw/aw001.shtml

Kiichiro, Y., Brown, L. F., and Detmar, M. (2001). Control of hair Growth and follicle size by VEGF-mediated angiogenesis. The Journal of Clinical Investigation. Retrieved June 21, 2016, from, http://www.jci.org/articles/view/11317

Kim, M. H., Kim, S. H. and Yang, W. M. (2014). Beneficial effects of astragaloside IV for hair loss via inhibition of fas/fas L-Mediated Apoptotic Signaling. PLoS One. 2014; 9(3): e92984. doi: 10.1371/journal.pone.0092984. Retrieved September 12, 2015, from, http://www.ncbi.nlm.nih.gov/pmc/articles/PMC3968031/

Klingman, A. M. (1961). Pathologic Dynamics of Human Hair Loss : I. Telogen Effluvium. *Arch Dermatol,* 83(2):175- 198. doi:10.1001/archderm.1961.01580080005001. Retrieved January 6, 2014, from,http://archderm.jamanetwork.com/article.aspx?articleid=526620

Klingman, A. M., and Strauss, J. S. (1956). The Formation of vellus hair follicles from human adult epidermis. The Journal of Investigative Dermatology, 27, 19–23; doi:10.1038/jid.1956.71. Retrieved October 23, 2015, from, http://www.nature.com/jid/journal/v27/n1/full/jid195671a.htm

Kraissl, C. J. (1951). The selection of appropriate lines for elective surgical incisions. Plastic and Reconstructive Surgery, 8(1):1-28. Retrieved September 20, 2015, from, http://www.gpnotebook.co.uk/simplepage.cfm?ID=x20131001203243685340

Lai Saha, M. and Chintamani, N. (2013). Bedside Clinics in Surgery: Long and Short Cases, Surgical Problems, X-rays, Surgical Pathology, Preoperative Preparations, Minor Surgical Procedures, Instruments, Operative Surg. 2nd edition. Jaypee Brothers Medical Publishers (P) Ltd. 4838/24 Ansari Road. Daryaganj, New Delhi 110 002 India.

Lam, S. (2012). Understanding recipient dominance in hair transplantation. Retrieved December 7, 2015, from,http://www.hairtx.com/eyebrow/understanding-recipient dominance-in-hair-transplantation/

Lam, S. M. and Williams, Jr., K. L. (2016). Hair transplant 360: Follicular Unit Extraction (FUE). Jaypee Brothers Medical Publishers (P) Ltd. 4838/24 Ansari

Road Daryaganj, New Delhi 110 002 India. ISBN-13: 978-9352500369 ISBN-10: 9352500369

Lamont, E. S. (1957). A plastic surgical transformation. West J. Surg. Obstet. Gynecol. 65(3): 164-165. Retrieved September 23, 2015, from,https://www.ncbi.nlm.nih.gov/pubmed/13443270

Lange-Ionescu, S. and Frosch, P. J. (1995). Complications of synthetic hair implantation. Hautarzt. 1995; 46:10–4. Retrieved August 1, 2016, from, http://www.ncbi.nlm.nih.gov/pubmed/7875965

Lanzafame, R. J., Raymond R Blanche, R, R., Chiacchierini, R. P., Kazmirek, E. R. and Sklar, J. A. (2014). The growth of human scalp hair in females using visible red light laser and LED sources. Lasers Surg Med, 46(8): 601–607. Retrieved January 10. 2016, from, https://www.ncbi.nlm.nih.gov/pmc/articles/PMC4265291/

Leavitt, M., Charles, G., Heyman, E. and Michaels, D. (2009). HairMax Laser Comb laser phototherapy device in the treatment of male androgenetic alopecia: A randomized, double-blind, sham device-controlled, multicentre trial. Clin Drug Investig. 2009;29(5):283-92. doi: 10.2165/00044011-200929050-00001. Retrieved August 23, 2015, from, http://www.ncbi.nlm.nih.gov/pubmed/19366270

Lee, H. J., Ha, S. J., Kim, D., Kim, H. O. and Kim, J. W. (2002) Perception of men with androgenetic alopecia by women and nonbalding men in Korea: how the nonbald regard the bald. Int J Dermatol 41: 867-869. Retrieved September 5, 2015, from, http://www.ncbi.nlm.nih.gov/pubmed/12492971

Lee, R. (2016). Anagen effluvium: causes and symptoms. Retrieved October 25, 2016, from, https://www.hairlosstalk.com/news/education/anagen-effluvium-causes-symptoms/

Lee, Won-Soo et al. (207). A new classification of pattern hair loss that is universal for men and women: Basic and specific (BASP) classification. Journal of the American Academy of Dermatology, Volume 57, Issue 1, 37-46. Retrieved January 29, 2017, from, http://www.jaad.org/article/S0190-9622 (07)00021-7/abstract? cc=y=

Lee-Daum, C. M. (2006). Self-regulation in the cosmetic industry: A Necessary Reality or a Cosmetic Illusion? LEDA at Harvard Law School. Retrieved August 2, 2015, from, https://dash.harvard.edu/bitstream/handle/1/8965615/Daum06.html?sequence=2

Leyden, James et al. (1999). Finasteride in the treatment of men with frontal male pattern hair loss. J Am Acad Dermatol. 1999 Jun;40(6 Pt 1):930-7. Retrieved October 16, 2014, from, http://www.ncbi.nlm.nih.gov/pubmed/10365924

Lillie, R. D. (1957). Metal reduction reactions of the melanins: Histochemical studies. Journal of Histochemistry and Cytochemistry. 5 (4): 325–33. Retrieved December 20, 2016, from, https://www.ncbi.nlm.nih.gov/pubmed/13463306

Lindsey, H. (2008). Off-label hair growth. NBCUniversal 2008. Retrieved August 25, 2016, from, http://www.nbcnewyork.com/news/health/Off-Label_Hair_Growth.html

LoPresti, P., Papa, C. M. and Kligman, A. M. (1968). Hot comb alopecia. Archives of dermatology, 1968. Sept; 98(3):234-8. Retrieved October 20, 2015, from, https://www.ncbi.nlm.nih.gov/pubmed/5673883

Lucky, A. W., Piacquadio, D. J., Ditre, C. M., Dunlap, F., Kantor, I. Pandya, A. G., Savin, R. C. and Tharp, M. D. (2004). A randomized, placebo-controlled trial of 5% and 2% topical minoxidil solutions in the treatment of female pattern hair loss. J Am Acad Dermatol, 50(4):541-53. Retrieved January 10, 2016, from, https://www.ncbi.nlm.nih.gov/pubmed/15034503

Ludwig E. (1977). Classification of the types of androgenetic alopecia (common baldness) occurring in the female sex. Br J Dermatol, 97 (3):247-54. Retrieved July 2, 2015, from, http://www.ncbi.nlm.nih.gov/pubmed/921894

Lynch, A. (2015, January 29). Scientists believe they have discovered a cure for baldness. Retrieved January 8, 2016, from, http://metro.co.uk/2015/01/29/scientists-believe-they-have-discovered-a-cure-for-baldness-5041177/#ixzz3wmDRr220

Lynfield, Y. L. (1960). Effect of pregnancy on the human hair cycle. Journal of Investigative Dermatology (1960) 35, 323–327; doi:10.1038/jid.1960.127.

Retrieved October 15, 2013, from, http://www.nature.com/jid/journal/v35/n6/full/jid1960127a.html

MacKenzie, D. (2012). Rosacea may be caused by mite feces in your pores. Retrieved January 12, 2015 from, https://www.newscientist.com/article/dn22227-rosacea-may-be-caused-by-mite-faeces-in-your-pores

Marechal, E. R. (1977). New treatment for seborrheic alopecia: The Ligature of the Arteries of the Scalp. J Natl Med Assoc. Oct; 69(10): 709–71. Retrieved September 1, 2015, from, http://www.ncbi.nlm.nih.gov/pmc/articles/PMC2536995/

Marginean, C. O., Melit, L.E., Sasaran, M. O., Marginean, R., and Derzsi, Z. (2021). Rapunzel Syndrome— An Extremely Rare Cause of Digestive Symptoms in Children: A Case Report and a Review of the Literature. Frontiers in Pediatrics. Retrieved April 8, 2022, from, https://www.frontiersin.org/articles/10.3389/fped.2021.684379/full#:~:text=Rapunzel%20syndrome%20is%20an%20extremely,stages%2C%20it%20is%20usually%20asymptomatic.

Matthews, K. (2008). Stem Cell Research: A Science and Policy Overview. Retrieved January 20, 2016, from, http://www.ruf.rice.edu/~neal/temp/ST%20Policy/index/SCBooklet/stemcell-intro-0208.pdf

Mayse, K. (2010). Premature balding in men. Retrieved January 12, 2015, from, http://www.livestrong.com/article/155175-premature-balding-in-men/

McAndrews, P. J. (2012). Hairmeds.com. Frequently asked questions about minoxidil. Placing minoxidil on a wet scalp. Retrieved April 23, 2016, from, http://hairmeds.com/questions_minoxidil.htm

McAndrews, P. J. (2004). Causes of Hair Loss. American Hair Loss Association. Retrieved March 23, 2016, from, https://www.americanhairloss.org/women_hair_loss/causes_of_hair_loss.html

McDonald, K. A., Shelley, A. J., Colantonio, S., and Beecker, J. (March 1, 2017). Hair pull test: Evidence-based update and revision of guidelines. Journal of the American Academy of Dermatology (JAAD). VOLUME 76, ISSUE 3, P472-477. Retrieved April 26, 2022, from, https://www.jaad.org/article/S0190-9622(16)30892-1/fulltext

Menton, D. (2007, July 4). The amazing human hair. Retrieved January 20, 2016, from, https://answersingenesis.org/human-body/the-amazing-human-hair/

Messenger, A. G. and Rundegren, J. (2004). Minoxidil: Mechanisms of Action on Hair Growth. Retrieved December 13, 2015, from, http://www.medscape.com/viewarticle/470297

Mester, E., Szende, B. and Tota, J. G. (1967). Effect of laser on hair growth of mice. Kiserl Orvostud. 1967; 19:628–631. Retrieved December 23, 2015, from, https://www.ncbi.nlm.nih.gov/pubmed/5732466

Milner. Y., Sudnik, J., Filippi, M., Kizoulis, M., Kashgarian, M., and Stenn, K. (3003). Exogen, shedding phase of the hair growth cycle: characterization of a mouse model. J Invest Dermatol. 2002 Sep;119 (3):639-44. Retrieved January 20, 2016, from, http://www.ncbi.nlm.nih.gov/pubmed/12230507

Mohebi, P. (2016). FUE v. Strip hair transplantation. Retrieved September 21, 2016, from, http://parsamohebi.com/hair-transplant/follicular-unit-transplant-fut/fue-vs-strip-hair-restoration/

Montagna, W. R. and Uno, H. (1968). The phylogeny of baldness. Retrieved August 10, 2015, from, http://journal.scconline.org/abstracts/cc1968/cc019n03/p00173-p00185.html

Montagna, W. R. and Uno, H. (1968). Baldness in nonhumans Primates. J. Soc. Cosmetic Chem. 19, 173-185. Retrieved March 12, 2013, from, http://pdfstori.com/pdf/33578_baldness-in-nonhuman-primates

Montagna, W. R. and Ellis, R. A. (1958). The biology of hair growth. Publisher: Academic Press, New York and London. Retrieved January 12, 2015, from, http://www.amazon.com/Biology-Growth-MONTAGNA

Morishima, C. (N.D.). Chika Morishima's Introduction to Amino Acids. Ajinomoto. Eat Well, Live Well. Retrieved April 21, 2022, from, https://www.ajinomoto.com/aboutus/amino-acids/how-amino-acids-can-solve-the-worlds-health-and-nutrition-challenges

Morris, J. M., and Mahesh, V. B. (1963). Further observation of the syndrome, "Testicular Feminization." Am J Obstet Gynecol, 87:731-48. Retrieved February 12, 2014, from, http://www.ncbi.nlm.nih.gov/pubmed/14085776

Morrisey, B. (2016, March 14). Lanugo and eating disorders. Retrieved March 20, 2016, from, http://www.eatingdisorderexpert.co.uk/lanugoandeatingdiso- ers html

Mowszowicz, I., Melanitou, E., Doukani, A., Wright, F., Kuttenn, F., and Mauvais-Jarvis, P. (1983). Androgen binding capacity and 5[alpha]-reductase activity in pubic skin fibroblasts from hirsute patients. Journal of Clinical Endocrinology and Metabolism, 56: 1209-1213. Retrieved February 10, 2014, from, http://www.ncbi.nlm.nih.gov/pubmed/6841558

Mowszowicz, I. (1989). Antiandrogens mechanisms and paradoxical effects. Ann. Endocrinol. (Paris). 50 (3): 50(3):189–99. Retrieved September 12, 2015, from, https://www.ncbi.nlm.nih.gov/pubmed/2530930

Münster, U., Nakamura, C., Haberland, A., Jores, K., Mehnert, W., Rummel, S., Schaller, M., Korting, H. C., Zouboulis, Ch. C., Blume-Peytavi, U. and Schäfer-Korting, M. (2005). RU 58841-myristate--prodrug development for topical treatment of acne and androgenetic alopecia. Pharmazie. 60(1):8-12. Retrieved August 23, 2015, from, https://www.ncbi.nlm.nih.gov/pubmed/15700772

Mysore, V. (2010). Controversy: Synthetic Hairs and their Role in Hair Restoration? Int J Trichology. 2010 Jan-Jun; 2(1): 42–44. doi: 10.4103/0974-7753.66913. Retrieved August 5, 2016, from, http://www.ncbi.nlm.nih.gov/pmc/articles/PMC3002411/

Mysore, V. (2012). Finasteride and sexual side effects. Indian Dermatol Online J. 2012 Jan-Apr; 31): 62–65. doi: 10.4103/2229-5178.93496. Retrieved November 24, 2016, from, https://www.ncbi.nlm.nih.gov/pmc/articles/PMC3481923/

Ngan, V. (2005). Demodex. DermNet New Zealand: All about skin. Retrieved January 20, 2016, from, http://www.dermnetnz.org/topics/demodex/

Naito, A., Sato, T., Matsumoto, T., Takeyama, K., Yoshino, T., Kato, S., Ohdera, M. (2008) Dihydrotestosterone inhibits murine hair growth via the androgen receptor. Br J Dermatol;159(2) Epublic med. Retrieved October 15, 2014, from, http://onlinelibrary.wiley.com/doi/10.1111/j.13652133.2008.08671.x/abstract?user Is Authenticated=false & denid Access Customized Message=; Retrieved December 12, 2015, from, http://www.ncbi.nlm.nih.gov/pubmed/18547308

National Alopecia Areata Foundation (2015). Alopecia Areata. Retrieved November 21, 2015, from, https://www.naaf.org/alopecia-areata

Nishimura, E. K., Granter, S. R., and Fisher, D. E. (2005). Mechanisms of hair graying: Incomplete Melanocyte Stem Cell Maintenance in the Niche. Retrieved July 23, 2016, from, http://science.sciencemag.org/content/307/5710/720.full

Nishiyama, T., Ikarashi, T., Hashimoto, Y., Suzuki, K., and Takahashi, K. (2006). Association between the dihydrotestosterone level in the prostate and prostate cancer aggressiveness using the Gleason score. J Urol., 176(4 Pt 1):1387-91. Retrieved August 17, 2016, from, https://www.ncbi.nlm.nih.gov/pubmed/16952639

Newman, T. (2015). DHT (Dihydrotestosterone): What Is DHT's role in male pattern baldness? Retrieved February 3, 2015, from, http://www.medicalnewstoday.com/articles/68082.php

Nieves, A., and Garza, A. L. (2015). Does prostaglandin D2 hold the cure to male pattern baldness. Retrieved July 20, 2016, from, http://www.ncbi.nlm.nih.gov/pmc/articles/PMC3982925/

Norwood, O.T. (1975). Male pattern baldness: classification and incidence. South Med J. 1975 Nov; 68(11):1359-65. Retrieved September 22, 2013, from, http://www.ncbi.nlm.nih.gov/pubmed/1188424

Novak, M. A. and Meyer, J. S. (2009). Alopecia: Possible causes and treatments, particularly in captive nonhuman primates. Comp Med. 59(1): 18-26. Retrieved July 27, 2016, from, http://www.ncbi.nlm.nih.gov/pmc/articles/PMC2703143/

Nobelprize.org. (N.D.). The Nobel Prize. Joshua Lederberg Biographical. Retrieved April 25, 2016, from, https://www.nobelprize.org/prizes/medicine/1958/lederberg/biographical/ https://www.nobelprize.org/prizes/medicine/1958/summary/

Nusbaum, B. P. (2004). Techniques to reduce pain associated with hair transplantation: optimizing anesthesia and analgesia. Am J Clin Dermatol. 2004; 5(1): 9-15. Retrieved July26, 20016, from, http://www.ncbi.nlm.nih.gov/pubmed/14979739

O'Donnell, B. P., Sperling, L. C., and James, W. D. (1992). Loose Anagen Hair Syndrome. Int'l Journal of Dermatology. Retrieved April 25, 2022, from, https://onlinelibrary.wiley.com/doi/abs/10.1111/j.1365-4362.1992.tb03248.x

Okuda, S. (1939) Clinical and experimental study transplantation of living hairs. Jan J Dermatol Urol. 46: 135 138. Retrieved December 19, 2015, from, http://www.ishrs.org/content/okuda-papers-0

Olsen, E. A. (2001). Female pattern hair loss. Journal of the American Academy of Dermatology, vol. 45, supplement 3, pp. S70–S80, 2001. Retrieved October 12, 2013, from, http://www.jaad.org/article/S0190-9622(01)86748-7/abstract

Olsen, E.A., Hordinsky, M., Whiting, D., Stough, D., Hobbs, S., Ellis, M. L., Wilson, T. and Rittmaster, R. S. (2006). The importance of dual 5alpha-reductase inhibition in the treatment of male pattern hair loss: results of a randomized placebo-controlled study of dutasteride versus finasteride. J Am Acad Dermatol., 55(6):1014-23. Retrieved September 25, 2014, from, https://www.ncbi.nlm.nih.gov/pubmed/1711021

Orentreich, N. (1959). Autographs in alopecia and other selected dermatological conditions. Ann NY Acad. Sci. 83: 463. Retrieved April 5, 2014, from, http://onlinelibrary.wiley.com/doi/10.1111/j.17496632. 1960.tb40920.x/abstract; jsessionid=934F887F 2A79C85EB7C10BF910EF07D.f03t02

Orentreich, D. and Orentreich, N. (1995). Androgenetic alopecia and its treatment, a historical view. In: Unger W. P., editor. Hair transplantation. 3rd ed. New York: Marcel Dekker; pp.133. Retrieved December 12, 2015, from, http://www.ncbi.nlm.nih.gov/pmc/articles/PMC1113949/#B27

O'Sullivan, R. L., Keuthen, N. J., Christenson, G. A., Mansueto, C. S., Stein, D. J. and Swedo, S. E. (1997). Trichotillomania: behavioral symptom or clinical syndrome? Am J Psychiatry. 1997 Oct; 154(10):1442-9. Retrieved August 12, 2015, from, http://www.ncbi.nlm.nih.gov/pubmed/9326829

Passot, R. (1931). Cosmetic surgery and its results. Paris: G. Doin et Cie.

Pathomvanich, D. and Imagawa, K. (2010). Restoration surgery in Asians. Springer Tokyo Berlin Heidelberg New York. ISBN-13:9784431996583 e-ISBN: 9784431996590

Peters, D.H., and Sorkin, E.M. (1993) Finasteride. A review of its potential in the treatment of benign prostatic hyperplasia. Drugs Jul; 46(1):177-208. Retrieved October 15, 2014, from, http://www.ncbi.nlm.nih.gov/pubmed/7691505

Petrow, V. (1986). The dihydrotestosterone (DHT) hypothesis of prostate cancer and its therapeutic implications. Prostate. 9(4): 343-61. Retrieved August 21, 2016, from, https://www.ncbi.nlm.nih.gov/pubmed/3537993

PFSfoundation.org. (2013). Post-finasteride syndrome: overview. Retrieved February 15, 2016 from, http://www.pfsfoundation.org/post-finasteride-syndrome-overview/ Piccardi, N. and Manissier, P. (2009). Nutrition and nutritional supplementation. Dermato endocrinol. 2009 Sep-Oct; 1(5): 271–274. Retrieved October 23, 2014, from, http://www.ncbi.nlm.nih.gov/pmc/articles/PMC2836433/

Pickart, L. (2002). Copper peptides for tissue regeneration, specialty chemicals 2002 (October) pages 29-31. Retrieved October 12, 2015, from, http://www.skinbiology.ca/main.php?p=543

Pickart, L. (2003). Reversing skin aging with copper peptides, Body Language Dermatol. 2003 (April) pages 12-13. Retrieved November 12, 2015, from, http://www.skinbiology.ca/main.php?p=543 Pickart, L., Vasquez-Soltero, J. M. and Margolina, A. (2015). GHK peptide as a natural modulator of multiple cellular pathways in skin regeneration. Biomed Res Int. 2015; 2015: 648108. Published online 2015 Jul 7. doi: 10.1155/2015/648108. Retrieved January 2, 2016, from, https://www.ncbi.nlm.nih.gov/pmc/articles/PMC4508379/

Piérard-Franchimont, C. and Piérard, G. E. (2001). Teloptosis, a turning point in hair shedding biorhythms. Dermatology 2001;203(2):115-7. Retrieved September 7, 2015, from http://www.ncbi.nlm.nih.gov/pubmed/11586007

Rather, P. A. and Iffat Hassan, I. (2014). Human demodex mite: The Versatile Mite of Dermatological Importance. Indian Journal of Dermatology; 2014,

Volume:59 Issue:1 Page: 60-66 Retrieved December 20, 2016, from, http://www.eijd.org/article.asp?issn=00195154;year=2014;volume=59;issue=1;spage=60;epage=66;aulast=Rather#

Rahimi-Ardabili, B., Pourandarjani, R., Habibollahi. P. and Mualeki, A. (2006). Finasteride induced depression: a prospective study. BMC Clinical Pharmacology. 6: 7. doi:10.1186/1472-6904-6-7. PMC 1622749free to read. PMID 1702677. Retrieved October 10, 2015, from, https://www.ncbi.nlm.nih.gov/pmc/articles/PMC1622749/

Rajput, R. J. (2010). Controversy: is there a role for adjuvants in the management of male pattern hair loss? J Cutan Aesthet Surg, 3(2):82-6. Retrieved July 24, 2016, from, http://www.ncbi.nlm.nih.gov/pubmed/21031065

Rashid, R. M. and Thomas, V. (2010). Androgenic pattern presentation of scarring and inflammatory alopecia. J Eur Acad Dermatol Venereol, Retrieved December 23, 2015, from, http:// www.ncbi.nlm.nih.gov/pubmed/20059630

Rassman, W. R., Pak, J.P. and Kim, J. (2013). Scalp micro-pigmentation: A Useful Treatment for Hair Loss. Facial Plast Surg Clin North Am. 2013 Aug;21(3):497-503. doi: 10.1016/j.fsc.2013.05.010. Retrieved December 2, 2016, from, https://www.ncbi.nlm.nih.gov/pubmed/24017991/

Rebora, A. and Guarrera, M. (2002). Kenogen: A new phase of the hair cycle? Dermatology. 2002;205(2):108-10. Retrieved September 2, 2016, from, http://www.ncbi.nlm.nih.gov/pubmed/12218222

Replicel.com (2017). DSC cell therapy. Treatment for Androgenetic Alopecia. RCH-01 Development Status. Retrieved December 23, 2016, from, http://replicel.com/product-pipeline/rch-01-hair-regeneration/

Ries, G. and Hess, R. (1999). Retinol: Safety considerations for its use in cosmetic products. J Toxicol. Cutaneous Ocul. Toxicol, 18:169–185. Retrieved October 16, 2015, from, http://www.tandfonline.com/doi/abs/10.3109/15569529909044238

Rinaldi, F., Sorbellini, E., and Coscera, T. (2011). The role of platelet rich plasma to control anagen phase: Evaluation in vitro and in vivo in hair transplant and hair treatment. Int J Trichology. 2011 Jul; 3(Suppl1): S14–S15. Retrieved January 2, 2016, from, https://www.ncbi.nlm.nih.gov/pmc/articles/PMC3171854/#top

Rogers, N. E. and Avram, M. R. (2008). Medical treatments for male and female pattern hair loss. Journal of the American Academy of Dermatology. 59 (4): 547–566. doi: 10.1016/j.jaad.2008.07.001. Retrieved August 2, 2015, from https://www.ncbi.nlm.nih.gov/pubmed/18793935

Rook, A. (1975). Hair II racial and other genetic variations in hair form. Br J Dermatol. 1975 May;92(5):599-600. Retrieved October 10, 2014, from, http://www.ncbi.nlm.nih.gov/pubmed/1100091

Rosebrook, J. (2016). You can't repair damaged hair: But Here's What You Can Do. Retrieved November 2, 2016, from, http://www.mindbodygreen.com/0-23804/you-cant-repair-damaged-hair-but-heres-what-you-can-do.html

Rose, P. T. (2015). Hair restoration surgery: challenges and Solutions. Clin Cosmet Investig Dermatol. 2015; 8: 361–370. Retrieved October 29, 2016, from https://www.ncbi.nlm.nih.gov/pmc/articles/PMC4507484/

Rossi, S. (2004). Australian Medicines Handbook. Adelaide: Australian Medicines Handbook. ISBN 0-9578521-4-2

Rossi, A., Cantisani, C., Scarnò, M., Trucchia, A., Fortuna, M. C., Calvieri, S. (2011). Finasteride, 1 mg daily administration on male androgenetic alopecia in different age groups: 10-year follow-up. Dermatologic Therapy 24(4): 455-461. doi:10.1111/j.15298019.2011. 01441.x. ISSN13960296 PMID 21910805. Retrieved December 12, 2014, from, http://finasteridesyndrome.blogspot.com/p/dht-role.html

Rouzaud, F., Kadekaro, A. L., Abdel-Malek, Z. A., and Hearing, V. J. (2005). MC1R and the response of melanocytes to ultraviolet radiation. Mutat Res. 2005; 571:133-52. Retrieved July 22, 2016, from, http://www.ncbi.nlm.nih.gov/pubmed/15748644 http://www.scielo.br/scielo.php?script=sci_nlinks&pid=S0365-0596201300010007600005&lng=en

Rushton, D. H., de Brouwer, B., de Coster, W. and van Neste, D. J. (1993). Comparative evaluation of scalp hair by phototrichogram and unit area trichogram analysis within the same subjects. Acta Derm Venereol. 1993 Apr; 73(2):150-3. Retrieved August 2, 2014, from, http://www.ncbi.nlm.nih.gov/pubmed/8103267

Rushton, D. H. (2002). Nutritional factors and hair loss. Clin Exp Dermatol 27: 396-404. Retrieved July 26, 2016, from, http://www.ncbi.nlm.nih.gov/pubmed/12190640

Said, H. M. (2009). Cell and molecular aspects of human Intestinal biotin absorption. J Nutr. 2009 Jan; 139(1): 158–162. doi: 10.3945/jn.108.092023.Retrieved October 12, 2015, from, https://www.ncbi.nlm.nih.gov/pmc/articles/PMC2646215/

Saitoh, M., Uzuka, M. and Sakamoto M. (1970). Human hair cycle. J Invest Dermatol 1970; 54:65- 81. Retrieved October 21, 2015, from, http://www.bioline.org.br/pdf?dv06083

Saleh, D., Naga, S., Yarrarapu, S., Cook, C. (2021). National Library of Medicine. Retrieved April 29, 2022, from, https://www.ncbi.nlm.nih.gov/books/NBK534854/#:~:text=Hypertrichosis%20is%20defined%20as%20excessive,hairs%20in%20androgen%2Ddependent%20sites.

Sampayo, J. N., Gill, G. J. and Lithgow, G. J. (2003). Oxidative stress and aging—the use of superoxide dismutase/catalase mimetics to extend lifespan. Biochem Soc Trans. 2003 Dec; 31(Pt 6):1305-7. Retrieved November 2, 2014, from, https://www.ncbi.nlm.nih.gov/pubmed/14641049

Sandler, R. (1961). Gesichtsponkte Zur Sogenannten Glatzen Operation; or Aspects to the so-called balding operation, Hautarzt 12: 516.

Sattur, S. S. (2011). A Review of surgical methods (excluding hair transplantation) and their role in hair loss management today. J Cutan Aesthet Surg. 2011 May-Aug; 4(2): 89–97. Doi: 10.4103/0974-2077.85020. Retrieved September 12, 2014, from, http://www.ncbi.nlm.nih.gov/pmc/articles/PMC3183735/#ref1

Savin, R. C. (1992). A method for visually describing and quantitating hair loss in male pattern baldness. J Invest Dermatol, 98:604. Vol. 98, No. 4, pp. 604-604). 350 main street, Malden, MA 02148 USA: Blackwell Publishing Inc.

Schallreuter, K. U., Mohammed, A. E., Salem, E. L., Holtz, S. and Panske, A. (2013). Basic evidence for epidermal H2O2/ONOO-mediated oxidation/nitration in segmental Vitiligo is supported by repigmentation of the skin and eyelashes after reduction of epidermal H2O2 with topical NB-UVB-activated pseudocatalase PC-KUS. Retrieved July 23, 2015, from, http://www.fasebj.org/content/early/2013/04/29/fj.12-226779.abstract?sid=07d5a98a-313d-4c1d-86c1-edff6332d1d1

Schultheiss, D., Knöner, W., Kramer, F. J. and Jonas, U. (1998). Johann Friedrich Dieffenbach (1792-1847) as the founder of plastic surgery. His contribution to maxillofacial surgery. Mund Kiefer Gesichtschir. 1998 Nov;2(6):309-15. Retrieved October 23, 2015, from, http://www.ncbi.nlm.nih.gov/pubmed/9881000

Schwartz, R. A. (2015, May 4). Anagen Effluvium. Retrieved November 21, 2015, from, http://emedicine.medscape.com/article/1073488-overview#a6

Schwartz, J. I., Van Hecken, A., De Schepper, P.J., De Lepeleire I.,Lasseter, K.C., Shamblen, E.C., Winchell, G.A., Constanzer, M.L., Chavez, C.M., Wang, D.Z., Ebel, D.L., Justice, S.J., Gertz, B.J. (1996). Effect of MK-386, a novel inhibitor of type 1, 5 alpha-reductase, alone and in combination with finasteride, on serum dihydrotestosterone concentrations in men. J Clin Endocrinol Metab, 81(8):2942-7. Retrieved April 20, 2014, from, http://press.endocrine.org/doi/abs/10.1210/jcem.81.8.876885? Journal Code=jcem. DOI: http://dx.doi.org/10.1210/jcem.81.8.8768856

Schweikert, H.U., and Wilson, J.D. (1974). Regulation of human hair growth by steroid hormones. I. Testosterone metabolism in isolated hairs. J Clin Endocrinol Metab, 38:811–819. Retrieved October 2, 2014, from, http://www.ncbi.nlm.nih.gov/pubmed/4823922?dopt=Abstract

Segrave, K. (1996). Baldness: A social history. Publisher: McFarland & Company May 31, 1996. ISBN-10: 0786401931 ISBN-13: 978-0786401932

Sharma, A. et al. (2019) Tretinoin enhances minoxidil response in androgenetic alopecia patients by upregulating follicular sulfotransferase enzymes. Dermatol Ther 2019 May;32(3):e12915. doi: 10.1111/dth.12915. Epub 2019 Apr 23. Retrieved March 16, 2022, from, https://pubmed.ncbi.nlm.nih.gov/30974011/

Shein, M. (1909). Relation between baldness and the growth of the cranium and scalp. Gvogyaszat (Budapest) 49: 484.

Shetty, S., Krishnaveni, J. and Pavai, A. (2013). Trichotillomania with gastric trichobezoar. Ann Gastroenterol, 26(3): 255. Retrieved August 2, 2015, from, http://www.ncbi.nlm.nih.gov/pmc/articles/PMC3959449/

Shiell, R. C. (2008). A review of modern surgical hair restoration techniques. J Cutan Aesthet Surg. 2008 Jan; 1(1): 12–16. doi: 10.4103/0974-2077.41150. Retrieved November 29, 2015, from, http://www.ncbi.nlm.nih.gov/pmc/articles/PMC2840892/

Shiell, R. C. and Kossard, S. (1990). Problems associated with synthetic fibre implants for hair replacement ("NIDO" process) Med J. 152:560. Retrieved August 2, 2016, from, http://www.ncbi.nlm.nih.gov/pubmed/2338937

Siah, T. W., and Harries, M. J. (2014). Anterolateral Leg Alopecia: Common but Commonly Ignored. Int'l Journal of Trichology. Retrieved March 28, 2022, from, https://www.ncbi.nlm.nih.gov/pmc/articles/PMC4154156/

Singh, M. K. and Avram, M. (2014). Persistent sexual dysfunction and depression in finasteride users for male pattern hair loss: a serious concern or red herring? The Journal of clinical and aesthetic dermatology. 7 (12): 51–5. PMC 4285451free to read. PMID 25584139. Retrieved October 6, 2014, from, https://www.ncbi.nlm.nih.gov/pmc/articles/PMC4285451/

Sonthalia, S., Daulatabad, D. and Tosti, A. (2015). Hair restoration in androgenetic alopecia: Looking Beyond Minoxidil, Finasteride and Hair Transplantation. Journal of Cosmetology & Trichology. Retrieved September 5, 2016, from, http://www.omicsonline.org/open-access/hair-restoration-in-androgenetic-alopecia-looking-beyond-minoxidil-finasteride-and-hair-transplantation-jctt1000105.php?aid=68395

Sood, A. (2013). Guide to stress-free living. Mayo Foundation for Medical Education and Research (MFMER). Published by Da Capo Press 1st Ed. ISBN: 978-0-7382-1713-3 e-Book

Stamatiadis, D., Bulteau-Portois, M. C. and Mowszowicz, I. (1988). Inhibition of 5α-reductase activity in human skin by zinc and azelaic acid. British Journal of Dermatology. Retrieved December 29, 2016, from, http://onlinelibrary.wiley.com/doi/10.1111/j.1365-2133.1988.tb03474.x/abstract

Stenn, H. (2005). Exogen, the shedding phase of the hair cycle. Retrieved February 5, 20015 from, http://nahrs.org/InTheNews/RecentNews/Exogen.aspx

Stern, A. (March 2, 2022). How much is the cost of a hair transplant in Turkey? The Jerusalem Post. Retrieved April 15, 2022, from, https://www.jpost.com/special-content/how-much-is-the-cost-of-a-hair-transplant-in-turkey-699102

TattooPro (2021). 21 Tattoo Statistics & Trends in 2021: A Primer Into the Tattoo Industry. Retrieved March 23, 2022, form, https://www.tattoopro.io/blog/tattoo-industry-statistics/

Tauber, H. (1939). Alopecia prematura and its surgical treatment. J. Ceylon BR: Brit MA, 1939, 36:237-242.

Taylor, P. J. (2008). Big head? Bald head! Skull expansion: alternative model for the primary mechanism of AGA. Med Hypotheses. 2009 Jan.72(1):23-8. Doi: 10.1016/j.mehy.2008.07.048. Retrieved August 12, 2014, from, http://www.ncbi.nlm.nih.gov/pubmed/18789604

Tillmanns, H. (1894). Principles of Surgery and Surgical Pathology: A Text-Book of Surgery. D. Appleton and Co. Retrieved December 18, 2015, from, http://babel.hathitrust.org/cgi/pt?id=nnc2.ark:/13960/t3bz6vt0; view=1up; seq=7

Tobin, D. J., Paus, R. (2001). Graying: Gerontobiology of the hair follicle pigmentary unit. Retrieved December 12, 2015, from, http://www.ncbi.nlm.nih.gov/pmc/articles/PMC2938584/

Thoemmes, M. (2014). Ubiquity and diversity of human associated demodex mites. PLOS ONE. 9 (8): e106265. doi: 10.1371/journal.pone.0106265. PMC 4146604Freely accessible. PMID 25162399. Retrieved December 23, 2015, from, https://www.ncbi.nlm.nih.gov/pubmed/25162399

Torjesen, P. A. and Sandnes, L. (2004). Serum testosterone in women as measured by an automated immunoassay and an RIA. Clinical Chemistry. 50 (3): 678; author reply 678–9. Retrieved October 29, 2014, from, https://www.ncbi.nlm.nih.gov/pubmed/14981046

Tosi, A., Misciali, C., Piraccini, B. M., Peluso, A. M. and Bardazzi, F. (1994). Drug-induced hair loss and hair growth. incidence, management, and avoidance. Retrieved July 16, 2016, from, http://www.ncbi.nlm.nih.gov/pubmed/8018303

True, H. R. and Dorin, J. R. (2014). Hypopituitarism and hair loss: What you should know. Retrieved October 29, 2016, from, http://www.truedorin.com/blog/2014/09/03/hypopituitarism-and-hair-loss-what-148782

Trüeb, R. M. (2005). Aging of hair. Journal of cosmetic dermatology. Retrieved January 6, 2015, from, http://onlinelibrary.wiley.com/doi/10.1111/j.1473-2165.2005.40203.x/abstract; jsessionid=23CEDA07FFBE38912182E440D57EFB1C.f04t03? userIsAuthenticated=false&deniedAccessCustomisedMessage=

Trüeb, R. M. (2015). The Difficult hair loss patient: Guide to Successful Management of Alopecia and Related Conditions. Springer, 2015. ISBN 9783319197012 Pg. 95.

Tsatmali, M., Ancans, J., Thody, A. J. (202). Melanocyte function and its control by melanocortin peptides. J Histochem Cytochem. 2002; 50:125-33. Retrieved August 12, 2016, from, http://www.scielo.br/scielo.php?script=sci_nlinks&pid=S0365-05962013000100076000 11&lng=en http://www.ncbi.nlm.nih.gov/pubmed/11799132

Uebel CO, da Silva JB, Cantarelli D, Martins P. The role of platelet plasma growth factors in male pattern baldness surgery. Plast Reconstr Surg, 118:1458–66, Retrieved October 23, 2014, from, https://www.ncbi.nlm.nih.gov/pubmed/17051119

Uemura, M., Tamura, K., Chung, S., Honma, S., Okuyama, A., Nakamura, Y., and Nakagawa, H. (2007). Novel 5α-steroid reductase (SRD5A3, type-3) is overexpressed in hormone-refractory prostate cancer. Cancer Science Volume 99, Issue 1, pages 81–86, January 2008. Article first published online: 6 Nov

2007. DOI: 10.1111/j.1349-7006.2007.00656. x. Retrieved January 6, 2015, from, https://www.ncbi.nlm.nih.gov/pubmed/17986282

Unger, M. G. and Unger, W. P. (1978). Management of alopecia of the scalp by a combination of excision and transplantation. J Dermatol Surg Oncol, 4:670–2. Retrieved November 1, 2014, from, https://www.ncbi.nlm.nih.gov/pubmed/701586

Unger, W. P. (1994). Delineating the safe donor area for hair transplanting. The American Journal of Cosmetic Surgery 11:239–243. Retrieved December 6, 2015, from, https://en.wikipedia.org/wiki/Hair_transplantation#cite_note-9

Uno, H. and Kurata, S. (1993). Chemical agents and peptides affect hair growth. J Invest Dermatol. 101(1 Suppl):143S-147S Retrieved August 2, 2015, from, http://www.ncbi.nlm.nih.gov/pubmed/8326148

Urysiak-Czubatka, I., Kmiec, M. L. and Broniarczyk-Dyta, G. (2014). Assessment of the usefulness of dihydrotestosterone in the diagnostics of patients with androgenetic alopecia. Postepy Dermatol Alergol, (4):207-15. doi: 10.5114/pdia.2014.40925. Epub. Retrieved January 20, 2016, from, https://www.ncbi.nlm.nih.gov/pubmed/?term=Urysiak-Czubatka%20I%5BAuthor%5D&cauthor=true&cauthor_uid=25254005

U.S. Patent Database. (n.d.). Results of Search in US Patent Collection db for: hairpiece Retrieved October 23, 2016, from, http://patft.uspto.gov/netacgi/nphParser?Sect1=PTO2&Sect2=HITOFF&p=1&u=%2Fnetahtml%2FPTO%2Fsearchbool.html&r=0&f=S&l=50&TERM1=hairpiece&FIELD1=&co1=AND&TERM2=&FIELD2=&d=PALL

Vallis, C. P. (1964). Surgical treatment of the receding hairline: Report of a case. Retrieved August 3, 2015 from, http://journals.lww.com/plasreconsurg/Citation/1964/03000/srgical_treatment_of_the_receding_hairline_.6.aspx

Van Neste, D. J. and Rushton, D. H. (1997). Hair problems in women. Clin Dermatol. 1997; 15:113–25. Retrieved October 12, 2015 from, http://www.ncbi.nlm.nih.gov/pubmed/9034660

Van Neste, D. and Tobin, D. J. (2004). Hair cycle and dynamic interactions and changes associated with aging. Micron, 35:193–200. Retrieved December 20, 2015, from, https://www.ncbi.nlm.nih.gov/pubmed/15036274

Venning, V. A. and Dawber, R. P. (1988). Patterned androgenic alopecia in women. J Am Acad Dermatol, 18 (5 Pt1):1073-7. Retrieved December 20, 2015, from, http://www.ncbi.nlm.nih.gov/pubmed/3385027

Walsh, P. C., Hutchins, G.M. & Ewing, L. L. (1983). Tissue content of dihydrotestosterone in human prostatic hyperplasia is not supra normal. J Clin Invest, 72(5):1772-1777. Retrieved December 2, 2015, from, http://www.jci.org/articles/view/111137

Ward, A. (October 3, 2014). Guinter Kahn, dermatologist, 1934-2014. Physician who was first to fertilize lazy male hair follicles. Retrieved March 18, 2022, from, https://www.ft.com/content/cc8601a4-497d-11e4-8d68-00144feab7de

Weihua, Z., Lathe, R., Warner, M., and Gustafsson, J. A. (2002). An endocrine pathway in the prostate, ERbeta, AR, 5alpha-androstane-3beta,17beta-diol, and CYP7B1, regulates prostate growth. Proc Natl Acad Sci U S A. 2002 Oct 15;99(21):13589-94. Epub. Retrieved August 2, 2015, from, https://www.ncbi.nlm.nih.gov/pubmed/12370428

Whiteman, D. C., Parsons, P. G. and Green, A, C. (1999). Determinants of melanocyte density in adult human skin. Arch Dermatol Res, 291:511–6. Retrieved November 2, 2015, from, https://www.ncbi.nlm.nih.gov/pubmed/10541882

Whiting, D. A. and Olsen, E. A. (2008). Central centrifugal cicatricial alopecia. Dermatol Ther, 21(4):268-78. doi: 10.1111/j.1529-8019.2008.00209. x. Retrieved October 15, 2015, from, https://www.ncbi.nlm.nih.gov/pubmed/18715297

Whiting, D. A. (2011). How real is senescent alopecia? A histopathologic approach. Clin Dermatol, 29(1):49-53. doi: 10.1016/j.clindermatol.2010.07.007. Retrieved September 3, 2014, from, http://www.ncbi.nlm.nih.gov/pubmed/21146732

Wigs.com (2016). The Differences between human hair & synthetic hair. Retrieved December 28, 2016 from, https://www.wigs.com/pages/the-differences-between-human-hair-synthetic-hair

Wilhelmi, B. J., Blackwell, S. J., Phillips, L. G. (1999). Langer's lines: to use or not to use". Plast. Reconstr. Surg. 104 (1): 208–14. Doi: 10.1097/00006534-199907000-00032. PMID 10597698. Retrieved October 15, 2015, from, http://www.ncbi.nlm.nih.gov/pubmed/10597698

Wolf, B. R. (1998). Surgical hair restoration. Retrieved October 16, 2016, from, https://www.wolfhair.com/learning-center/hair-loss-why/articles-by-dr-wolf/langers-lines/

Wolf, P., Nghiem, D. X., Walterscheid, J. P. (2006). Platelet-activating factor is crucial in psoralen and ultraviolet A-induced immune suppression, inflammation, and apoptosis. Am J Pathol. 2006 Sep;169(3):795-805. Retrieved October 14, 2015, from, http://patient.info/doctor/PUVA#ref-1

Wolfram, L. J. (2003). Human hair: a unique physicochemical composite. J Am Acad Dermatol 2003; 48: S106–114. Retrieved February12, 2015, from, http://www.ncbi.nlm.nih.gov/pubmed/12789162

Wolff, K., Goldsmith, L.A., Katz, S. I., Gilchrest, B. A., Paller, A. S. and Leffell, D. J. (2008). Fitzpatrick's dermatology in general medicine (7th Ed). The McGraw-Hill Companies, Inc., New York 2008, pg 2397.

Wolff, K., Johnson, R. A. and Suurmond, D. (2009). Disorders of hair follicles and related disorders. In Fitzpatrick's color atlas and synopsis of clinical dermatology, 6th ed. (ed. Wolff K, et al.). McGraw-Hill, New York

Wong, C. (2015). Biotin for hair growth. Retrieved August 3, 2016, from, https://www.verywell.com/biotin-for-hair-growth-89236

Wong, A. C. and Mak, S. T. (2011). Finasteride-associated cataract and intraoperative floppy-iris syndrome. Journal of Cataract & Refractive Surgery. 37 (7): 1351–1354. doi: 10.1016/j.jcrs.2011.04.013. Retrieved October 10, 2015, from, https://www.ncbi.nlm.nih.gov/pubmed/21555201

Wood, J. M., Decker, H., Hartmann, H., Chavan, B., Rokos, H., Spencer, J. D., Hasse, S., Thornton, M. J., Shalbaf, M., Paus, R., and Schallreuter, K. U. (2009). Senile hair graying: H2O2 mediated oxidative stress affect human hair color by blunting methionine sulfoxide repair. Retrieved July 23, 2016, from, http://www.fasebj.org/content/23/7/2065.short

Yamana, K., Labrie, F., Luu, -The V (January 2010). Human type 3 5α-reductase is expressed in peripheral tissues at higher levels than types 1 and 2 and its activity is potently inhibited by finasteride and dutasteride. *Hormone Molecular Biology and Clinical Investigation* 2 (3). Retrieved August 2, 2014, from, Doi:10.1515/hmbci.2010.035. Retrieved December 20, 2015, from, http://www.ncbi.nlm.nih.gov/pubmed/25961201

Yildiz, B.O., Bolour, S., Woods, K., Moore, A., and Azziz, R. (2009, 2010). Visually scoring hirsutism. Hum Reprod Update. 2010 Jan-Feb. 16(1):51-64. Retrieved February 12, 2015, from, https://humupd.oxfordjournals.org/content/early/2009/06/30/humupd.dmp024.full http://www.ncbi.nlm.nih.gov/pmc/articles/PMC2792145/

Yang, C., Todorova Chen, W., , A., Khuzaei, S. A., Chiu, H. C., Worret, W. I., and Ring, J. (2010). Hair Loss in Elderly Women. Eur J Dermatol, 20 (2), 145-51. Retrieved March 22, 2020, from https://pubmed.ncbi.nlm.nih.gov/20172841/ DOI: 10.1684/ejd.2010.0828

Yang, R., and Xu, X. (2013). Isolation and culture of neural crest stem cells from human hair follicles. J Vis Exp, (74). Doi: 10.3791/3194. Retrieved Sept 23, 2014, from, http://www.ncbi.nlm.nih.gov/pubmed/23608752

Young, E. (2012). Everything you never wanted to know about the mites that eat, crawl, and have sex on your face. Science for the curious Discover. Retrieved January 23, 2016, from, http://blogs.discovermagazine.com/notrocketscience/2012/08/31/everything-you-never-wanted-to-know-about-the-mites-that-eat-crawl-and-have-sex-on-your-face/

Young, S. N. (2009). L-Tyrosine to alleviate the effects of stress? J Psychiatry Neurosci v.32(3); PMC1863555. Retrieved August,3, 2016 from, http://www.ncbi.nlm.nih.gov/pmc/articles/PMC1863555 Zappacosta, A. R. (1980). Reversal of baldness in patient receiving minoxidil for hypertension. *N Engl J Med* 303: 1480-1. Retrieved December 12, 2015, from, http://www.medscape.com/viewart

Zari, J., Adolmajid, F., Massod, M., Vahid, M. and Yalda, N. (2008). Evaluation of the relationship between androgenetic alopecia and demodex infestation. Indian J Dermatol. 2008; 53(2): 6467.doi: 10.4103/0019-5154.41647. Retrieved January 12, 2016, from, https://www.ncbi.nlm.nih.gov/pmc/articles/PMC2763723/

Zlotogorski, A., Panteleyev, A. A., Aita, V. M., Christiano, A. M. (2002). Clinical and molecular diagnostic criteria of congenital atrichia with papular lesions. J Invest Dermatol. Retrieved April 30, 2022, form, https://pubmed.ncbi.nlm.nih.gov/11982770/

Index

C

D

G

H

I

J

K

L

M

N

O

P

Q

R

S

T

U

V

W

X

Y

Z

About the Author

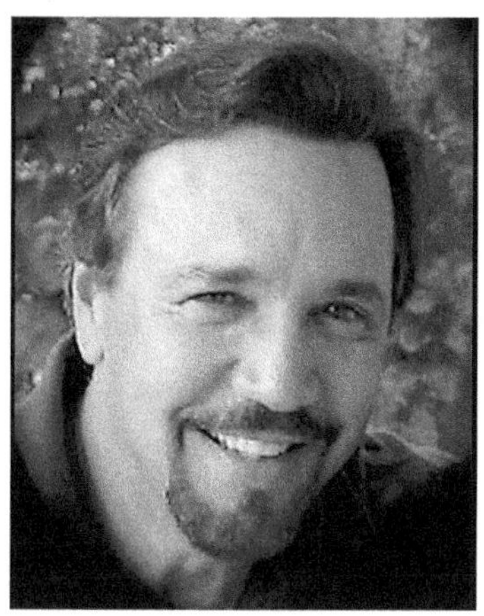

Gustavo J. Gomez, Ph.D., is a multi-award-winning author who concentrates on writing medical and business books that are detailed, comprehensive, and meticulously researched to bring to market books with actionable information readers can use. Gustavo has been a successful entrepreneur, businessman, educator, inventor, healthcare executive, and consultant for the past thirty-five years. His academic background encompasses degrees in health sciences and business administration. This broad-ranging educational background has made him quite versatile, achieving numerous successes in the healthcare and business fields.

To learn more about the author, please visit his:

Official author's website: https://www.gustavojgomez.com

Amazon author's page: https:// www.Amazon.com/author/gustavojgomez

Printed in the USA
CPSIA information can be obtained
at www.ICGtesting.com
CBHW080906080824
12842CB00010B/411